Autonomy, Rationality, and Contemporary Bioethics

OXFORD PHILOSOPHICAL MONOGRAPHS

Other titles in this series include

Everything, more or less: A defence of generality relativism
J. P. Studd

Five Modes of Scepticism: Sextus Empiricus and the Agrippan Modes
Stefan Sienkiewicz

Vagueness and Thought
Andrew Bacon

Visual Experience: A Semantic Approach
Wylie Breckenridge

Discrimination and Disrespect
Benjamin Eidelson

Knowing Better: Virtue, Deliberation, and Normative Ethics
Daniel Star

Potentiality and Possibility: A Dispositional Account of Metaphysical Modality
Barbara Vetter

Moral Reason
Julia Markovits

Category Mistakes
Ofra Magidor

The Critical Imagination
James Grant

From Morality to Metaphysics: The Theistic Implications of our Ethical Commitments
Angus Ritchie

Aquinas on Friendship
Daniel Schwartz

The Brute Within: Appetitive Desire in Plato and Aristotle
Hendrik Lorenz

Autonomy, Rationality, and Contemporary Bioethics

Jonathan Pugh

OXFORD
UNIVERSITY PRESS

OXFORD
UNIVERSITY PRESS

Great Clarendon Street, Oxford, OX2 6DP,
United Kingdom

Oxford University Press is a department of the University of Oxford.
It furthers the University's objective of excellence in research, scholarship,
and education by publishing worldwide. Oxford is a registered trade mark of
Oxford University Press in the UK and in certain other countries

First Edition published in 2020

Published in the United States of America by Oxford University Press
198 Madison Avenue, New York, NY 10016, United States of America

British Library Cataloguing in Publication Data
Data available

Library of Congress Control Number: 2019949400

ISBN 978–0–19–885858–4

For my parents, Chris and Amy, and my god-daughter Grace

Contents

Acknowledgements

I would like to begin by thanking the Uehiro Foundation on Ethics and Education. I am extremely humbled by their generous support of both myself, and the Oxford Uehiro Centre for Practical Ethics as a whole, where I was lucky enough to write this book.

I would also like to thank the Wellcome Trust for funding the doctoral research that formed the basis of this book, as well as St Anne's College, and the Philosophy Department at the University of Oxford for their support throughout my time at Oxford. As well as providing me with a generous scholarship, travel grants from the college and the department also enabled me to present my research at a number of international conferences.

Whilst I would not have been able to embark on this project without the generous financial support detailed above, money will only get you so far. My work on this project would not have been possible if I had not been lucky enough to receive the support and advice of a large number of people.

First, I would like to express my deep appreciation for the time and effort of my doctoral supervisors Prof. Julian Savulescu and Prof. Roger Crisp. Prof. Savulescu was instrumental in persuading me to embrace a completely new topic in my doctoral research when I first moved to Oxford. His belief in my abilities at this early stage gave me the confidence to stretch myself in my research, and this has undoubtedly enabled me to become a far better philosopher. He also provided me with invaluable advice on numerous written drafts of my doctoral thesis (and other work), as well as providing me with numerous professional opportunities.

Prof. Crisp has also been extremely generous with his time and expertise over the course of my research. I thoroughly enjoyed our supervision discussions, and I learnt a huge amount from them; I often left his office trying to get my head around a devastating criticism of a claim that I had naively assumed to be self-evident! I shall also remember Prof. Crisp's kind words of encouragement when I was trying to publish my first academic papers. All in all, there is little else that a student could hope for from their two supervisors. I am sincerely grateful to them both, as well as to my thesis examiners Prof. Jeff McMahan and Prof. Walter Sinnott-Armstrong.

I also owe huge thanks to Peter Momtchiloff at Oxford University Press, who has been a patient and highly engaged editor. He also found two readers to review the book who both provided a number of extremely useful comments on earlier versions of the manuscript. The published version of the book owes a great deal to their insightful comments, and I benefited a great deal from their time and effort. I am extremely grateful to them both. Needless to say, all of the book's remaining deficiencies are solely my responsibility.

Over the course of writing this book, two people who have had a huge influence on me sadly passed away. Much of the theoretical material in this book is grounded by the seminal work of Derek Parfit, and I was lucky enough to share some correspondence with him over the course of my doctoral studies. It will be no surprise to those who knew Derek well that he not only provided extensive insightful comments on my drafts, but that he was also forthcoming with advice when I was unsure that I would be able to continue a career in medical ethics beyond my DPhil. It is a source of considerable regret that I was not able to send him a completed version of this book, and to let him know how important his words of encouragement were.

The second person I would like to mention in this regard is someone who I never met personally. I did, however, over the last decade attend numerous concerts where Scott Hutchison showcased his incredible musical talent, as a member of the band 'Frightened Rabbit'. Scott tragically took his own life in 2018, and his family have since launched a mental health charity named 'Tiny Changes' in his honour. Tiny Changes aims to raise awareness about young people's mental health and to advance understanding of mental illness. This is a hugely important issue for society, and also, of course, for medical ethics. In Scott's memory, I will be sending proceeds I receive for this book to this important charity.

I reserve my deepest gratitude for my family. They have been a source of love, strength, and support throughout this project. As former medics, my mum and dad have undoubtedly had a huge influence on my interest in applied ethics. Not only that, but they have taken such interest in my work that they now often pose far more difficult questions to me than many philosophers! This is also true of my brother Chris. As a fellow academic, albeit in a different discipline, he has been a huge source of inspiration to me, and I doubt that I would have had the courage to embark on a doctoral thesis in the absence of his fine example; he is, as always, a trail-blazer. With his wife Amy, he has also been instrumental in keeping my philosophy rooted in the 'real world' and as far as possible from the ivory tower—it is the best place for it.

Introduction

Personal autonomy is often lauded as a key value in contemporary Western bioethics.[1] Indeed, on their widely endorsed 'four principles' approach to biomedical ethics, Beauchamp and Childress propose that the principle of respect for autonomy is one of four fundamental principles of biomedical ethics (alongside the principles of beneficence, non-maleficence, and justice).[2] The concept of autonomy is also commonly understood to undergird the doctrine of informed consent, a doctrine that is invoked ubiquitously in contemporary bioethics.

In light of this, it should come as little surprise that considerations of autonomy are salient in a wide array of contemporary bioethical questions. To take just a small sample, debates about the moral permissibility of euthanasia,[3] gene-editing,[4] so-called 'sin taxes',[5] mandatory vaccination policies,[6] markets for human organs,[7] genome screening,[8] and involuntary psychiatric treatment[9] all turn to a significant extent on arguments about personal autonomy. Furthermore, the emergence of new neurotechnologies that can modulate neural circuits associated with thought, behaviour, and mood are raising important new questions about autonomy and its value in contemporary bioethics.[10]

[1] For example, see Gillon, 'Ethics Needs Principles—Four Can Encompass the Rest—and Respect for Autonomy Should Be "First among Equals"'; Beauchamp and Childress, *Principles of Biomedical Ethics*; Smith, 'The Pre-Eminence of Autonomy in Bioethics'. However, for non-Western perspectives of autonomy's value, see Yang, 'Serve the People'; Kara, 'Applicability of the Principle of Respect for Autonomy'; Foster, *Choosing Life, Choosing Death*, 11.

[2] Beauchamp and Childress, *Principles of Biomedical Ethics*.

[3] Brock, 'Voluntary Active Euthanasia'; Velleman, 'A Right of Self-Termination?'

[4] Habermas, *The Future of Human Nature*; Pugh, 'Autonomy, Natality and Freedom'.

[5] Barnhill and King, 'Ethical Agreement and Disagreement about Obesity Prevention Policy in the United States'; Green, 'The Ethics of Sin Taxes'.

[6] ; Grzybowski et al., 'Vaccination Refusal'.

[7] Annas, 'Life, Liberty, and the Pursuit of Organ Sales'; Rippon, 'Imposing Options on People in Poverty'; Jaycox, 'Coercion, Autonomy, and the Preferential Option for the Poor in the Ethics of Organ Transplantation'.

[8] Andorno, 'The Right Not to Know'; Harris and Keywood, 'Ignorance, Information and Autonomy'.

[9] Dickenson, 'Ethical Issues in Long-Term Psychiatric Management'; Rudnick, 'Depression and Competence to Refuse Psychiatric Treatment'; Tan et al., 'Competence to Make Treatment Decisions in Anorexia Nervosa'.

[10] Maslen, Pugh, and Savulescu, 'The Ethics of Deep Brain Stimulation for the Treatment of Anorexia Nervosa'; Kraemer, 'Authenticity or Autonomy?'; Sharp and Wasserman, 'Deep Brain Stimulation, Historicism, and Moral Responsibility'; Pugh et al., 'Brainjacking in Deep Brain Stimulation and Autonomy'.

Autonomy, Rationality, and Contemporary Bioethics. Jonathan Pugh, Oxford University Press (2020). © Jonathan Pugh.
DOI: 10.1093/oso/9780198858584.001.0001

How we conceive of autonomy has highly significant practical implications. If an individual is deemed to be autonomous with respect to a decision, then that decision is often taken to have considerable weight in bioethical discussions. For instance, it is widely accepted that if a patient has made an autonomous decision to refuse treatment, then this decision typically ought to be respected, even if we believe that this decision is contrary to the patient's best interests. In contrast, if an individual is not autonomous with respect to a decision that will have harmful consequences for them, then it is far less clear that this decision ought to be respected. This is of course a descriptive, rather than prescriptive point at this stage; however, it is undeniable that autonomous persons are typically understood to have a considerable (although not complete) sphere of authority over self-regarding matters in Western bioethics. To use Ranaan Gillon's memorable phrase, although the four principles of biomedical ethics are (in theory) meant to have equal weight, the principle of autonomy is commonly understood to be 'first amongst equals'.[11]

As such, in developing a theory of autonomy, we are walking a tightrope between two errors, each with a significant cost.[12] Most obviously, a theory of autonomy might be deficient because it renders the standards of autonomy too demanding. An overly demanding conception of autonomy would lead to 'false negative' judgements that would serve to deny decision-making authority to individuals whose decisions should warrant respect. However, a theory of autonomy can also be deficient if it fails to make the standards of autonomy sufficiently demanding. Such a theory would lead to 'false positive' judgements that would grant authority to potentially harmful decisions, without the justificatory evaluative force of autonomy.

Accordingly, there is a great deal at stake in trying to develop an adequate understanding of autonomy. Yet, autonomy is an ambiguous concept that has lent itself to a plethora of different uses in moral philosophy.[13] Indeed, the ambiguity of the concept has led contemporary bioethicists to reach divergent conclusions about bioethical issues (such as those listed above) in which autonomy related concerns are salient. Moreover, abstract philosophical discussions about autonomy in a broadly metaphysical sense are often divorced from the concerns about autonomy that are raised by the clinical realities of medical decision-making in practical contexts.

In particular, there has been considerable disagreement amongst theorists about the relationship between autonomy and concepts such as rationality and freedom. Over the course of the development of bioethics, the claim that there is an important relationship between autonomy and rationality has sometimes been treated as quite uncontroversial, and perhaps even obvious. Nonetheless, as I shall go on to explain, a number of theorists have vehemently objected to the apparent inherent elitism of supposing that rationality lies at the heart of autonomy.

[11] Gillon, 'Ethics Needs Principles—Four Can Encompass the Rest—and Respect for Autonomy Should Be "First among Equals"'.

[12] Herring and Wall make a similar observation in Herring and Wall, 'Autonomy, Capacity and Vulnerable Adults', 698.

[13] See Arpaly, *Unprincipled Virtue*, 118–25 and Dworkin, *The Theory and Practice of Autonomy*, 3–6 for surveys of the different understandings of autonomy in the philosophical literature.

Furthermore, this ambiguous treatment of rationality and autonomy is also reflected to some extent in medical law. On the one hand, the recent Montgomery ruling governing standards of disclosure in cases of medical negligence in England and Wales explicitly appeals to the concept of rationality in outlining its standards of information disclosure; information is deemed to be material if a 'reasonable person' in the patient's position would be likely to attach significance to that information, or if the doctor should reasonably be aware that the particular patient would be likely to attach significance to it.[14] In contrast, it is instructive to compare this feature of medical law in England and Wales to Lord Donaldson of Lymington's famous judgment that competent patients have an absolute right to choose whether to consent to medical treatment, regardless of whether '. . . the reasons for making the choice are rational, irrational, unknown or even non-existent'.[15]

Whilst not contradictory, these two features of medical law certainly evidence something of a tension regarding the relationship between rationality and autonomy. The tension is exemplified even more clearly when we contrast the Donaldson judgment with the approach to mental capacity enshrined in the 2005 Mental Capacity Act of England and Wales. This approach seems to implicitly incorporate considerations of rationality in claiming that mental capacity requires the ability to 'weigh' information that is relevant to a treatment decision. Indeed, in a recent case, judge Jackson J concluded that an individual suffering from anorexia nervosa lacked capacity to refuse treatment because her:

> . . . obsessive fear of weight gain makes her incapable of weighing the advantages and disadvantages of eating in any meaningful way . . . The need not to gain weight overpowers all other thoughts.[16]

Cases such as these raise a descriptive legal question of whether patients do have an absolute legal right to make even irrational decisions concerning consent to treatment (as Donaldson contends). Yet they also raise the moral question of whether they *ought* to have such a right. I shall explore this question in more detail later in the book. At this point though, I simply observe that the tensions alluded to above arguably reflect deeper ambiguities in medical law, philosophy, and bioethics about what we mean to capture when we invoke the concept of rationality, and how different conceptions of rationality are understood to relate to autonomy and its value.

My aim in this book is to outline a more fully developed account of how we may plausibly understand one conception of rationality to play a significant role in an account of autonomy that can be usefully invoked in bioethics. In doing so, I shall attempt to unite some disparate threads in the literature on different aspects of autonomy, and seek to present a unified theory of the concept, one that can elucidate the relationship between autonomy, rationality, and freedom, and the nature of forms of influence that can subvert autonomy. In this introductory chapter, I shall

[14] Montgomery (Appellant) v. Lanarkshire Health Board (Respondent) (Scotland). See also Canterbury v. Spence (464 F.2d 772) 1972.

[15] Re T (Adult: Refusal of Medical Treatment).

[16] Re E (Medical Treatment Anorexia) EWHC 1639 (COP) at [49].

make some preliminary remarks about the nature of autonomy broadly construed, and delineate what has been termed the 'standard view' of autonomy in the bioethical literature. I shall conclude by explaining the framework that I shall adopt in developing my own rationalist account of personal autonomy.

1. Introducing Autonomy

The term 'autonomy' is derived from the Greek 'autos' (self), and 'nomos' (law); as such, the concept that the term 'autonomy' aims to capture seems to be, broadly speaking, the property of self-government.[17] Accordingly, as a preliminary observation, we might say that in investigating the nature of autonomy, we are investigating what it is for an agent to be self-governing.

Even this formulation might be understood to be making an important presumption, since it assumes that autonomy is a property of *agents*. Although Gerald Dworkin has averred that this is one of the few claims that autonomy theorists agree upon,[18] in developing what has come to be seen as the standard account of autonomy in bioethics, Beauchamp and Childress primarily focus their discussion of autonomy as a property of choices or actions rather than agents.[19] I shall argue below that these differences in our understanding of what autonomy is a property of more plausibly reflect a distinction between autonomy in a *local* sense, and autonomy in a *global* sense. For the purposes of this preliminary discussion, I shall assume that autonomy is a property of agents, and that a choice can be autonomous only in a derivative sense, in so far as it is made by an agent who is autonomous with respect to it.

What then is it for an agent to be self-governing? Immanuel Kant famously claimed that in order to be autonomous, an agent must be governed by her *noumenal* self, that is, the self as it is conceived as a member of the transcendent realm of pure reason, and not the self as a member of the phenomenal realm, in which it is subjected to external causes according to Kant's dualist metaphysics. It is worth noting three features of the Kantian account, as it is commonly understood.[20] First, on Kant's view, the autonomous agent is not moved to act by their desires; on the contrary, this would be the paradigm of heteronomy on the Kantian account, since desires represent contingent external causes on the will in Kant's metaphysics.[21] Second, autonomy is an inherently *moral* concept for Kant, since on his view pure reason demands that agents act in accordance with the Categorical Imperative. Third, autonomy is a property that undergirds the unique value of human life on the Kantian view; as autonomous agents, humans are understood to have dignity, a non-fungible objective value beyond mere price.

Onora O'Neill has set out a detailed account of the role that Kantian autonomy can play in bioethics, in particular how such 'principled autonomy' can provide the basis

[17] Dworkin, *The Theory and Practice of Autonomy*, 12. [18] Ibid., 6.

[19] Beauchamp and Childress, *Principles of Biomedical Ethics*, 102.

[20] These are at least features of Kant's account on orthodox understandings of his view. For an alternative see Herman, *The Practice of Moral Judgment*.

[21] See Hill, *Autonomy and Self-Respect*, 30.

for our interpersonal obligations, and in turn a framework for human rights.[22] However, as O'Neill points out, the conceptions of autonomy that many bioethicists invoke in their discussions are decidedly un-Kantian, instead taking their lead from John Stuart Mill's views regarding liberty and individuality.[23] *Pace* Kant, many contemporary theorists understand an agent to be autonomous if they direct their decisions in the light of their own desires, without the controlling influence of others;[24] notice that on this understanding, an autonomous agent's desires can have non-moral content.

O'Neill suggests that contemporary admirers of personal autonomy in bioethics '...crave and claim Kantian credentials'.[25] Whether or not this is true of others, I want to quite clearly state that, despite my interest in the role of rationality in autonomy, I neither crave nor claim Kantian credentials for the theory that I shall develop here. As I shall explain in more detail below, in this book I shall be interested in a Millian, rather than Kantian understanding of autonomy and its relation to rationality.

Before setting the Kantian approach aside though, it is worth noting that Kant's is a *substantive* account of autonomy, in so far as it stipulates that the choices of autonomous agents must have certain (on Kant's account, *moral*) content. According to substantive accounts of autonomy, an agent is not autonomous '...unless she chooses in accord with certain values'.[26] We may contrast substantive accounts of autonomy with *procedural* accounts; according to procedural accounts, the question of whether an agent is autonomous with respect to a particular decision depends on the manner in which they came to make that decision. The precise details of the sort of decision procedures that are indicative of autonomous decision-making will differ from theory to theory; however, the key point is that procedural theories do not claim that the autonomous agent's choices must have a particular *content*.

In this book, I shall develop a procedural theory of autonomy. There has admittedly been a revived interest in substantive theories of autonomy in recent years.[27] As I suggested above, Kant believed that autonomy requires that agents act in accordance with pure reason, and that this implies a substantive account of autonomy, in so far as reason demands that agents act in accordance with universalizable moral maxims. In contrast, modern-day philosophers who endorse substantive accounts have accepted a metaphysical claim that Kant denies here, namely that acting in accordance with one's desires can be compatible with autonomous agency. Instead, they have rejected procedural theories for other reasons. For instance, some feminist philosophers reject procedural theories on the basis that agents who make their choices in accordance with such theories might still lack autonomy because their

[22] O'Neill, *Autonomy and Trust in Bioethics*; see also Velleman, 'A Right of Self-Termination?'; Secker, 'The Appearance of Kant's Deontology in Contemporary Kantianism'.

[23] O'Neill, *Autonomy and Trust in Bioethics*, 30.

[24] Taylor, *Practical Autonomy and Bioethics*, xiii.

[25] O'Neill, *Autonomy and Trust in Bioethics*, 30; see also Foster, *Choosing Life, Choosing Death*, 7–8.

[26] Friedman, *Autonomy, Gender, Politics*, 19.

[27] For an insightful discussion of this development, see Dive and Newson, 'Reconceptualizing Autonomy for Bioethics'.

choices are guided by values that have been determined by oppressive patriarchal norms that run contrary to the very value of autonomy.[28]

The debate on this point has important implications for the role that autonomy can play in practical debates. One obvious example is the ethics of cosmetic procedures. If one holds the view that a woman's desire for a beautifying cosmetic procedure is merely an artefact of the influence of a pervasive and oppressive societal ideal,[29] then one might deny that a woman can be autonomous with respect to that desire, no matter how much she personally endorses it. Others have argued that procedural theories are inadequate because they do not rule out the possibility of individuals qualifying as autonomous when they decide on the basis of pathologies that distort their values and beliefs.[30] Consider, for instance, the patient suffering from severe and enduring anorexia nervosa who strongly endorses her desire to avoid weight-gain, whilst understanding that her disordered eating behaviour may have fatal consequences.

Problematic cases such as these have prompted some theorists to endorse substantive accounts that stipulate that there are normative restrictions, grounded by objective moral norms or prudential values,[31] upon what autonomous agents can desire; for instance, such theories might claim that an autonomous agent cannot choose a life of servitude[32] or one of self-destruction.[33] Despite this revived interest in substantive theories, I shall not directly consider them in this book. In order to justify this narrower focus, it is prudent to highlight what I take to be the main issue facing these theories. The crux of the debate between procedural and substantive theories lies in the importance (or lack thereof) of the individual's subjective understanding of their own desires and values. On substantive accounts of autonomy, one cannot be autonomous with respect to those of one's choices that fail to comply with certain norms, even if one does not endorse those norms, or the values they imply. Yet, even at a pre-theoretical level, this seems somewhat jarring; autonomy, it seems, should allow for the possibility that agents can reach different views about value, and that part of being autonomous is choosing to act in accordance with one's own beliefs about value, even if those beliefs are not universally shared.

The significance of acting in accordance with one's own values is something that John Stuart Mill stresses in his discussion of the importance of what he termed 'individuality', when he claims:

> If a person possesses any tolerable amount of common sense and experience, his own mode of laying out his existence is the best not because it is the best, but because it is his own mode.[34]

[28] Stoljar, 'Autonomy and the Feminist Intuition'; Westlund, 'Selflessness and Responsibility for Self'; Griffiths, *Feminisms and the Self*; Nedelsky, 'Reconceiving Autonomy'. See also Oshana, 'Personal Autonomy and Society'.

[29] For a detailed discussion of the beauty ideal, see Widdows, *Perfect Me*.

[30] Pettit and Smith, 'Backgrounding Desire'; Ciurria, 'A Virtue Ethical Approach to Decisional Capacity and Mental Health'.

[31] Although I believe that autonomy should be conceived as a value-neutral concept, I accept that it must also be a value-utilizing concept, as will become clear in my discussion. For more on this distinction, see Meyers, 'The Feminist Debate Over Values in Autonomy Theory'.

[32] See Benson, 'Freedom and Value'.

[33] Nordenfelt, *Rationality and Compulsion*.

[34] Mill, *On Liberty*, 131.

Mill's claim here is not simply that individuals are in a privileged epistemic position with regards to what mode of existence will be best for them, although this is also a claim that he endorsed.[35] Rather, Mill's broader claim is that even if we were to concede that a third party is in a better epistemic position with regards to the question of what is in another person's interests, there is still significant value in the individual herself making her *own* decisions about her life, even if these decisions are not the best for her from a third-party perspective.

Reflecting on this passage reveals a reason to be wary of substantive theories of autonomy in bioethics. The worry it raises is that such accounts threaten to subsume the notion of autonomy into considerations of purely objective morality or well-being. This, however, would overlook the fundamental thought motivating procedural accounts of autonomy, namely that the individual's acting in accordance with their own understanding of the good is integral to that which we value in the concept labelled 'autonomy', and, moreover, that considerations of autonomy can be distinguished from purely objective norms of morality and well-being.[36] Of course, this is not a knock-down objection to substantive theories;[37] such theorists would surely respond to the above observations by arguing that those values that are congruous with oppressive norms are not truly 'the agent's own', even if she cannot perceive that this is so. However, I take this general issue to be sufficient to motivate an enquiry into alternative procedural accounts of autonomy that take seriously the thought that the salience attributed to personal autonomy is grounded by a concern to live a life of one's own; a concern to live a life that is *valued* by oneself, rather than simply construed as one that is lived in accordance with that which is *valuable*.

In spite of my dismissal of substantive theories, the criticisms raised by opponents of procedural theories are genuine concerns. The procedural theory that I shall develop shall aim to engage with these issues, and will aim to be compatible with at least some of the elements that have motivated substantive theories of autonomy. First, the theory that I shall endorse is compatible with a broadly relational view of the autonomous agent. However, contrary to some substantive theorists, I do not believe that these relational influences must undermine procedural autonomy, even if they lead an agent to endorse values that reflect oppressive norms. I shall say more about this in Chapter 3. Second, the rationalist account that I shall develop shall draw on an account of rationality and the good that grants the possibility of impersonal goods, and denies relativism about the good.[38] Third, by outlining a detailed account of rationality and its relationship to well-being, I shall explain how the procedural theory that I develop can respond to cases of 'pathological values' raised by supporters of substantive theories. Finally, in Chapter 9, I shall suggest that there is considerably more overlap between the concepts of autonomy and well-being than is

[35] Ibid., 140.

[36] Frankfurt makes a similar objection in Frankfurt, *Necessity, Volition, and Love*, 130–5. See also Haworth, *Autonomy*, 156–7 and Noggle, 'Autonomy and the Paradox of Self-Creation', 96.

[37] For deeper refutation of substantive theories, see Friedman, *Autonomy, Gender, Politics*, 19–25; Christman, *The Politics of Persons*, 138–9.

[38] As Ciurria points out, concerns about relativism can plausibly motivate a move towards substantive theories. See Ciurria, 'A Virtue Ethical Approach to Decisional Capacity and Mental Health'.

often taken to be the case in procedural theories. This somewhat complicates our understanding of both the prudential value of autonomy, and how we ought to conceive of the principles of beneficence and autonomy in medical ethics.

In the next section, I shall consider what an adequate procedural theory of autonomy should aim to achieve, and suggest that procedural theories pertain to one of two dimensions of autonomy.[39]

2. The Decisional Dimension of Autonomy

Given the diverse array of approaches to the concept of autonomy, it seems unlikely that we will be able to capture the essence of autonomy by attempting to unite all the disparate accounts into one single theory. Rather, as Neil Levy suggests, it seems that in attempting to provide an adequate theory of autonomy we must 'restrict the range of meanings that we attribute to the word'.[40]

In this book, I shall be interested in the concept of autonomy in bioethics. From the outset, it should be acknowledged that this focus shall unavoidably influence my understanding of the concept, given the role that it plays in this specific context. To illustrate the significance of specifying the context in which I shall be discussing autonomy, consider the fact that theorists who are interested in autonomy as a broader social ideal have often suggested that one can only qualify as autonomous with respect to one's life-choices if one has a range of qualitatively different choices available.[41] Whilst it may be important to stress the necessity of adequate opportunities for autonomous agency in a broad social context, in bioethics we may often be interested in the autonomy of individuals who are facing severely restricted choice sets. For instance, we may be interested in what might affect the autonomy of a patient who faces a choice between certain death and undergoing an invasive medical procedure. This is not to deny that the breadth of an individual's choice set can matter. Rather the point here is that focusing on autonomy in the bioethical context means that it may be appropriate to set different thresholds for satisfying the minimum conditions for autonomy in this context, which may not translate straightforwardly to the use of the concept in other contexts.

Accordingly, in this book, I shall understand the concept of autonomy to denote a particular capacity to which we attribute value in bioethical contexts, and that we mean to invoke with respect to two particularly salient concerns:

[39] There are of course other ways of cutting the autonomy pie. Recently, Catriona Mackenzie has suggested that there are three dimensions of autonomy in Mackenzie, 'Three Dimensions of Autonomy'. Her dimensions of self-determination and self-government roughly map onto what I call below the decisional and practical dimensions of autonomy. Mackenzie also postulates a third dimension of self-authorization pertaining to an individual's regarding oneself as having the *normative authority* to be self-determining and self-governing. Notably, though, Mackenzie suggests that it is a mistake to believe that this is a necessary condition of self-government (Mackenzie, 'Three Dimensions of Autonomy', 35). Furthermore, we may note that self-authorization is plausibly less of a concern in bioethics than in broader social contexts given the widely accepted normative authority of individual decision-making, and the various instruments through which that is facilitated, most notably through robust consent procedures.

[40] Levy, 'Autonomy and Addiction', 429.

[41] For example, see Raz, *The Morality of Freedom*; Hurka, 'Why Value Autonomy?'; see also Mackenzie's discussion of self-determination, 'Three Dimensions of Autonomy'.

(i) Is an agent making her own decisions about what to do?
(ii) Is an agent able to act on the basis of those decisions?[42]

In view of the first concern, a theory of autonomy must be able to explain what it is for an agent to make their own decisions. I shall refer to this dimension of autonomy as 'the decisional dimension of autonomy'. In this section, I shall explain that the decisional dimension of autonomy incorporates elements that pertain to two different senses of voluntariness. In the next section, I shall turn briefly to the second concern outlined above, according to which autonomy, on the understanding that I shall employ, is an inherently practical concept.

To begin this discussion of the decisional dimension of autonomy with a methodological point, we should note that an adequate account ought to reflect at least some of our pre-theoretical intuitions about which agents are autonomous. Of course, it would be a mistake to claim that an adequate theory of autonomy should be able to justify *all* of our pre-theoretical intuitions about which agents might appropriately be deemed to be autonomous in bioethical contexts. After all, it may be possible to debunk some of these intuitions. However, it seems plausible to claim that we should aim for a reflective equilibrium between theory and our robust intuitions in our thinking about autonomy.[43]

According to what I shall call the 'standard view' of this dimension of autonomy in bioethics,[44] an agent is autonomous with respect to an action, including an act of making a decision, if it is performed:

(1) intentionally,
(2) with understanding,
and
(3) without controlling influences that determine their action.[45]

The standard account sets out conditions that *constitute* an agent's autonomy with respect to their decisions. As Friedman notes, we can distinguish such conditions from those conditions that may be causally necessary for the realization of autonomous choices and actions.[46] In the biomedical context, the second kind of conditions will be spelled out in theories of decision-making competence or capacity. In the first part of the book though, I shall be concerned with conditions of the first kind—those that constitute the agent's autonomy with respect to their decisions.

The standard account of autonomy implicitly reflects a distinction that Aristotle draws between two types of non-voluntary action at the beginning of Book III of the *Nicomachean Ethics*.[47] Here, Aristotle claims that an action can be thought to be non-

[42] For a similar understanding, see Brock, *Life and Death*, 28.

[43] See also Dworkin, *The Theory and Practice of Autonomy*, 9.

[44] Rebecca Walker refers to this as the standard view of autonomy per se in bioethics. I agree with this sentiment, but suggest that this account only captures the decisional dimension of autonomy. See Walker, 'Respect for Rational Autonomy', 340.

[45] Beauchamp and Childress, *Principles of Biomedical Ethics*, 103. See also Faden and Beauchamp, *A History and Theory of Informed Consent*, ch. 7.

[46] Friedman, *Autonomy, Gender, Politics*, 4.

[47] In the interests of accurate exegesis, it should be acknowledged that Aristotle's discussion of the voluntary here is situated within an examination of virtue, and is motivated, not by considerations of

voluntary if it is either performed from reason of ignorance, or if the action takes place by force, in such a manner that the moving principle of the action is most appropriately understood to be 'external' to the agent.[48] Conditions (1) and (3) of the standard account above can primarily be understood to reflect this latter sense of voluntariness, whilst condition (2) primarily reflects the former (although deception represents a form of controlling influence that can be understood to determine action by adversely affecting the patient's understanding). The standard account of autonomy thus understands the concept of autonomy to incorporate both of these senses of voluntariness.

It is generally accepted that conditions (1) and (2) of the standard account are necessary conditions of autonomy. For instance, although there may be considerable debate about how we should cash out the details of what sort of understanding autonomy requires, the basic thought that autonomous choice requires some minimum degree of understanding is uncontroversial. As Savulecu and Momeyer write in discussing the relevance of true beliefs to evaluative choice, 'we cannot form an idea of what we want without knowing what the options on offer are like'.[49]

However, the standard account becomes more controversial when we consider condition (3). The main inadequacy of the standard account in this regard is that it fails to offer a sufficient account of the sorts of influences that can undermine our decisional autonomy. Contra the standard account, the mere fact that an influence can be understood to 'determine action' is not sufficient to establish that the influence in question undermines autonomy.[50] To claim otherwise would be to beg the question against compatibilist views of autonomy of the sort that I shall consider in the first two chapters of this book. On these compatibilist theories, autonomy is understood to be compatible with the truth of causal determinism; on these views, not all forms of determining influence are understood to undermine autonomy. Moreover, as relational theories of autonomy correctly point out, autonomous decision-makers are relationally situated beings, and will thus be subject to unavoidable but legitimate influences.[51]

In Aristotle's discussion of the sense of voluntariness under consideration, he claims that actions are forced in the relevant sense when their cause is in the 'external circumstances', and when the agent contributes nothing.[52] Whilst this may seem like a natural way to draw the relevant distinction between internal and external moving forces of action, it is not an adequate approach for understanding voluntariness in a bioethical context. The reason for this is that on this Aristotelian understanding, the

autonomy, but rather by the thought that voluntariness is a necessary condition of praiseworthiness and blameworthiness. See Meyer, 'Aristotle on the Voluntary'. It might be argued that conditions of voluntariness undergirding ascriptions of praiseworthiness may differ from those undergirding the validity of consent. See Wertheimer, 'Voluntary Consent', 239.

[48] Aristotle, *Nicomachean Ethics*, 1110a. Note that acting from ignorance or forced action is only sufficient for non-voluntariness for Aristotle. In order for the action to qualify as *involuntary*, the agent must also be pained by the action or regret it afterwards. See Aristotle, 1110b18–20.

[49] Savulescu and Momeyer, 'Should Informed Consent Be Based on Rational Beliefs?', 283.

[50] For a similar criticism, see Walker, 'Medical Ethics Needs a New View of Autonomy', 601.

[51] Ploug and Holm, 'Doctors, Patients, and Nudging in the Clinical Context—Four Views on Nudging and Informed Consent', 30.

[52] Aristotle, *Nicomachean Ethics*, 1110b.

decision to comply with a coercive threat should be understood as voluntary, in so far as the moving principle of compliance lies within the agent herself.[53] However, this approach runs contrary to the widespread view that coercion undermines voluntariness in bioethical contexts.

Naturally then, the standard account of autonomy in bioethics rejects the Aristotelian understanding of coercion and voluntariness, instead explicitly claiming that coercion is a controlling influence that can determine action. It also suggests that other forms of external influence such as manipulation and deception undermine autonomy, in addition to forms of internal influence including '... conditions such as debilitating disease, psychiatric disorders, and drug addiction'.[54]

However, the standard account lacks a unified explanation of what it is that makes these forms of influence controlling in the sense that undermines the voluntariness of an agent's decision, and *a fortiori*, their decisional autonomy. Those who defend the standard view simply stipulate that coercion, non-rational persuasion, and manipulation can all render putative acts of autonomy void,[55] whilst other influences (such as rational persuasion) are paradigmatic examples of influences that are compatible with autonomy.[56] Yet, even if we assume that these stipulations are correct, it seems that an adequate theory of autonomy should be able to explain how and why these forms of influence undermine autonomy; listing examples of internal and external controlling influences is not satisfactory and instead appears to be simply ad hoc.[57]

Even more problematically though, in some cases the standard account's conception of the forms of controlling influence that undermine autonomy seems misguided. For instance, although Beauchamp and Childress suggest that psychiatric disease can undermine autonomous choice, it is far from clear that patients suffering from such diseases must lack autonomy with respect to their choices, particularly if they identify and positively endorse their choice to act in certain ways. More generally, Rebecca Walker expresses scepticism about the standard account's condition of controlling influences because the fact that an action is controlled does not entail that the individual lacks autonomy with respect to it. As she points out, some paradigmatic examples of autonomous choice involve decisions to do things that are highly controlled, in the sense that they are necessitated by moral or emotional commitments such as love. What seems to matter in these cases is not the fact that an action is controlled per se, but rather '... the sources of that control and the reasons why those sources necessitate the action'.[58] Accordingly, she claims that the standard

[53] Aristotle is initially somewhat ambivalent about this claim. He starts by noting that such decisions are 'mixed' with regards to voluntariness (*Nicomachean Ethics*, 1110a 12–20). Ultimately, though, he concludes that such decisions should be understood to be voluntary, even if they do not appropriately occasion blame (*Nicomachean Ethics*, 1110b 1–9).

[54] Beauchamp and Childress, *Principles of Biomedical Ethics*, 138.

[55] Ibid., 139.

[56] Nelson et al., 'The Concept of Voluntary Consent', 7–8.

[57] The criterion of intentionality offers little assistance here. The criterion merely states that intentional action amounts to the agent acting in accordance with a plan proposed for the execution of an action, corresponding to the actor's own conception of the act in question. Nelson et al., 'The Concept of Voluntary Consent', 10.

[58] Walker, 'Medical Ethics Needs a New View of Autonomy', 602.

accounts' requirement of the absence of controlling influences is a requirement of the wrong sort, at least when those controls are 'internal'.

What we need then is to develop a theory about what sorts of control are compatible with autonomy and which are not. One way in which it is possible to develop such a theory is to draw on legalistic approaches to voluntariness, and to develop an account of controlling influence grounded by the moral significance of the illegitimate, intentional control of third parties.[59] However, such theories adopt a narrow conception of voluntariness that overlooks an important point captured by the standard account, namely that non-agential forces (such as debilitating disease) can plausibly be construed as undermining voluntariness in some cases.

In view of this, the alternative strategy that I shall adopt in order to supplement the standard account in this regard shall be to draw on the philosophical literature concerning autonomy, rationality, and authenticity. I shall suggest that the standard account of autonomy should be supplemented with a rationalist authenticity condition, which can explicate what it is for an agent's motivating desire to be 'external' to the self in the manner that may aptly be construed to undermine the second sense of voluntariness identified in the Aristotelian distinction. Further, by reflecting on the role that rationality plays in autonomy, we will be able to offer a deeper justification for why certain forms of *external* controlling influence undermine autonomy. Crucially though, whilst I have identified the standard view of autonomy as having broadly Aristotelian roots, the theory that I offer here departs from both the standard view and an Aristotelian conception of voluntariness in emphasizing the role of rationality in the relevant sense of voluntariness.[60]

To close this section I shall illustrate two cases in which agents seem to face internal impediments to making decisions in the light of their own desires and values, impediments that philosophical accounts of authenticity may serve to illuminate, and which the legalistic approach to voluntariness neglects. To begin, we may observe that being autonomous cannot always simply be a matter of 'doing what one wants to do'. Such sheer independence will often not be sufficient for autonomous agency, since one's motivating desire might be an impostor on one's will.[61] To illustrate, consider the following example:

[59] Appelbaum, Lidz, and Klitzman, 'Voluntariness of Consent to Research'; see also Wertheimer, 'Voluntary Consent'. This sort of account also seems to be implicit in Taylor, *Practical Autonomy and Bioethics*; Bublitz and Merkel, 'Autonomy and Authenticity of Enhanced Personality Traits'.

[60] Although Aristotle acknowledges that rational choice is obviously voluntary, he notes that voluntariness is a broader notion, since non-rational agents can act in voluntary ways, even though they cannot choose voluntarily (Aristotle, *Nicomachean Ethics*, 1111b7–10). Furthermore, he notes that non-rational feelings are also a part of human nature, and that it would thus be odd to class them as involuntary (Aristotle, *Nicomachean Ethics*, 1111b3–4). Although my account is broadly compatible with the elements of truth in these statements (truths that are contingent on particular understandings of rationality), I am not intending to provide an Aristotelian conception of autonomy here. For a broadly Aristotelian conception that can be invoked in medical ethics, see Radoilska, *Aristotle and the Moral Philosophy of Today* (*L'Actualité d'Aristote en Morale*).

[61] As David Velleman has pointed out, it is possible to formulate examples of motivating desires that an individual lacks agential authority over, but which are not deviant in the sense that they are compulsive. See Velleman, 'What Happens When Someone Acts?', 474. For further discussion of construing autonomy as sheer independence, see O'Neill, *Autonomy and Trust in Bioethics*, 26–7.

> Jane is a drug addict. She is aware that her addiction is jeopardizing her ability to maintain her career and family, aspects of her life that she values. However, she continues to take drugs knowing that this will destroy her career and her marriage. Although Jane continues to take drugs, she feels alienated from her action whenever she does so; she believes that it is not a reflection of what she really wants.[62]

It seems that part of the reason that Jane is not self-governing is that she is moved to act by a desire from which she feels alienated. We might say that her motivating desire is thus 'inauthentic' in some sense; it does not reflect what Jane truly wants. Although I use the example of drug addiction to illustrate an 'inauthentic' desire, there are various medical conditions that could cause an agent to be alienated from their desires in this manner. For instance, some (although clearly not all) sufferers of psychiatric disorders might be understood as being motivated by a desire that they feel alienated from when they engage in self-harming behaviour. Furthermore, my use of this particular example should not be understood to imply that *all* addicts lack autonomy in the manner that Jane does;[63] it is rather an illustrative example of how one individual might plausibly lack autonomy.

Of course, an advocate of the standard account might point out that Beauchamp and Childress stipulate that drug addiction is an internal form of controlling influence that undermines autonomy. However, as I suggested above, without a deeper account of *why* drug addiction in particular threatens autonomy, this observation lacks explanatory power; in contrast, a theory of authenticity and its role in autonomous agency, could plausibly give us a deeper explanation of why drug addiction and psychiatric disorders may represent forms of internal control that undermine autonomy. Furthermore, it is possible to construct cases that raise a similar problem for the standard account that do not involve pathological behaviour. For example, Rebecca Walker describes the case of a woman named Desiree who feels an impulsive desire to undergo cosmetic surgery, despite the fact that she herself strongly believes that this is an immoral practice, and that women should be accepted 'as they are'.[64] Like Jane, Desiree is plausibly not self-governing because her motivating desire is 'inauthentic' in some sense.[65]

These cases both suggest that in order for an agent to be autonomous, they must bear a certain sort of relation to the motivational states that give rise to their decisions and actions. Procedural theorists tend to cash this out by claiming that agents are only autonomous with respect to their motivating desires if they carry out some sort of reflection on these desires to ensure their authenticity to the agent. In carrying out such reflection on one's motivating desires, it is believed that agents can have a greater degree of assurance that those desires are in some way 'their own', and not

[62] This is adapted from Frankfurt's example of the unwilling addict in Frankfurt, 'Freedom of the Will and the Concept of a Person', 12.

[63] For accounts of how addiction can be compatible with autonomy, see Foddy and Savulescu, 'Addiction and Autonomy'; Foddy and Savulescu, 'A Liberal Account of Addiction'.

[64] Walker, 'Medical Ethics Needs a New View of Autonomy', 598. Walker has two further examples that speak against the standard account.

[65] Substantive theorists might claim that Desiree lacks autonomy even if she endorses her desire for cosmetic surgery, and does not hold the belief that it is immoral.

merely the outcome of determining forces of the sort that serve to undermine autonomy.

I propose that the above discussion suggests that an adequate theory of decisional autonomy will incorporate what we may term a *reflective element* that captures what it is for an agent to make decisions in accordance with her own desires and values. This dimension reflects the second Aristotelian senses of voluntariness discussed above, pertaining to actions that are motivated by forces that are in some sense 'internal' to the self. This can be understood as a primary explanandum of procedural theories of the decisional dimension of autonomy.

A second explanandum pertains to the criterion of understanding, which reflects the first sense of voluntariness identified in the Aristotelian distinction. I shall refer to this as the 'cognitive element' of decisional autonomy. Whilst considerations relevant to the cognitive element shall arise in the first three chapters, I shall consider this element in much more detail in my discussion of informed consent in Chapter 6. Henceforth, when I intend to refer to agents who meet the conditions pertaining to both of these elements of a procedural theory of autonomy, I shall say that such agents are 'autonomous' with respect to their decision, on that theory. In turn, when I intend to refer to agents who meet only the conditions pertaining to a theory of the reflective element of decisional autonomy, I shall say that such agents are reflectively autonomous.

Many of the questions that I shall consider in my investigation of the decisional dimension of autonomy have also been understood as pertaining to the concept of moral responsibility, rather than autonomy. This is a by-product of the fact that these two concepts have often been conflated in the philosophical literature.[66] I lack the space here to consider the extent to which these two concepts differ. However, it is prudent to warn the reader against extrapolating the arguments that I shall make regarding autonomy to the concept of moral responsibility, and the questions that these theorists are seeking to answer. Where possible, I shall restrict my discussion of autonomy to works that ostensibly discuss autonomy as opposed to moral responsibility.

Bioethicists should similarly take care not to simply extrapolate philosophical theories of moral responsibility and autonomy to the bioethical context without reflecting on the role that these concepts might be playing in different contexts. Theories developed in the philosophical sphere are often designed to answer a narrow set of questions about internal control, without attending to issues relating to the cognitive element of decisional autonomy, or the practical dimension of autonomy I introduce below. Accordingly, they may not be well-placed to answer the questions that are the primary concern of medical ethicists. Nonetheless, bioethicists who reject the standard view of autonomy have appealed (either implicitly or explicitly) to a diverse range of philosophical theories of both autonomy and moral responsibility, often without acknowledging important philosophical objections to

[66] See Fischer, 'Recent Work on Moral Responsibility', 98 for discussion of this point. For attempts to differentiate the two concepts, see Oshana, 'The Misguided Marriage of Responsibility and Autonomy'; McKenna, 'The Relationship between Autonomous and Morally Responsible Agency'.

these theories.[67] Moreover, the standard view itself explicitly eschews reference to what I have termed the reflective element of autonomy due to concerns that it would render autonomous decision-making too demanding, and so risk the first error that I identified at the beginning of this introductory chapter.

Accordingly, once we have decided to leave the standard account behind, there is still a significant amount of work for bioethicists to do to develop their thinking about autonomy beyond the theories of the concept developed in the philosophical sphere. Having introduced what I have called the decisional dimension of autonomy, and its cognitive and reflective elements, let me now turn to what I shall call the practical dimension of autonomy. This is a distinct, but importantly related part of how we might understand the concept of autonomy in bioethics, and a dimension that has been somewhat neglected in the philosophical sphere.

3. The Practical Dimension of Autonomy

Philosophers who write on the concept of autonomy sometimes purport to provide a comprehensive analysis of autonomy by giving an account of the decisional dimension of autonomy. Still others consider only the reflective element of this dimension.[68] However, meeting conditions pertaining to decisional autonomy is not sufficient for autonomy *in toto* on the understanding of autonomy that I am invoking here. Autonomy, on this understanding, involves not only being able to make decisions on the basis of one's own desires and values, but also being able to *act* in accordance with those decisions (or to otherwise have those decisions realized) in some minimal sense.

This sort of understanding of autonomy is implicit in the bioethical application of the principle of respect for autonomy. The principle of respect for autonomy incorporates a positive obligation that enjoins us to facilitate an agent's ability to make an autonomous decision; however, it also incorporates a negative obligation not to restrain the autonomous *actions* of others.[69] For instance, the principle might enjoin us to respect a patient's decision to refuse a treatment that is necessary for saving her life. In view of this negative obligation, we can be accused of undermining another agent's overall autonomy if we obstruct their pursuit of an end that they have chosen to pursue (in accordance with the conditions of a theory of decisional autonomy). Accordingly, this negative obligation implies that autonomy can be understood as having a *practical* dimension, pertaining to the agent's ability to act effectively in pursuit of their ends.

[67] For a limited sample, Doorn, 'Mental Competence or Capacity to Form a Will' endorses a Frankfurtian hierarchical approach; for a bioethical endorsement of historical approaches, see Juth, 'Enhancement, Autonomy, and Authenticity'; Sharp and Wasserman, 'Deep Brain Stimulation, Historicism, and Moral Responsibility'. DeGrazia, *Human Identity and Bioethics*, 95–106 endorses a hybrid of these two approaches. Kihlbom, 'Autonomy and Negatively Informed Consent', 147 endorses a coherentist approach. Walker, 'Respect for Rational Autonomy' endorses a rationalist account.

[68] See Oshana, 'Personal Autonomy and Society', 83–6, for an analysis of this tendency in the philosophical literature.

[69] Beauchamp and Childress, *Principles of Biomedical Ethics*, 107.

I shall further defend this view in Chapter 3. However, I introduce the practical dimension here because I shall use the distinction between the decisional and practical dimensions of autonomy to frame my overall theoretical discussion of the nature of autonomy. Crucially, I am not claiming that we should recognize this dimension of autonomy simply because we need to be able to make sense of the negative obligation incorporated into the principle of respect for autonomy. I shall claim that neglecting to incorporate a practical dimension into our overall theory of autonomy actually leads to an impoverished view of the nature of decisional autonomy. For the purposes of this introductory chapter though, I suggest that an adequate theory of autonomy *in toto* for use in bioethical contexts must incorporate conditions pertaining to both the decisional and practical dimensions of autonomy.

With this in mind, we can present a conceptual map of autonomy in the following way (see Figure 1).[70] In the interests of completeness, this diagram reflects a claim that I have not yet defended, namely that the practical dimension of autonomy incorporates both positive and negative freedoms. I shall defend this claim in Chapter 5.

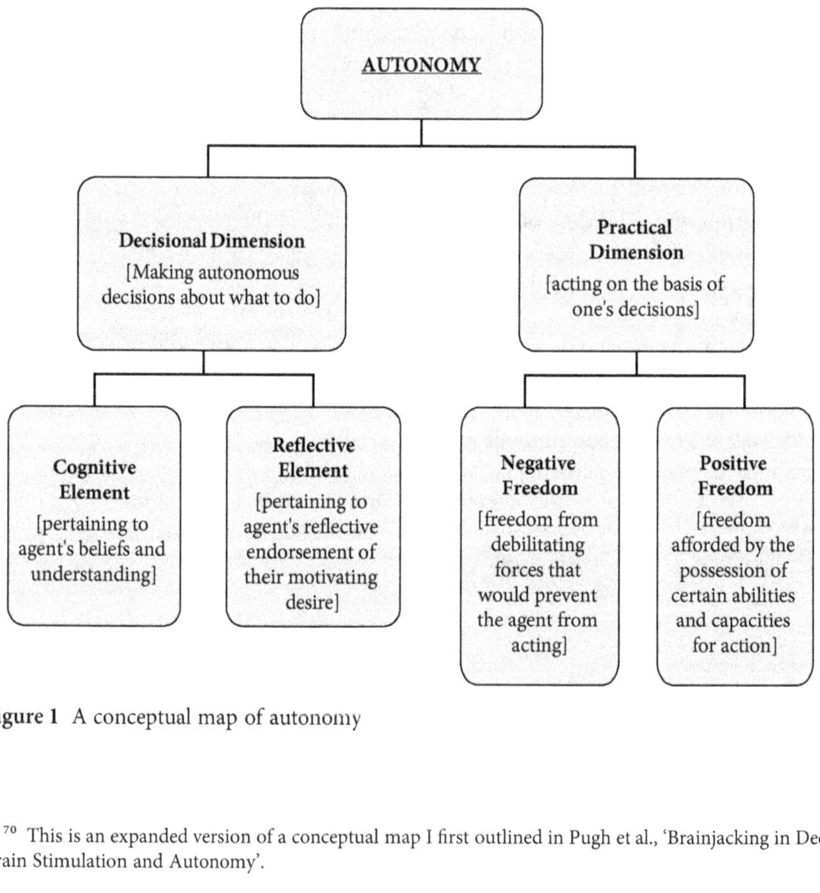

Figure 1 A conceptual map of autonomy

[70] This is an expanded version of a conceptual map I first outlined in Pugh et al., 'Brainjacking in Deep Brain Stimulation and Autonomy'.

4. Local and Global Autonomy

I have delineated an understanding of autonomy that frames the concept in terms of both a decisional and practical dimension. To conclude this introductory chapter, I shall explain the distinction between local and global autonomy that I shall also use throughout my discussion.[71]

Our interest in being self-governing seems to stem from our interest in being in charge not only of our individual decisions and acts, but also of our diachronic projects, and indeed, our own lives. Accordingly, when we consider the question of whether an agent is autonomous, it is possible to ask this question at both a global and local level. Conceived as a global concept, autonomy is:

> ...a feature that evaluates a whole way of living one's life (that) can only be assessed over extended portions of a person's life.[72]

Dworkin claims that autonomy is intuitively only a global concept, on the basis that it is odd to claim that people can switch back from autonomy to non-autonomy over short periods of time.[73] I do not share this intuition; it is not at all clear why it must be odd to suppose that an agent might be autonomous with respect to a particular decision but not to another one shortly after. This is particularly true in bioethical discussions of informed consent; for instance, it seems plausible that a physician could ensure that a patient was able to autonomously consent to some intervention by adequately informing them about the nature of the intervention, but fail to do so for another intervention shortly after. Moreover, it is widely acknowledged that decision-making capacity should be treated as specific to particular decisions. Indeed, as I shall suggest below, this perhaps partly explains why the standard account of autonomy treats autonomy as a property of particular decisions and actions, rather than persons per se. However, I see no reason to deny that both conceptions can be coherent. We can conceive of autonomy as a global property, but we can also conceive of it as a *local* property that an agent instantiates in a specific time-slice with respect to particular acts and decisions.[74]

The question of whether an agent is locally autonomous is perhaps less complex than the question of whether an agent is globally autonomous. Although it might be clear how to assess an agent's autonomy with regards to a particular decision in a certain specified set of circumstances, it is not immediately clear how we are to evaluate a person's autonomy as a feature that pertains to extended portions of their life, given the varied circumstances which 'a significant portion of one's life' can include.

One plausible way in which we might assess an agent's global autonomy is to consider whether the agent lives in accordance with diachronic plans of her own choosing, where a diachronic plan is understood to stipulate long-term goals that serve to guide the individual's local decision-making. These diachronic plans may

[71] Meyers draws the same distinction using the terms episodic and programmatic autonomy. See Meyers, *Self, Society, and Personal Choice*, 48–9.

[72] Dworkin, *The Theory and Practice of Autonomy*, 16. [73] Ibid.

[74] Christman, 'Autonomy and Personal History', 3.

vary in length; for example, in a biomedical context, we may say that a patient might have a diachronic plan to overcome some health problem, and that they may make local decisions that will have an effect on their pursuit of that long-term goal. However, some diachronic plans may cover the agent's whole life. Furthermore, it seems that some diachronic plans may be of more importance to the agent than others; typically, it seems that an agent's life-plans concerning her career and family will often be central to the agent's sense of 'who she is', whilst other diachronic plans, such as finishing an enjoyable TV series say, may not represent goals that are particularly central to the agent's self-conception.

There has been little discussion concerning how we should understand the relationship between global and local autonomy. On one view, it might be claimed that global autonomy arises as a result of the aggregate of instances of local autonomy over a person's life.[75] I shall not employ this sense of global autonomy here, since it seems plausible to claim that some instances of local autonomy can serve to *undermine* the pursuit of global commitments. Suppose an agent values two mutually exclusive diachronic goals, such as living a healthy lifestyle and becoming a gourmand. She continually changes her mind about which goal to prioritize. Here, it seems that the agent might make a locally autonomous decision to act in pursuit of one goal that will threaten the successful fulfilment of the other competing goal. The mere fact that the agent might be autonomous with respect to each of her local decisions does not seem to contribute to her global autonomy in this case, because her locally autonomous decisions to act in pursuit of alternating competing goals undermines her ability to successfully pursue *either* of them.

In stressing the importance of diachronic plans to global autonomy, I am not claiming that an agent's life must be unified by a certain single set of static diachronic plans throughout her life.[76] Clearly, people, and their circumstances, change over time, and people may change their diachronic plans accordingly. However, it seems that at least some threshold level of stability is required, so that the agent has sufficient time to commit to long-term goals that can confer an intelligible diachronic purpose to her decisions and actions. Furthermore, the nature of the way in which we change our plans is important. If an agent is to maintain their global autonomy despite a significant change in their plans, then they must be locally autonomous with respect to their decision to change their plans.

I mentioned above that Beauchamp and Childress' primary focus on autonomy as a property of choices rather than agents belies a failure to acknowledge the distinction between local and global autonomy; I am now in a position to explain this point. Beauchamp and Childress claim that the reason why autonomy should not be understood as a property of agents in a bioethical context is that:

> ...even autonomous persons with self-governing capacities sometimes fail to govern themselves in particular choices... [and] some persons who are generally not capable of autonomous decision-making can, at times, make autonomous choices.[77]

[75] Ibid. [76] Raz, *The Morality of Freedom*, 37 raises this concern.
[77] Beauchamp and Childress, *Principles of Biomedical Ethics*, 102.

Pace Beauchamp and Childress, these cases do not demonstrate that autonomy should not be conceived of as a property of persons; rather, these cases just show the importance of distinguishing local and global autonomy. With respect to the first case, there is no reason to think that a person's failure to make a locally autonomous decision must necessarily undermine their status as a globally autonomous person; indeed, I shall suggest in Chapter 9 that sacrificing our local autonomy with regards to a particular decision might sometimes be necessary for facilitating our global autonomy. Furthermore, we can also claim that a person might lack the capacities that are necessary to autonomously form and execute diachronic plans, and yet claim that they can be locally autonomous with respect to simple, synchronic decisions. As such, I shall claim that autonomy is a property of persons, and that a person's desires, intentions, actions, and decisions are autonomous in a *derivative* sense; they are, I suggest, things that an agent can be autonomous '*with respect to*'.

Conclusion

I have attempted to map some of the contours of a plausible pre-theoretical understanding of autonomy, in preparation for the theoretical analysis that I shall undertake in the following chapters. In Chapter 1, I shall outline four distinctions concerning rationality that shall play an integral role in my discussion of the relationship between rationality and autonomy. In Chapter 2, I shall go on to outline how considerations of rationality can be incorporated into a plausible account of decisional autonomy. In Chapters 3 and 4, I explain how this rationalist approach can allow for a deeper understanding of how and why deception, manipulation, and coercion serve to undermine autonomy.

In Chapter 5, I turn to defend the inclusion of conditions pertaining to the practical dimension of autonomy in an overall theory of autonomy in bioethics, and consider the relationship between freedom and autonomy, and how we might seek to enhance autonomy. I also claim that considerations of the practical dimension of autonomy provide crucial insights about the beliefs that are central to the cognitive element of decisional autonomy. Building on this analysis, in Chapter 6 I consider the ramifications that my theory has for the justification and elements of informed consent. In doing so, I further flesh out how we might understand the boundaries of the cognitive element of decisional autonomy. In Chapter 7, I turn to the implications of a rationalist theory of autonomy for the related question of decision-making capacity, and respond to prominent anti-paternalist objections to such theories of autonomy. In Chapter 8, I further develop this discussion by considering decision-making capacity in the context of decisions to refuse life-saving treatment. Finally, in Chapter 9, I consider the prudential value of autonomy, and its relation to well-being.

1

Four Distinctions Concerning Rationality

As I pointed out in the introductory chapter, bioethicists and medical lawyers frequently invoke the language of rationality in their discussions of autonomy. However, they often do so without fully explicating the understanding of rationality they mean to invoke, or the nature of its relationship to autonomy. This is problematic because different understandings of rationality and its relationship to decisional autonomy can lead to contrasting conclusions about the sorts of decisions that qualify as autonomous in bioethical contexts.

To illustrate, consider the much-discussed question of whether a Jehovah's Witness who refuses a life-saving blood transfusion can be said to be making a 'rational decision'. It seems that a case can be made for both the interpretation that the decision is rational, and the interpretation that it is irrational, depending on the sense of rationality that one invokes. On the one hand, given that the Jehovah's Witness believes that they will be unable to enjoy eternal bliss in the afterlife if they receive a blood transfusion, it seems in one sense rational for them to refuse the life-saving transfusion; it is quite rational to prefer eternal bliss over living for the remainder of one's mortal lifespan. On the other hand, we might question whether the Jehovah's Witness can rationally believe that they will not receive eternal bliss in the afterlife if they receive the transfusion; on this reading, there seems to be a good case for claiming that their decision is irrational.

I will consider the autonomy of individuals who refuse life-saving treatment in greater detail in Chapter 8. However, I mention this example here to illustrate how different assumptions regarding the nature of rationality can easily creep into bioethical discussions. Crucially, these assumptions can have hugely important effects if one also holds that decisional autonomy requires that one makes rational decisions, or that one acts on the basis of rational desires. Indeed, similar questions about rationality and autonomy will arise in cases in which individuals either choose to act (i) in ways that others believe are contrary to their best interests (which might include, for example, individuals deciding to engage in unhealthy behaviours like smoking), or (ii) on the basis of dubious beliefs (such as certain anorexic patients who refuse food on the basis of a belief that they are overweight, despite the fact that they are really dangerously underweight).

Accordingly, in order to develop an adequate rationalist account of decisional autonomy, it is imperative to first be clear about the understanding of the nature of rationality that one is invoking, and its relationship to autonomy. My task in the

Autonomy, Rationality, and Contemporary Bioethics. Jonathan Pugh, Oxford University Press (2020). © Jonathan Pugh.
DOI: 10.1093/oso/9780198858584.001.0001

following two chapters is to delineate an understanding of the nature of rationality, and how it should be understood to relate to decisional autonomy. To begin to do so, in this chapter I shall elucidate four key distinctions concerning the nature of rationality. In doing so, I shall draw on Derek Parfit's recent work on the nature of rationality, and join him in endorsing an objectivist account of reasons.

Although the discussion of this chapter concerns somewhat technical philosophical distinctions, it is, I believe, impossible to begin a conversation about the role that rationality plays in autonomy without having an adequate grasp of the distinctions that I shall outline here. Indeed, I believe that a failure to grasp these distinctions, and the conflation of quite distinct concepts is responsible for a number of important confusions about the role of rationality in autonomy, as I shall go on to explain in later chapters. Once we are clear about the nature of what an objectivist account of reasons entails, I will be able to explain how it may be used to supplement existing rationalist theories of autonomy in bioethics and philosophy, so that they can overcome important criticisms. This shall be my task in Chapter 2.

With this motivation in mind, I shall outline four distinctions in this chapter. The first distinction, between theoretical and practical rationality, concerns the different norms of rationality governing beliefs and desires. The second, between real and apparent reasons, concerns whether our beliefs about our practical reasons map onto reason-giving facts that actually obtain in the world. The third, between objectivism and subjectivism about reasons, concerns the fundamental *source* of all of our practical reasons, that is, what it is that ultimately grounds our having a reason to want or do something. The fourth, between personal and impersonal reasons, concerns the different kinds of facts that ground practical reasons on objectivist theories. Accordingly, these distinctions focus on progressively narrower features of particular conceptions of rationality.

It should be noted that there is very little consensus in the philosophical literature regarding the precise terms that one should use to capture these distinctions about rationality. For instance, what I am calling theoretical rationality is sometimes called epistemic rationality, and the distinction I follow Parfit in drawing between objectivism and subjectivism about reasons significantly (although perhaps not completely) overlaps with some understandings of what has been called internalism and externalism about reasons. However, rather than get bogged down in questions of semantics and exegesis here, I shall instead have to be somewhat stipulative in my choice of terms, and simply choose to follow some philosophers rather than others in my framing of the discussion below. To be clear though, it is the distinctions that matter, and not the terms we use to describe them.

1. Theoretical and Practical Rationality

Whilst beliefs and desires are both kinds of mental states, it is common for philosophers to distinguish them on the basis of what has been called their 'direction of fit'.[1] Since it is generally the case that the aim of a belief is for it to be true, a belief can

[1] Humberstone, 'Direction of Fit'.

be said to be successful if it fits the world as it is. If I hold a false belief, then I should seek to change my belief so that it better fits the world. In contrast, generally the aim of a desire is to realize the object of the desire. Like belief then, a desire is successful if it fits the world, but in the case of an unrealized desire the flaw does not lie in the desire. Rather, one should keep the desire and attempt to change the world to fit it; a desire's 'direction of fit' thus differs from that of a belief.[2]

Rationality can be partly construed as a set of norms that govern these different mental states. *Theoretical* rationality relates to the set of norms that govern how we come to form and sustain our beliefs.[3] These norms may involve, among other things, being responsive to evidence in sustaining one's beliefs, drawing logical implications from matters of fact and probability, and holding broadly consistent and coherent sets of beliefs.[4] To illustrate a failure of theoretical rationality in the medical context, consider the following example (from Savulescu and Momeyer) of a patient who is deciding whether to undergo an operation, and reasons as follows:

(1) There is a risk of dying from anaesthesia. (true)
(2) I will require an anaesthetic if I am to have this operation. (true)
Therefore, if I have this operation, I will probably die.[5]

This patient comes to hold an irrational belief because, due to a failure in logical reasoning, they have derived a false conclusion from the true beliefs in (1) and (2).

There is thus an important relationship between the theoretical rationality of our beliefs, and their truth. In following the norms of theoretical rationality, we come to form and sustain rational beliefs that are more likely to be successful, in the sense that they are more likely to be true; they are more likely to 'fit the world'. Conversely, failures of theoretical rationality will often lead to false beliefs. This is clearest in the case of many delusions and confabulations; whilst delusions and confabulations typically (but not necessarily) amount to false beliefs, they represent particularly pernicious kinds of false belief because they are typically based on underlying failures of theoretical rationality.[6]

However, it is important to notice the limits to this relationship. First, theoretical rationality does not *guarantee* the truth of our beliefs. In some cases, we can form a

[2] Platts, *Ways of Meaning*, 257.

[3] I use the terminology of theoretical rationality in accordance with existing rationalist theories of autonomy that employ this terminology. Notably, Derek Parfit, whose work I will draw on substantially in this chapter, refers to what I am terming theoretical rationality as 'epistemic rationality' (Parfit, *On What Matters*). It is also worth noting that although Parfit claims it is possible to distinguish theoretical (epistemic) rationality and practical rationality by appealing to considerations pertaining to the different 'directions of fit' of these mental states, he believes that it is better to draw the distinction in another way. He claims that the deeper distinction between the two lies in the fact that we respond to practical reasons with voluntary acts, whilst our responses to theoretical (epistemic) reasons are non-voluntary (Parfit, *On What Matters*, 118). However, for my purposes, nothing of great significance turns on the way in which we draw this distinction.

[4] For other discussions of norms of theoretical rationality in bioethics, see Walker, 'Respect for Rational Autonomy'; Savulescu and Momeyer, 'Should Informed Consent Be Based on Rational Beliefs?'

[5] Savulescu and Momeyer, 'Should Informed Consent Be Based on Rational Beliefs?', 283.

[6] Bortolotti, *Delusions and Other Irrational Beliefs*.

false belief in a manner that nonetheless meets the requirements of theoretical rationality. Suppose you go to your kitchen, turn the tap and collect the forthcoming liquid in a glass. It would be theoretically rational for you to believe the liquid in the glass is safe to drink, given your previous experience of drinking water from the tap, and the coherence of this belief with your various other beliefs. However, it might still be the case that the liquid is not safe to drink; perhaps, unbeknownst to you, the water supply has been contaminated today. In this example, your belief that the liquid in the glass is safe to drink is false, even though you formed it in a theoretically rational manner.

Second, theoretical irrationality does not preclude one's beliefs from being true. For instance, there can be cases in which delusions do not concern false beliefs. Fulford and Radilowska offer the example of an individual suffering from 'Othello' syndrome, which involves the persistent belief that one's spouse is being unfaithful. They note that it is quite possible for an individual to manifest this belief in a manner that fails to adhere to norms of theoretical irrationality, even if it happens to be true.[7] This is an example in which an individual's doxastic justification (i.e. the agent's justification for believing his wife is being unfaithful) is divorced from propositional justification (i.e. that which actually provides a sufficient reason to believe the proposition in question).[8] Whilst theoretical rationality does not guarantee the truth of our beliefs, abiding by norms of theoretical rationality helps to ensure that one's doxastic justification for a belief will align with its propositional justification, and make it more likely that one's beliefs will be true.

Whilst theoretical rationality pertains to the rationality of your beliefs, *practical* rationality pertains to the rationality of what we *do*, or the desires that move us to action.[9] On one prominent approach, practical rationality might be understood to derive from theoretical rationality. On the view under consideration, a desire is understood to be rational if it is *causally dependent* upon beliefs that the individual has attained in a theoretically rational manner. Indeed, some discussions of rationality and autonomy seem to implicitly rely on this sort of view.[10] However, although it is true that many of our desires causally depend on our beliefs, merging the two forms of rationality in this way is problematic. As Derek Parfit argues, an individual's theoretical irrationality need not transmit to her *practical* rationality in the way that the view I am considering here implies.

[7] Fulford and Radoilska, 'Three Challenges from Delusion for Theories of Autonomy'.

[8] Turri notes that it is widely claimed that if p is propositionally justified for S in virtue of S's having reason(s) R, and S believes p on the basis of R, then S's belief that p is doxastically justified. For a discussion and rejection of this view, see Turri, 'On the Relationship between Propositional and Doxastic Justification'.

[9] This phrasing implicitly adopts the Humean view of motivation, according to which desires are necessary for motivation. Whilst this view is not universally accepted, the rationalist theories of autonomy I survey in the next chapter are phrased in terms of 'rational desires' rather than the rationality of other motivational states. Accordingly, I shall follow these theorists in adopting this Humean assumption regarding the role of desires in practical reasoning.

[10] For example, Julian Savulescu claims that a necessary condition of autonomy is that one acts on the basis of a rational desire, which in turn is a desire that one holds on the basis of an evaluation that is grounded in theoretically rational beliefs. See Savulescu, 'Rational Desires and the Limitation of Life Sustaining Treatment'.

To see why, compare two cases. First, suppose that Alice holds the irrational belief that smoking will improve her health, and that she forms a desire to smoke on the basis of this belief. In light of my discussion above, we may say that Alice is theoretically irrational here because she holds the belief that smoking will improve her health, despite the overwhelming evidence she has against the veracity of this claim.[11] However, her desire to smoke *given that she has that belief* can plausibly be described as practically rational. One might explain this by claiming that Alice wants 'what, if (her) beliefs were true, (she) would have strong reason to want'.[12]

Alice's case is thus a counterexample to the claim that causal dependence on a rational belief is a *necessary* condition for the rationality of a desire. Consider now a case that suggests that casual dependence on rational beliefs is also not *sufficient* to establish the rationality of a desire. Suppose that Rosie holds the rational belief that smoking will damage her health, and that she forms the desire to smoke *on the basis* of this belief that it will damage her health.[13]

Some philosophers might deny the claim that Rosie is being practically irrational here. They might claim that desires for particular ends are not an appropriate target of rational assessment; we can only assess the rationality of the beliefs upon which these desires depend, and the rationality of acting in certain ways as a means to those ends. I shall consider this sort of view in the next section, where I discuss subjectivism about reasons.

In contrast to this view, I suggest that it is plausible to claim that Rosie is practically irrational here, despite the fact that her desire causally depends on a rational belief. The reason for this is that, *certeris paribus*, Rosie's belief that smoking will damage her health plausibly gives her a strong reason not to want to smoke. Of course, there may be other reasons that do count in favour of smoking (perhaps Rosie finds it pleasurable; perhaps she may even want to die prematurely). These other reasons might even outweigh the reasons against smoking. I will consider this point later. However, the more basic point about practical rationality that I am highlighting here is that, Rosie's forming a desire to smoke *as a result of the belief that it will damage her health in isolation* can plausibly be understood to involve a breakdown in practical rationality, and one that is not attributable to an underlying irrational belief.

In order to fully support this interpretation, I need to explain what it is for a consideration to count as a practical reason. I shall elaborate on this over the course of this chapter. For now though, I shall make the more general observation that the problem in Rosie's case is that her rational belief causes a desire that is not *justified* by the content of that belief; her desire to want to smoke is not a rational response to the belief that smoking is bad for her health. More generally, some of our desires can be aberrant in a sense that denotes irrationality because they causally depend on entirely irrelevant (yet rational) beliefs, or even (rational) beliefs that contra-indicate the desire in question, like Rosie's desire to smoke. In short, the fact that a rational belief *causes* a desire does not entail that the belief *justifies* the desire in question, in the sense that it provides rational grounds for having the desire.[14]

[11] Parfit, *On What Matters*, 115. [12] Ibid., 113. [13] Ibid., 115. [14] Ibid., 112.

Rather than claim that the rationality of a desire is conditional on the rationality of the belief upon which it depends, we should instead claim that it is the *content* of these beliefs that matters when we are thinking about whether a desire is rational.[15] That is to say, the relevant question for practical rationality is whether we have a reason to want the object of a particular desire, given our beliefs. Naturally, this raises the question of what kinds of beliefs are relevant to establishing that we have a reason to want the object of a particular desire. This question concerns a distinction between what Parfit calls subjectivism and objectivism about reasons. Prior to turning to that distinction, it is first important to be clear about the difference between real and apparent practical reasons.

2. Apparent and Real Practical Reasons

When we are deciding what to do, we typically tend to lack epistemic access to a number of important facts. In such scenarios, we have to decide how to act on the basis of the reasons that we understand ourselves as having *given* our beliefs. However, when our beliefs are false, our understanding of what we have reason to do may not map onto reality. As such, in assessing our practical reasons, and in thinking about the relationship between autonomy and practical rationality, it is essential to distinguish what we have 'real' reasons to do (notwithstanding our beliefs), from what we have 'apparent' reasons to do, given our beliefs. In some cases, the two can come apart, and we can have very strong 'real' reasons to refrain from some course of action, despite the fact that we may have very good *apparent* reasons to do that thing.

This is best illustrated by way of example. Recall my earlier example of turning on the tap in your kitchen, and setting about to drink the liquid in your glass. Suppose that the liquid that you believe to be potable water, is (unbeknownst to you) actually acid.[16] Here, you have a strong reason to *not* drink the liquid in the glass; it will kill you. We may say that you have a *real* reason here, one that is not dependent on what you believe. However, because you lack epistemic access to facts about what is in the glass (the contaminated liquid looks exactly the same as water, and you have no other cause to doubt that it is safe), and because you believe that drinking the liquid will serve as a means to an end that you value (quenching your thirst), we may say that you have an 'apparent reason' to drink the liquid. Whether or not an agent's apparent reasons amount to 'real' reasons (that is, the reasons that do, as a matter of fact obtain) depend on the truth status of the beliefs upon which the apparent reason causally depends. If the beliefs are *true*, the apparent reason will also be a real reason; if not, the apparent reason is 'merely apparent'.[17]

Since we typically make our decisions without complete information about our decision-making context, questions about the role that practical rationality plays in

[15] Ibid., 113.

[16] I adapt this from Williams, *Moral Luck*, 102. Notice that Williams uses this example in defence of a subjectivist view about reasons. For Parfit's specific comments on Williams' view, see Parfit, *On What Matters*, 65 and 77.

[17] Parfit, *On What Matters*, 35.

autonomous decision-making should be understood to pertain to apparent rather than real reasons. Drawing this distinction can enable a rationalist theory of autonomy to avoid some important confusions, as I shall explore in the next chapter.

3. Subjectivism and Objectivism about Reasons

The two theories about reasons that I consider in this section are theories about the *source* of our practical reasons, that is, what gives us reasons to do or to want certain things.

According to Parfit's conception of subjectivism about reasons, our practical reasons are always grounded by some set of our (perhaps hypothetical) present desires and aims. There are of course more complex versions of this basic view. For instance, some subjective theories might stipulate that only some of our desires can ground reasons; for instance, it might be claimed that our desires can only ground reasons if they are based on true beliefs, or perhaps if they are the desires that we would have if we were aware of all the relevant available information. These details about different subjective theories need not concern us here; what matters for my purposes is the fundamental thought underlying subjective theories, namely, the claim that all of our practical reasons are grounded by our desires. The relative strength of one's practical reasons on this view will thus be a function of the strength of the desire upon which the reason depends.

To illustrate, on a subjectivist account, if I harbour only one desire, which is to engage in a boring and meaningless activity, such as counting the blades of grass on my lawn every day, I thereby have a reason to do this; it is practically rational for me to count the blades of grass every day. Simply wanting to do something can create practical reasons. On more basic subjectivist accounts, simply desiring a very bad outcome, perhaps one that involves you suffering severe harm unnecessarily, can create a practical reason for one to act in ways that will bring about this outcome. If these desires are also adequately informed, or if they are the desires that we would have if we were aware of all the relevant information, then these desires would also create practical reasons on more complex subjective theories. David Hume famously captured the essence of the subjectivist view of practical reason in his claim that, ''tis not contrary to reason to prefer the destruction of the whole world to the scratching of my finger'.[18]

On subjectivist accounts then, our beliefs have a somewhat limited role in practical rationality. The beliefs that are relevant to establishing that I have a reason to do something (or to want something) are my beliefs about the means that are necessary to realize my more fundamental desires. I do not need to have any evaluative *beliefs* about the value of the object of my desires in order to be rational in pursuing them. The subjectivist can of course claim that I may need to have some kind of pro-attitude towards them; but that is not the same as believing that the object is good. Notice then that the subjectivist will have difficulty in explaining why Rosie

[18] Hume, *A Treatise of Human Nature*. I am not claiming here that the subjectivist is committed to a Humean conception of desires, as is sometimes thought to be the case. See Persson, *The Retreat of Reason*, 125 for discussion.

(in the example from the previous section) is in any sense practically irrational if she starts smoking.

In contrast, objectivism about reasons denies that an individual's desires fundamentally ground her practical reasons; rather it is evaluative facts about the *object* of the agent's desire that provide her with reasons to act. In outlining his objectivist account, Parfit claims that there are facts that make certain outcomes worth pursuing that '... give us reasons both to have certain desires or aims, and to do whatever we can to fulfil them'.[19] More specifically, an outcome may be understood as worth pursuing for a particular person if '... there are certain facts that give this person self-interested reasons to want this event to occur'.[20] We may also note that outcomes can be worth pursuing for reasons other than prudential ones concerning what is in our own interest. For instance our reasons may be moral or aesthetic; alternatively, they might concern the well-being of others. For the sake of brevity and simplicity, I shall frame my discussion of practical rationality in the majority of this book in terms of prudential reasons. However, we should not overlook the possibility of other rational grounds; in particular, our other-regarding reasons are a corollary of the relational nature of autonomy, a point to which I shall return in the next chapter.

On the objectivist account then, it would only be rational for me to count the blades of grass in the above example if there were facts about performing that activity that make it *worth* my pursuing it; does it, for instance, give me pleasure? Further, I would have no reason to cause myself harm (like Rosie) that did not serve as a means[21] to some further end that I *did* have reason to care about. This is true *even if* (like Rosie) I harboured a desire to cause myself such harm.

Unlike the subjectivist account then, the mere fact that I harbour a desire for some outcome does not itself render behaviour aimed at achieving the object of the desire rational. Rather my actions to realize a desire (and indeed the desire *itself*) are rational when there are facts about the object of the desire that make it worth pursuing. I shall say more about what it is for an object of a desire to be worth pursuing below.

Despite this considerable difference between subjectivism and objectivism, there is some overlap between the two. Most saliently, the objectivist account is compatible with the thought that some of our reasons can be grounded by our desires in a *derivative* sense. Let us suppose that being healthy is something that I believe to be worth pursuing, and that I form a desire to be healthy in response to this belief about the value of health. This is a rational desire on the objectivist account. We might say that this rational desire to be healthy now gives me a reason to do a number of other things that are instrumental to remaining healthy, such as exercising and eating well. However, the fact that this desire to be healthy is grounding my reasons to exercise and eat well does not mean that the desire is grounding a practical reason in the same way that subjectivism about reasons claims. The difference here is that for the objectivist, the normative force of these reasons is not fundamentally derived from the desire to be healthy itself (as the subjective account would claim); rather, on the

[19] Parfit, *On What Matters*, 45. [20] Ibid., 41.

[21] Or that did not constitute a foreseeable side-effect.

objectivist view, the normative force of these reasons is fundamentally derived from the facts that gave me the reason to desire being healthy in the first place.

The subjectivist and the objectivist can thus agree that a fundamental norm of practical reasoning is that we have reasons to do things that are necessary to realizing our desire for a certain end to obtain. However, they disagree about what fundamentally grounds these reasons. For the subjectivist, the mere fact that I desire the end in question is sufficient; for the objectivist, I only have a reason to do the things that are necessary to realizing my desire if the desire is *itself* rationally grounded by facts about the value of the object of my desire. I only have a reason to exercise if it is rational to want the end to which exercising serves as a means, in this case, being healthy (let us suppose). Crucially, on this view, if objectivism is true, it must apply fundamentally to *all* of our practical reasons.[22]

This may seem a somewhat technical distinction about the nature of practical rationality. However, it can have important practical upshots in medical ethics. Consider, for example, an individual who is suffering from severe and enduring anorexia nervosa. Many sufferers of this disease hold theoretically irrational beliefs about their weight, but they need not; some sufferers understand that they are dangerously underweight, yet harbour a desire to maintain a low weight, a desire that trumps all others. If such a patient refuses food, then it seems that the subjectivist is committed to the claim that such a patient is being practically rational; refusing food is a necessary means to achieving the end of maintaining low weight, the end that the patient most strongly desires (and one that she may hold whilst being aware of relevant information, having deliberated, and despite knowing that this desire is threatening her life). In contrast, on the objectivist approach, the rationality of the patient's desire to refuse food depends on whether the patient's desire to maintain low weight is a response to a belief that there are facts about low weight that make it valuable, or worth pursuing. I shall consider this objectivist interpretation further later in this chapter, and also in Chapter 8.

There is a considerable debate in philosophy about whether we should endorse subjectivism or objectivism about reasons. On the one hand, objectivists argue that there are clearly some things that we have reasons to want or do, irrespective of either our actual inclinations, or even what our fully informed inclinations might hypothetically be. For example, one of Parfit's own main arguments in defence of an objectivist account is that on subjectivist theories, we have no basis for explaining why an agent who has no desire to avoid a period of agony in the future after ideal deliberation is being practically irrational; this, Parfit claims, is surely implausible, terming this objection to subjectivist theories 'The Agony Argument'.[23] In response, the subjectivist may be sceptical of the claim that the objectivist can succeed in providing justifiable criteria for explaining why we have a reason to want or avoid certain things (such as agony) that do not appeal to the agent's desires.[24]

[22] This is the conclusion of Parfit's All or Nothing Argument. Parfit, *On What Matters*, 102–8.

[23] Parfit, *On What Matters*. The Agony Argument against subjectivism is also supplemented by Parfit's Incoherence Argument (Parfit, *On What Matters*, 108–15).

[24] For the classic defence of subjectivism, see Williams, *Moral Luck*, 101–13. For further discussions, Velleman, 'The Possibility of Practical Reason'; Brewer, 'The Real Problem with Internalism About

I cannot hope to resolve this long-standing dispute here. However, I believe that the objectivist view that Parfit has developed can provide rationalist theories of autonomy with the conceptual apparatus to respond to problems facing existing rationalist accounts of autonomy. I shall spell out further details of Parfit's objectivist account over the course of this chapter, though I shall not provide a detailed defence of objectivism over subjectivism about reasons. I direct the interested reader to Parfit's own powerful and to my mind persuasive arguments in this regard.[25] In the next chapter I shall also suggest that subjectivism about reasons is ill-suited to serve as the basis for a rationality criterion of autonomy.

Having assumed that objectivism is true, and before turning to a final distinction between different kinds of reason that objectivism about reasons can accommodate, let me conclude this discussion with some comments about the relative strength of our reasons on the objectivist account. The relative strength of our practical reasons on the objectivist account depends on the relative value of the objects of our desires, rather than the strength of the desires themselves (as per the subjectivist account). If we believe that the object of one desire is more valuable than the object of another desire, then we have stronger reason to realize the former. Parfit also offers some further terminology that is useful for comparing the relative strength of reasons on the objectivist account. He writes:

> If our reasons to act in some way are stronger than our reasons to act in any of the other possible ways, these reasons are *decisive*, and acting in this way is what we have *most reason* to do. If such reasons are much stronger than any set of conflicting reasons, we can call them *strongly* decisive.[26]

Accordingly, some possible act of ours would be:

> *rational* if we have beliefs about the relevant facts whose truth would give us sufficient reasons to act in this way,
> what we *ought rationally* to do if these reasons would be decisive,
> *less than fully rational* if we have beliefs whose truth would give us clear and decisive reasons not to act in this way,
> and
> *irrational* if these reasons would be strongly decisive.[27]

I believe we should also add the following definition to Parfit's list, for reasons that shall become clear in the following chapter. We may say that an act is *arational*, if we choose to perform it without believing that there are any particular facts that speak in favour of or against the act in question; our mere whims on this definition would be arational, rather than irrational.

Reasons'; Goldman, 'Desire Based Reasons and Reasons for Desires'; Sobel, 'Parfit's Case Against Subjectivism'; Sobel, 'Subjective Accounts of Reasons for Action'; Korsgaard, *The Sources of Normativity*; Manne, 'Internalism about Reasons'.

[25] Parfit, *On What Matters*, Part One. For criticism, see Smith, 'Parfit's Mistaken Meta-Ethics'.

[26] Parfit, *On What Matters*, 32. [27] Ibid., 34.

With these comments about the relative strength of different reasons on the objectivist account, I now want to consider a final distinction about different kinds of reason that might obtain on the objectivist account.

4. Personal and Impersonal Reasons

Subjectivism and objectivism about reasons have different implications for the kinds of practical reasons that are possible. Since the subjectivist claims that desires fundamentally ground our practical reasons, and we only have practical reason to act in ways that serve as a means to achieving the outcomes we desire, a practical reason would only ever be universally applicable if every existing person held a desire for the same outcome. Only then would everyone have the same practical reason to do what it takes to bring about that outcome. However, it is not clear that this would often be the case;[28] to slightly improvise on Hume's remark above, some people might prefer the destruction of worlds to finger-scratching.

In contrast, the claim that there are some universally applicable practical reasons is readily compatible with the objectivist account. Recall that the objectivist claims that our practical reasons are grounded by the value of the objects of our desires. It is now time to consider what it is for a consideration to count as a practical reason in this sense. One important way in which an outcome may be understood as worth pursuing for a particular person is if '. . . there are certain facts that give this person self-interested reasons to want this event to occur'.[29] In turn, 'self-interested reasons' are reasons provided by facts concerning the person's well-being.[30]

Whilst there are a number of different kinds of facts and considerations that can ground practical reasons, the kind that is most salient for a discussion of personal autonomy are these facts about well-being.[31] Naturally, this raises the question of what sort of facts might concern a person's well-being. Again following Parfit, theories of well-being are commonly classified into one of the following three types, as schematized below:

> *Hedonistic Theories*—What would be best for someone is what would make their life happiest.
> *Desire-Fulfilment Theories*—What would be best for someone is what, throughout their life, would best fulfil their desires.
> *Objective List Theories*—Certain things are good or bad for us, whether or not we want to have the good things, or to avoid the bad things.[32]

[28] Such reasons would be grounded by what Ingmar Persson terms intersubjective values, values that as an empirical matter of fact are shared by all persons. Persson argues that there are evolutionary reasons for thinking that there may be some significant intersubjective values, such as concern for one's future well-being. See Persson, *The Retreat of Reason*, 102–3. Michael Smith notably defends a the view that fully informed individuals would hold the same set of desires if they were formed in that (counterfactual) condition. Smith, *The Moral Problem*. For criticism, see Joyce, *The Myth of Morality*.

[29] Parfit, *On What Matters*, 41. [30] Ibid., 39–40.

[31] Recall that moral and aesthetic facts might also plausibly ground practical reasons.

[32] Parfit, *Reasons and Persons*, Appendix I.

I mentioned above that Parfit's Agony argument is taken to offer strong support to objectivism about reasons. However, in accepting this argument, we are accepting the claim that well-being incorporates objective elements. Even if we do not want to avoid some period of future agony despite having full awareness of the relevant facts, we still have a reason to avoid future agony.[33] The thought implicit in this argument is that we all have some self-interested reason to avoid agony because it is simply bad for us (in the prudential sense associated with well-being) to be in the conscious state of having a sensation that we dislike, regardless of our desires.

The terminology of 'objective elements' to describe this feature of well-being is widespread; however, in the context of a discussion concerning objectivism about reasons in the broader context of rationalist theories of autonomy, it is somewhat unfortunate. The reason for this is that this terminology lends itself to an important confusion between objective elements of well-being, and objectivism about reasons. However, the two are quite distinct; although objectivism about reasons allows for the possibility that practical reasons can be grounded by so-called 'objective values', it also allows for the possibility of reasons that are grounded by *other* facts about well-being. Moreover, contrary to what is commonly assumed, objectivism about reasons is compatible with the claim that reasons grounded by so-called 'objective values' need not trump all others.

I believe this confusion is rife in discussions of rationality and autonomy, and undergirds some prominent objections to rationalist theories of autonomy. In order to avoid this confusion as far as possible, I shall abandon the terminology of 'objective values' to describe the things that are postulated to be good for us, whether or not we want to have them. For want of a better term, I shall instead use the term 'impersonal goods' to refer to these goods, and call the practical reasons they ground our 'impersonal reasons'.[34]

The first thing to note about impersonal reasons is that they have somewhat limited scope. The sorts of goods that are typically postulated as impersonal goods are often quite abstract; for instance, one might claim that pleasure is an impersonal good. Yet, even on a theory of well-being that incorporates *only* impersonally good ends, agents may differ with regards to what they have self-interested *instrumental* reasons to want. Suppose our theory of well-being suggests that we all have a reason to pursue a certain final outcome, let us say pleasure; I shall follow Parfit in terming this latter form of reason a 'telic reason', that is a reason to pursue a particular end. Even on the assumption that agents have a self-interested telic reason to want to be in the conscious state of having a pleasurable experience, agents will achieve this same goal in very different ways. For example, if the sensation of eating ice-cream were pleasurable for Ben, then this fact would give Ben a self-interested reason to want to

[33] Parfit, *On What Matters*, 73–82.

[34] This choice of terminology is also not ideal, since Parfit himself uses the term 'impersonal' to describe a type of goodness that contrasts with goodness for a *particular* person. Parfit, *On What Matters*, 41. However, a somewhat confusing choice of terminology is unavoidable, since Parfit also uses other terms that one could plausibly use to clearly make the distinction that I draw above for other purposes. For example, he uses the term 'impartial reasons' to refer to reasons that we have to care for *anyone's* well-being. Ibid., 40. Furthermore, he uses the term 'objective' to refer to the theory that facts concerning the objects of our desires give us reasons. Ibid., 45.

eat ice-cream; however, if the sensation of eating ice-cream were painful for Chris (say because he has toothache), Chris would have a self-interested reason not to eat ice-cream. They would have different instrumental reasons that are grounded by the same sort of telic, impersonal, reason.

However, as I shall discuss in greater detail in Chapter 9, objectivism about reasons is also compatible with accounts of well-being that incorporate *subjective* elements. I shall call those reasons that are understood to depend on facts concerning subjective elements of well-being, including those contingent facts about what particular individuals have *instrumental* reasons to want in order to achieve impersonal goods, their '*personal* self-interested reasons'. Notice though, that what I call both impersonal and personal practical reasons are still objectivist reasons; they are grounded by claims about the *value* of their objects, and not by the mere fact that the objects are desired (as *per* subjectivism about reasons).

This distinction has important implications for how we assess the relative strength of our practical reasons. Accepting the claim that there are impersonal goods does not entail that there is also an impersonal *ranking* of such goods. Such a claim would have the unpalatable implication that the strength of our practical reasons would be determined by where the object of a particular telic desire appears on this hypothetical impersonal ranking of goods. Although this view is sometimes implicitly assumed to be an implication of objectivist theories, they need not have this implication. In addition to the fact that individuals can have personal reasons of the sort that I described above, rational agents can disagree to a significant extent about the *weight* they assign to different impersonal goods.

Indeed, Parfit himself is absolutely clear on this point. Although he is a champion of what I have called impersonal reasons, he also claims that, '[t]hough there are truths about the relative strength of different reasons, these truths are often very imprecise',[35] and that:

> ...there are many intrinsically good ends, but no ends have supreme value. Nor are there precise truths about which ends are most worth achieving. We often have to choose between many good ends or aims, none of which is clearly better than the other, and in such cases there is no end that reason requires us to choose.[36]

To be clear then, objectivism about reasons is quite distinct from, and does not imply the claim that rationality demands acting in accordance with what is 'objectively most valuable', or what I would rather term is of 'highest impersonal value'.

It is difficult to overstate the importance of this particular distinction when talking about the relevance of rationality to autonomy. A failure to adequately distinguish objectivism about reasons from impersonal reasons, and/or an impersonal ranking of such goods and reasons can lead to three related objections to rationalist accounts of autonomy. First, the strongest objection that this conflation might lead to is that a rationalist approach to autonomy will essentially collapse into a substantive theory of autonomy. After all, if rationality requires choosing in accordance with one's strongest reasons, and the strength of one's reasons can be determined impersonally, then

[35] Parfit, *On What Matters*, 33. [36] Ibid., 100.

the claim that autonomous choice must be practically rational would amount to the claim that we must choose in accordance with this impersonal ranking of goods. To illustrate, suppose that we believe that on an impersonal ranking of goods, the pleasure that one gets from smoking and/or drinking will be outranked by the goods associated with health that these activities might jeopardize. On this view, one might easily draw the conclusion that someone who knows the relevant risks and benefits at stake cannot rationally and autonomously choose to smoke and/or drink. Yet this sounds suspiciously like a substantive account of autonomy.

The conflation between objectivism about reasons and the claim that rationality demands acting in accordance with what is 'objectively most valuable' might lead one to think that a rationalist account of autonomy will be doomed to fail for another reason. It might lead one to think that such a theory cannot accommodate the possibility that agents can be alienated from impersonal judgements about what they have most reason to do, and that such alienation undermines their autonomy. Third, and finally, one might take these so-called 'implications' of objectivism about reasons to lend support to a theory of rationalist autonomy grounded instead by subjectivism about reasons, and the problems that may be associated with these theories.

Fortunately, these problems can be circumvented by carefully drawing the distinctions I have outlined in this chapter. In the next chapter, I shall show how objectivism about reasons can be used to supplement existing discussions of rational autonomy in bioethics, so that they are able to overcome some prominent objections.

2

Rationality and Decisional Autonomy

With the preceding chapter's discussion in mind, I am now in a position to consider what role rationality might play in decisional autonomy. Recall that the standard account of autonomy in bioethics claims that decisions are only autonomous if they are made intentionally, with understanding, and in the absence of controlling influences. However, as I pointed out in the introduction, there are some cases in which our intuitions speak strongly in favour of the claim that an agent can lack autonomy with respect to their decision, even though it meets the conditions set out in the standard account. Moreover, the standard account lacks a deep explanation of what constitutes a controlling influence.

Recall Jane, the unwilling addict who acts on a compulsive desire to take drugs. If Jane's failure of autonomy here could be attributed to her being irrational in some sense, then this would provide some motivation for claiming that the standard account should be supplemented with a rationality condition that precludes these agents from being autonomous with respect to irrational decisions.[1] However, this strategy raises three important questions. First, we might ask whether *all* forms of irrationality preclude autonomous choice. Second, we might ask whether the rationality of a decision makes a positive contribution to an agent's autonomy with respect to it, or whether we should simply make the weaker negative claim that irrationality precludes autonomy. Finally, and most importantly, we might wonder whether we can say anything more to justify the general strategy of appealing to rationality conditions to supplement the standard account, other than the fact that it accords with our intuitions in certain paradigm cases.

I shall answer these questions in this chapter by outlining an account of the role that theoretical and practical rationality play in decisional autonomy. In doing so, I shall particularly contrast my view with Rebecca Walker's recent defence of a rationalist account of autonomy. Walker endorses a negative rationality criterion on autonomy, according to which both practical and theoretical irrationality preclude autonomous choice. However, she does not commit herself to the claim that rationality might positively contribute to the autonomy of a decision (although she does leave open that possibility).[2] Instead, she claims that the 'straightforward' explanation for why one cannot be autonomous with respect to an irrational choice is that '... choosing irrationally is choosing on the basis of an error'.[3]

[1] Walker, 'Respect for Rational Autonomy', 343. [2] Ibid., 344. [3] Ibid., 344.

Autonomy, Rationality, and Contemporary Bioethics. Jonathan Pugh, Oxford University Press (2020). © Jonathan Pugh.
DOI: 10.1093/oso/9780198858584.001.0001

Whilst I agree with Walker about the significance of both theoretical and practical rationality, I shall argue that we need a deeper explanation of the role that rationality plays in autonomy than she provides. In outlining my own account of this, I shall suggest that a deeper explanation points us towards the view that rationality makes a positive contribution to autonomy. I shall begin by explaining why autonomous decision-making requires some degree of theoretical rationality, before turning to consider practical rationality.

1. Theoretical Rationality and Autonomy

In the introduction, I claimed that the standard account of autonomy reflects Aristotle's distinction between two types of non-voluntary action. In particular, I suggested that the criterion of understanding in the standard account reflects Aristotle's claim that an action is non-voluntary if it is performed from reasons of ignorance. Understanding is thus crucial to our ability to make voluntary choices in this sense; as Savulescu and Momeyer rightly point out, 'we cannot form an idea of what we want without knowing what the options on offer are like'.[4] We may add to this that in some cases a person may fail to understand the significance of their choice because they do not understand certain key features of their alternatives.

The criterion of understanding thus implies that agents must hold at least some *true* (and not merely rational) beliefs about their alternatives if they are to make an autonomous decision in that particular choice context. Call these 'decisionally necessary' true beliefs. What sort of beliefs might qualify as decisionally necessary? This is a complex question that I shall only be able to answer once further theoretical claims are in place (in Chapter 5). Roughly here though, we may say that there are at least some true beliefs that an agent must hold if they are to be able to minimally draw accurate connections between their values and their available options, in the manner that autonomous decision-making seems to require. Crucially, this view does not entail the strong claim that autonomous decision-making requires that we *only* choose on the basis of true beliefs; this is implausibly strong, given that we often cannot know for certain whether our beliefs are true. This is most clearly the case with our beliefs about future states of events. However, this does not mean that there cannot be *any* true beliefs that an agent must hold in order to make an autonomous decision.

To give one example here, suppose that a patient decided to undergo a vasectomy without understanding that this procedure will render him infertile. It seems doubtful that such a decision could qualify as autonomous. The individual has no idea about the implications that the procedure will have for him; we can even go further and say that it is doubtful that the patient in this case is even consenting to a vasectomy at all if he lacks this understanding. In my view, the belief that a vasectomy will cause infertility is thus decisionally necessary; to make an autonomous decision, we must know what our options are like in some minimal sense. This is a corollary of

[4] Savulescu and Momeyer, 'Should Informed Consent Be Based on Rational Beliefs?', 283.

the Aristotelian claim that actions performed from reasons of ignorance are in an important sense non-voluntary.

I shall attempt to further flesh out the concept of decisionally necessary beliefs later in the book. Here though, I am interested in the point that the criterion of adequate understanding may not preclude all forms of ignorance that are inimical to decisional autonomy. One's decision may be grounded in reasons of ignorance even when one holds the relevant decisionally necessary true beliefs. The explanation for this is that an individual may be theoretically irrational with respect to the way in which they *use* this information.

One illustration of this is the example of the patient I raised in my initial discussion of theoretical rationality in the previous chapter, who infers that they are likely to die from a surgery involving anaesthesia. Indeed, Savulescu and Momeyer raised this case to defend the view that autonomy requires theoretical rationality.[5] To illustrate the point further, Walker provides an example of a woman, called Maureen, who has been diagnosed with HIV/AIDS, and who refuses medication that there is a strong evidence base to suggest will be statistically likely to dramatically increase her chances of survival. However, Maureen believes that her statistical chances of survival with and without treatment are irrelevant to her, simply because they do not affect the more basic fact of fate that it is either the case that she will die in the next ten years, or she will not. In short, although she understands the relevant information and the statistical evidence about the treatment, her other fatalistic belief prevents her from applying this evidence to her own case.[6]

One might argue that the individuals in both of these cases of theoretical irrationality would fail to qualify as autonomous even on the standard account of autonomy, because they do not truly understand the information relevant to their decision if they reason in these ways. I am not convinced that the standard account's criterion of understanding is intended to capture such forms of theoretical irrationality, but the point is somewhat moot for my purposes here.[7] The reason for this is that if an advocate of the standard account conceptualizes the understanding criterion in this way, then this amounts to the concession that autonomous choice is precluded by irrational beliefs.

So why should we think that theoretical irrationality undermines autonomy? Is it simply the case that theoretical irrationality only undermines autonomy, or can theoretical rationality make a positive contribution to decisional autonomy? Walker advocates the former view, and justifies this by adverting to the further claim that theoretical irrationality undermines autonomy because it entails that one chooses on the basis of an error. Of course, this will only be a satisfactory explanation if *all* errors undermine the autonomy of the choices to which they lead. Yet this seems unlikely; indeed, Walker herself denies this, since she denies that true beliefs are necessary for autonomy.[8] By her own lights, autonomy is compatible with choosing on the basis of *some* errors in belief, namely decisions based on rational but false beliefs. Moreover, as I noted in the previous chapter, failures of theoretical

[5] Savulescu and Momeyer, 'Should Informed Consent Be Based on Rational Beliefs?'

[6] Walker, 'Respect for Rational Autonomy', 347.

[7] For exegesis of the standard account on this point, see ibid., 349.

[8] Ibid., note 11.

rationality can be compatible with true beliefs, as was the case in the example of the Othello syndrome; why should we suppose this error undermines autonomous decision-making?

We might also observe that Walker's denial of the importance of true beliefs is somewhat in tension with her apparent endorsement of the standard account's criterion of understanding. As I suggested above, the criterion of understanding implies that some true beliefs may be necessary for decisional autonomy. I shall further support this view later in the book, but we can leave that support aside for the time being. The point I wish to make here is that if Walker's negative approach is to be convincing, then it needs to be supplemented with a deeper explanation of why she thinks *all* errors of theoretical rationality threaten autonomy (even in cases where they do not lead to false beliefs), an explanation which is also compatible with her commitment to the claim that autonomy is compatible with holding (rational) false beliefs.

Alternatively, one can endorse a different view of the relationship between theoretical rationality and autonomy, one which is compatible with the thought that autonomous decision-making requires that the individual holds at least *some* true beliefs. On this view, we should avoid the claim that autonomous choice is compatible with choosing on the basis of *only* false beliefs, or with *complete* ignorance about information that is crucial to one's choice, as Walker seems to imply. This view is implausibly strong, if there can be decisionally necessary beliefs.

The claim that an individual must hold some true beliefs in order to be autonomous with respect to a particular decision is implicitly defended by Julian Savulescu. Savulescu argues that a necessary condition of autonomy is that individuals make their decisions on the basis of rational desires. In turn he defines a rational desire as one that results from an evaluation of the alternatives available, according to which one option (say A) is better than the other (B). The evaluation must involve at least the following three elements:

(1) knowledge of relevant, available information concerning each of the states of affairs A and B,
(2) no relevant, correctable errors of logic in evaluating that information, and
(3) vivid imagination by P of what each state of affairs would be like for P.[9]

I agree with the spirit if not the precise letter of Savulescu's view. In view of the way in which I distinguished practical and theoretical rationality in the previous chapter, I am reluctant to claim that these are conditions of rational 'desires'. Instead, I suggest that condition (1) (and to some extent [3]) pertains to the kinds of true (and not merely rational) beliefs that individuals must have in order to make a locally autonomous decision. Condition (2) in contrast is a theoretical rationality condition on autonomy. However, we may also note that the language of 'evaluation' that Savulescu employs suggests that considerations of practical rationality also have an important role to play in his view, as I shall explore below.

[9] Savulescu, 'Rational Desires and the Limitation of Life Sustaining Treatment'.

On the alternative view that I am outlining here, theoretical rationality can positively contribute to autonomy because when we form and sustain our beliefs in a theoretically rational manner, our beliefs are more likely to be true. In some cases our decisional autonomy may be *enabled* by our holding certain true beliefs, if these beliefs are decisionally necessary. I shall attempt to offer a deeper explanation of why true beliefs matter for decisional autonomy in this way in Chapters 5 and 6.

We can also make a stronger claim about the relationship between theoretical rationality and autonomy. Abiding by the norms of theoretical rationality can be important not just because doing so makes it more likely that we will form *individual* true beliefs. Theoretical rationality is also indispensable for placing these true beliefs in their broader informational context, for how we understand the world and how it relates to what we value. It is rarely the case that our decisions simply concern one particular belief in isolation; rather, in order to adequately understand our decision-making context, we often have to consider the extent to which a particular belief coheres with our other beliefs, about both descriptive and evaluative features of the world. Theoretical irrationality can undermine our understanding in this broader sense, even when it is compatible with the truth of a particular belief.[10] This suggests that delusions of the sort considered in the previous chapter can undermine decisional autonomy in two ways. They can either involve holding a false belief about an element of one's choice that is in fact decisionally necessary (in ways that I shall explain in later chapters) or delusional states can involve ongoing violations of norms of theoretical irrationality that otherwise jeopardize the individual's broader understanding.[11]

But theoretical rationality may also be said to enhance our *practical* autonomy as well as enabling our decisional autonomy. If our beliefs are true, the apparent reasons that ground our decisions are more likely to track our real reasons (rather than merely apparent reasons).[12] I am not here claiming that decisional autonomy requires that we *must* choose in accordance with our real reasons; this would make autonomy far too demanding for reasons explored above. However, when the apparent reasons that ground our decisions are more likely to reflect our real reasons, it is more likely that we will be successful in realizing the object of our desires.

To conclude this discussion of theoretical rationality and autonomy, I agree with Walker that a plausible minimal theoretical rationality condition of decisional autonomy may be phrased in the negative. We may plausibly say that decisional autonomy minimally requires the absence of theoretical irrationality, in so far as such

[10] For similar reasons, we may also be concerned about instances where doxastic justifications of true beliefs do not align with their propositional justifications. Indeed, this is why we should be concerned about what Shlomo Cohen has called the Gettier problem of informed consent. See Cohen, 'The Gettier Problem in Informed Consent'.

[11] Notice that this claim is quite compatible with the thought that delusions can be beneficial in some regards. Bortolotti et al. go further and argue that the fact that delusions do not undermine the capacity to form self-narratives suggests that delusions are compatible with self-governance (Bortolotti et al., 'Rationality and Self-Knowledge in Delusion and Confabulation'). However, whilst I agree that something like a self-narrative condition is a plausible condition of autonomy, it is not a sufficient condition. For reasons that I have discussed here, delusions can undermine decisional autonomy in ways other than undermining the capacity to form a self-narrative.

[12] Savulescu and Momeyer, 'Should Informed Consent Be Based on Rational Beliefs?'

irrationality is likely to lead us to (i) fail to hold a particular decisionally necessary true belief and/or (ii) to render us unable to place our beliefs in a broader coherent informational context that bespeaks understanding.

Of course, this claim will only be convincing if it is aligned with a criterion of understanding that sets out conditions on the decisionally necessary beliefs that individuals must hold in order to be able to make a particular autonomous decision. Yet, going beyond the minimum threshold condition of theoretical rationality, we may say that theoretical rationality can also make a positive contribution to decisional autonomy, in so far as it makes it more likely that we will hold crucial true beliefs. Further, in light of my claims in the preceding paragraph, I shall suggest in the next chapter that certain true beliefs may be necessary for the practical dimension of autonomy, that is, for us to be able to act effectively in pursuit of our ends. In any case though, contra Walker, the explanation for the role that theoretical rationality plays in autonomy goes beyond the fact that choosing on the basis of irrational beliefs involves choosing on the basis of an error.

2. Practical Rationality and Autonomy

A condition of theoretical rationality cannot explain why Jane the unwilling addict lacks autonomy. Jane can clearly be theoretically rational when she is acting on the basis of a compulsive desire. But is she being practically rational? And does this matter for her autonomy?

Rebecca Walker argues that the answer to both of these questions is 'yes'. Walker distinguishes between two kinds of goals that agents can have. Sometimes a goal is 'contingently' true of a person, in the sense that it is just a goal a particular individual has or chooses.[13] She gives the example of a person called 'James' who is a healthy weight, and who decides he wants to lose 10 pounds.[14] Crucially, she claims that there is nothing necessarily rational or irrational about such goals. In contrast, she contends that other goals may be rationally necessary (such as 'living well') or prohibited (such as 'self-destruction') for 'us as human beings'.[15]

In turn, Walker claims that these different kinds of goals are associated with different norms of practical rationality. With respect to rationally necessary goals, she suggests that one can be practically irrational simply by virtue of 'failing to recognise and choose in accordance with these goals'.[16] In contrast, with respect to contingent goals, practical rationality pertains only to the agent's willing the means that are necessary to achieve their goal. Failing to adhere to either of these norms can be sufficient for practical irrationality. In turn, since practical irrationality involves choosing on the basis of an error, practical irrationality undermines autonomous choice on Walker's approach.

Jane is most plausibly understood as acting irrationally in the first sense that Walker identifies. Recall that Jane wants to return to live a normal family life, and she knows that her drug-taking is jeopardizing this. If we understand her desire to return to a normal family life as a contingent goal, then her failure of practical

[13] Walker, 'Respect for Rational Autonomy', 342. [14] Ibid., 343. [15] Ibid. [16] Ibid.

rationality is a failure of doing what is necessary to achieve her desired end. Walker's theory also allows for the possibility that an agent who *endorses* their desire to take particularly dangerous drugs could also qualify as being practically irrational, if one holds that the avoidance of self-destruction is a rationally necessary goal.

Walker's account can thus offer us an explanation of why Jane is practically irrational. However, I believe that some misunderstandings in her conception of practical rationality lead her to overlook some other potential forms of practical irrationality, and to overplay others. These problems arise in part because Walker seems to conflate the distinction between objectivism and subjectivism about reasons, with the distinction between what I have called personal and impersonal reasons. More specifically, she adopts a subjectivist approach about reasons when discussing what she calls our contingent goals, and an overly narrow form of objectivism about reasons to what she calls our rationally necessary goals. As well as leading to an incomplete understanding of what errors of practical rationality might involve, we may also note that Walker's approach here is problematic for a deeper theoretical reason. It is not the case that objectivism or subjectivism about reasons are the sorts of theory that are true of some reasons but not others; rather these theories are about the fundamental grounding of *all* of our reasons.[17]

Consider first our 'contingent goals'. Walker takes the subjectivist line that such goals are not appropriate targets of rational assessment. However, it is entirely possible to offer an objectivist interpretation of these goals, and the norms of practical rationality that should apply to them. Indeed, 'contingent goals' bear a striking similarity to goals that an agent might have grounded by what I have called her 'personal reasons'.

Subjectivists and objectivists about reasons agree that practical rationality can demand that we should do the things that are necessary to realizing our desires. In accordance with a subjectivist view about reasons, this is essentially the *only* norm of practical rationality that Walker suggests is relevant for our contingent goals. However, objectivists can also not only offer a deeper justification for *why* this norm should obtain, they can also claim that our contingent goals themselves can be targets of rational assessment, given their relation to what I have called our telic reasons. Our desires to act in ways necessary to bring about some desired end can nonetheless lack rational justification, if the desire for the end in question is not itself rational.

To illustrate these different failings of practical rationality, return to Walker's example of James. Is it true that we can say nothing about the rationality of James' desire to lose 10 pounds, as Walker claims? Perhaps not; for instance, the objectivist might claim that James' goal is only rational if he decides to pursue this goal in response to his belief that he has some (perhaps self-interested) reasons to lose weight. Yet it is entirely possible that James does not adopt the goal as a rational response to such beliefs; it may just be a mere whim that he can't explain. Perhaps closer reflection would reveal to James that he does not actually care about losing the extra 10 pounds; he is after all already a healthy weight, and it will take an extreme

[17] Recall that this is the conclusion of Parfit's All or Nothing Argument.

amount of effort to lose the extra weight. In this permutation, James' contingent goal is one that he sustains in an *arational* sense.

It is also worth noting that contingent goals can be adopted *irrationally*, as an irrational response to reason-giving facts. Suppose for instance that Helen is on the brink of dying of starvation and yet still desires to lose 10 pounds—the objectivist might say that this contingent goal is irrational for Helen, even though it may not be irrational for James. The explanation for this is that there are facts that give Helen very strong self-interested reasons to avoid even limited weight loss, reasons which do not apply to James who *ex hypothesi* is a healthy weight.

The preceding discussion suggests that whilst an agent is practically irrational when failing to will the means necessary to achieving a contingent goal, she can also be practically irrational if she has adopted the contingent goal irrationally. In such cases, the agent will believe that she has strongly decisive reasons not to want the contingent goal. Alternatively, we may say that she may have adopted the goal arationally, on the basis of a brute desire that does not reflect what she actually cares about. This raises the question of whether autonomy is incompatible with practical arationality as well as practical irrationality. I shall defend the claim that it is below.

Walker's assumption of subjectivism about reasons with respect to our contingent goals leads her to overlook these potential deficits of practical rationality. I shall now suggest Walker's version of objectivism about reasons regarding our necessarily rational goals leads her to overplay apparent failures of practical rationality, and puts her theory in danger of collapsing into a substantive account of autonomy. According to Walker, a failure to choose in accordance with a necessarily rational goal is sufficient to qualify as a failure of practical rationality. Yet this is too strong. Objectivism about reasons is not committed to the claim that goals must be rationally necessary in this sense; we can have competing personal and impersonal reasons, and the truths about the relative strength of these reasons are highly imprecise. On more plausible versions of objectivism about reasons, one can be practically rational but fail to choose in accordance with a particular impersonal reason that we have 'as humans', as long as one is choosing in accordance with some *other* reason.

Julian Savulescu and Richard Momeyer make an even stronger claim about the apparent compatibility of autonomy and practical irrationality in their discussion of the following case:

> Assume that the harms of smoking outweigh the benefits. Jim has good reason to give up smoking. However, he may choose to smoke knowing all the good and bad effects of smoking.[18]

Savulescu and Momeyer use this example to illustrate their claim that 'a person may autonomously choose some course which he or she has no good reason to choose'.[19] In discussing this example, Savulescu and Momeyer claim that Jim's choice in this situation would be irrational; however, it would be autonomous if it were grounded

[18] Savulescu and Momeyer, 'Should Informed Consent Be Based on Rational Beliefs?', 283.
[19] Ibid.

by rational beliefs. On this reading then, their position seems to be that autonomous choice is compatible with errors of practical rationality.

Prima facie, many of Savulescu and Momeyer's claims in response to this example are appealing. Indeed, to claim that Jim *cannot* autonomously choose to smoke in this example might be understood to come close to endorsing a substantivist understanding of autonomy. Moreover, it also seems plausible to claim that Jim's choice to smoke would be practically irrational. Despite this, once we further unpack the example, I do not believe that it shows that autonomy is compatible with *all* forms of practical irrationality.

Let me take the points of agreement first; Savulescu and Momeyer equate 'having a good reason' with what I have called having a 'real reason'. Recall that such reasons do not depend upon the agent's beliefs (unlike their 'apparent' reasons). I wholly agree that autonomous choice is quite compatible with making errors about our *real* reasons; to claim otherwise would be to make autonomy all but impossible given the fact that we typically lack epistemic access to reason-giving facts that actually obtain.

However, this example does not establish that autonomy is compatible with *all* kinds of practical irrationality, or that practical rationality has no bearing on decisional autonomy. Much depends on how we flesh out the case. We are told that Jim knows all the good and bad effects of smoking. We are also told to assume that the harms of smoking outweigh the benefits, and that Jim thus has a real reason to give up smoking. Crucially though, we are *not* told whether Jim himself *agrees* with this impersonal ranking of the reasons associated with the harms of smoking and the reasons associated with its hedonic benefits for Jim. Yet, this feature is integral to understanding if we should understand his choice to be irrational in the manner that matters for autonomy.

The claim that Jim *is* autonomous with respect to his choice to continue smoking has more intuitive appeal when we assume that he does *not* agree with this impersonal ranking of values. In that way, his choice to smoke is a reflection of his own personal judgement about the relative strength of the reasons associated with the alternatives available to him; he values the pleasure smoking gives him over the longevity it threatens. It may be that his assessment of the strength of these reasons differs from the way in which others weigh them. Yet, further argument would be required to show that Jim would be evidencing a failure in practical rationality if he were to weigh his reasons in this way, particularly given the imprecise truths governing the strength of the reasons associated with different goods. This is not to say that such an argument would not be forthcoming. One way in which Jim may nonetheless evidence irrationality in weighing his values in this way is if he prioritizes the pleasure from smoking now over additional years of life in the future just because of an irrational bias towards what happens to oneself in the near future than in the more distant future.[20] Crucially though, an argument to that effect is necessary to establish the absence of decisional autonomy.

[20] For discussion about the nature of this bias, see Parfit, *Reasons and Persons*; Persson, *The Retreat of Reason*, ch. 15.

In contrast to those who conflate objectivism about reasons with acting in accordance with impersonal standards about impersonal reasons, the truths about the relative strength of many of our reasons, including those associated with the goods of health and pleasure, are imprecise. There is room for reasonable disagreement about which reasons are stronger. In so far as irrationality denotes a failure to act in accordance with clear and decisive reasons, it is hard to see how one could qualify as being irrational for simply holding a different view about which reasons win out in these cases.

To press the point further, suppose that someone like Jim, let's say Jimmy, *does* endorse the judgement in question; he agrees that he has stronger reasons to stop smoking than to continue, given what he knows about its harms and benefits. Yet Jimmy continues to smoke. It now becomes far less intuitively appealing to suppose that Jimmy is autonomous with respect to his decision to smoke; his action does not flow from his own evaluative judgements about what he ought to do.

In short then, whilst I agree with Savulescu and Momeyer that autonomy is compatible with errors concerning one's 'real' reasons, we should treat with caution their claim that Jim can be practically irrational and yet still be autonomous with respect to his decision. Much depends on whether we judge Jim to be irrational by some impersonal ranking of the strength of his reasons, or whether we judge Jim to be irrational given his own judgement about the strength of his reasons. Interestingly, my interpretation of the case seems broadly compatible with Savulescu's earlier work, which I delineated in my discussion of theoretical rationality above. In this earlier work, Savulescu claims that autonomy requires deciding on the basis of 'rational desires', that is desires that arise from an *evaluation* that the individual carries out in accordance with certain conditions (outlined above). The important point for my purposes here though is that it is the agent *herself* who must evaluate her options, in accordance with her own beliefs about the good.

This latter point raises an important feature of the rational autonomy view that I am outlining. Theoretical and practical rationality are not entirely separate domains of rationality. In particular, with respect to our thinking about autonomy, they are interlinked in the following important way: If we believe that decisional autonomy requires both theoretical rationality and practical rationality, in the sense that autonomous decision-makers must choose in accordance with what they believe they have sufficient reasons to do, then consistency demands that autonomous agents should be theoretically rational with respect to their evaluative beliefs about the strength of their different practical reasons. They must be receptive to reasons to think that some things have value, even if they do not need to prioritize a particular value in their decision-making. This feature will become important below, as I shall suggest that some agents who are practically rational may nonetheless lack autonomy because they are theoretically irrational with respect to their beliefs about what is good or valuable.

An objectivist account of reasons can thus offer a more nuanced account of how agents can be practically irrational. I now turn to the deeper question of why failures of practical rationality should be understood to undermine autonomy. As I have explained, for Walker the explanatory buck stops at the mere fact that practical irrationality involves choosing on the basis of an error. I want to suggest that there are reasons for thinking that we should go deeper.

If one believes that errors of practical rationality undermine autonomy, and one also endorses objectivism about reasons (as I have assumed since Chapter 1), then one is committed to the claim that what matters for autonomy is acting in accordance with one's judgement about the relative strength of one's practical reasons. The deeper problem with simply saying that practical irrationality undermines autonomy because it involves choosing on the basis of an error, is that we still need an account of why we should trust that this aspect of our agency is the right place for the buck to stop with regards to autonomous decision-making. Why suppose that these judgements speak for us, or that they are the appropriate seat of self-government?[21]

To give a concrete example of the issue at stake here, Jillian Craigie has astutely observed that in some cases anorexic patients can express regret for their earlier refusals of treatment, and we may suspect that these patients' earlier decision-making suffered from a deeper kind practical irrationality. For some such patients, it is not the case that they were irrational because they failed to choose in accordance with what they valued (or what they desired); rather their regret for their earlier choices is grounded in the fact that they regret holding the values that undergirded their choices at the time of their decision, or for what they desired at that time.[22]

Craigie's example raises deep and important questions about the role of rationality in autonomy. I join her in believing that we can provide some of the answers to these questions by considering the positive role that practical rationality can play in a theory of decisional autonomy. It is not simply the case that practical irrationality undermines decisional autonomy because practical irrationality involves choosing on the basis of an error; rather, by fleshing out the objectivist approach to practical rationality that I have outlined here in certain ways, we can explain why our evaluative judgements about our rational desires can be the seat of autonomous decision-making. To make this argument, I will now consider how rationalist theories of autonomy have been developed in the wider philosophical literature concerning the philosophy of action. This, and my discussion of controlling influences in Chapter 3, will provide me with the necessary platform to engage with Craigie's discussion in more detail when I turn to the issue of rational competence in Chapter 8.

3. Values, Identification, and Authority

Questions concerning which aspect of our agency constitutes the source of our autonomy have been widely discussed in philosophy of action. In this section, I shall briefly trace the history of this discussion before defending the account I favour in the following section. Readers who already are familiar with the philosophical literature on autonomy and identification may wish to skip this section.

[21] Note that a similar problem will arise for subjectivist but with respect to why one's desires should play this role.

[22] Craigie, 'Competence, Practical Rationality and What a Patient Values'.

In an influential paper that has somewhat set the terms of the debate in this area, Harry Frankfurt sought to answer the question of why agents who act on compulsive desires (like Jane the unwilling addict) seem to lack freedom of the will.[23] The explanation for this, on Frankfurt's account, is that such agents do not *identify* with their motivating desires.

According to Frankfurt, conscious entities have 'first-order desires' to do or have certain things. Some of these desires are the ones that actually motivate them to act; for Frankfurt, it is these 'effective' first-order desires that constitute 'the will'.[24] So, on this view, if I have a desire to *x* and I end up *x*-ing, this particular first-order desire is effective, and thereby constitutes my will. In so far as we are creatures that have such first-order desires, nothing separates humans from other members of the animal kingdom. However, according to Frankfurt, 'persons' are unique in that they can also have 'second-order desires'; these desires are 'higher order' desires that have as their object a certain first-order desire.[25] Further, persons can have second-order *volitions*; such volitions are a particular species of second-order desire, defined by their object. The object of these volitions is that a particular first-order desire becomes *effective* in moving them to act.[26]

The relationship between the agent's effective first-order desires, and their second-order volitions is integral to freedom of the will for Frankfurt. He writes:

> ... it is in securing the conformity of his will to his second-order volitions ... that a person exercises freedom of the will.[27]

Frankfurt's approach can seemingly explain why being alienated from one's motivating desire can undermine autonomy. Recall the example of Jane from the introduction.[28] We can understand Jane as having two conflicting first-order motivating desires; she has an urge to take drugs, but she also harbours a desire not to do this. We can also understand her as having a second-order volition: for the latter first-order desire (to refrain from this behaviour) to constitute her will. Nonetheless, Jane's first-order desire to take drugs becomes effective; accordingly, she lacks autonomy with respect to her drug-taking on Frankfurt's approach. We may contrast Jane with another addict Beatrice who would be autonomous on Frankfurt's approach: suppose that Beatrice has only one first-order desire; she wants to take drugs. However, unlike Jane, suppose that Beatrice's second-order volition is that this desire *should* come to constitute her will. She embraces her addiction, and would reinstate her first-order desire to engage in this behaviour should it wane.[29]

The reason that Beatrice is autonomous with respect to her drug-taking on Frankfurt's approach is because her motivating desire is authentic to her in a way that Jane's is not. At least by the lights of his original theory, Beatrice's identification

[23] Frankfurt's intention in the work was to provide a theory of freedom of the will and its relation to personhood, rather than autonomy per se. However, this has not prevented many commentators regarding his theory as a prominent example of a theory of autonomy. Taylor is a notable exception. See his arguments against this interpretation in Taylor, *Practical Autonomy and Bioethics*, ch. 3.

[24] Frankfurt, 'Freedom of the Will and the Concept of a Person', 8. [25] Ibid., 10. [26] Ibid.

[27] Ibid., 15. [28] Introduction, 00.

[29] These examples correspond to Frankfurt's examples of the unwilling addict and the willing addict. Frankfurt, 'Freedom of the Will and the Concept of a Person', 12–15.

with her desire ensures that it is a reflection of what she really wants, or of the central elements of her 'true self'.

Given the controversial nature of 'the self',[30] it is perhaps apposite here to clarify the role that the concept is playing here.[31] On this understanding it is not merely a 'grammatical error'[32] to claim that agents have a self in some sense; rather the self can be understood as the metaphorical locus of the agent's 'character',[33] or of the psychological continuities that ground personal identity on some theories.[34] In holding that the self is something that both persists over time and can undergird the intelligibility of the agent's long-term diachronic plans, this understanding of the self is naturally not compatible with those theories that deny that the self can persist over long periods of time,[35] or in a diachronically continuous sense.[36] However, it is compatible with a number of claims that are incorporated into a diverse range of theories of the self. Most critically, it is not committed to the contentious claim that the self is static, or an extant metaphysical essence;[37] the true self can be construed to persist even if the elements that constitute it change over time, as long as the agent changes them in accordance with the sorts of procedure that procedural theories of autonomy seek to explicate.[38]

Frankfurt's theory has been highly influential, and it is still appealed to in bioethical discussions of autonomy. However, it faces a similar question to the one that I raised about rationalist theories of autonomy in bioethics at the end of the previous section. Why should we trust that our second-order volitions should serve as the proxy for the 'true self' and as the seat of self-governance? Here, it seems Frankfurt faces a choice between two unappealing alternatives. First, perhaps an *even higher* order volition authenticates one's second-order volitions as being one's own. However, this reply is problematic because it seems to lead inexorably to a regress

[30] For instance, Ekstrom writes '... in order to understand autonomous action ... we need a working conception of what constitutes the "self"' (Ekstrom, 'A Coherence Theory of Autonomy', 599). In contrast, Berofsky argues against conceiving of autonomous agency as that which proceeds from some extant metaphysical self. See Berofsky, *Liberation from Self.*

[31] For a deeper discussion of the role of the self in conceptions of authenticity, see Friedman, *Autonomy, Gender, Politics*, 3–29.

[32] Kenny, *The Self*, 4.

[33] Both Mill and Aristotle invoke the agent's character as a ground of choice in their discussions of individuality and voluntariness respectively. See Mill, *On Liberty*; Aristotle, *Nicomachean Ethics*, book III. See Meyer, 'Aristotle on the Voluntary' for a useful discussion of how character relates to voluntariness in Aristotle's theory of virtue.

[34] See Parfit, *Reasons and Persons* (Part Three) for a classic psychological theory of personal identity. Michael Bratman explicitly points out that the self-governing policies that undergird autonomy on his view are inextricably related to the agent's identity, since they concern plans that are constituted by psychological continuities. See Bratman, 'Planning Agency, Autonomous Agency', 41.

[35] For example, see Strawson's 'Pearl View of the Self' in Strawson, 'The Self', 424. For an explanation of how Strawson's and David Hume's seminal view differ, see Strawson, 'Hume on Himself'.

[36] For example, see Hume's exposition of his so-called 'Bundle Theory of the Self'; Hume, *A Treatise of Human Nature* (section entitled 'Of Personal Identity'). For a rejection of the Strawsonian and Humean approaches to the self, see Olson, 'There Is No Problem of the Self'.

[37] For criticism of this essentialist view, see DeGrazia, *Human Identity and Bioethics*, 233–4.

[38] For further discussion of this understanding of the self and how it functions in the kind of account of autonomy that I develop here, see Pugh, Maslen, and Savulescu, 'Deep Brain Stimulation, Authenticity and Value'.

of increasingly higher order conative attitudes. Alternatively, he might claim that at some level, a higher order desire cannot be authenticated, and does not require authentication.[39] However, this reply leads to what John Christman terms the *ab initio* problem,[40] since it implies that the authenticity of one's first-order desires can only be ensured by a second- (or higher) order desire that is not itself authentically the agent's. As Christman puts it, this would involve the claim that '. . . desires can be autonomous without foundations',[41] and this, he claims, renders the second response 'implausible'.[42]

One might suppose that the problem with Frankfurt's theory here is its over-reliance on non-cognitive elements as constituting the true self. One reason for doubting that our second-order volitions in particular can constitute the true self is that agents can, as Frankfurt concedes, form these desires in a capricious manner, and without any serious consideration.[43] If these volitions are thus 'blind or irrational'[44] impulses, then it is hardly surprising that they cannot serve as an appropriate seat of self-governance. In contrast, one might suppose that a rationalist theory would not fall foul of the same problem because reason allows us to identify the good in our evaluative judgements, and our rationally warranted desires are thus not blind impulses.[45]

Yet such appeals to the authority of 'rationality' will not be sufficient unless one discounts the possibility that agents could similarly be alienated from their values; why suppose that our values constitute the real self? This objection has more and less plausible variants. First, one might object that the prospect of alienation can arise because rationalist theories entail that the agent's values must track some objective good, and that they are thus unable to account for the undeniable fact that we '. . . sometimes place value on senseless or masochistic ends, that is, ends that have no objective value'.[46] However, my discussion of objectivism about reasons, real and apparent reasons, and the difference between personal and impersonal reasons should make it clear that a suitably nuanced theory of rationalist autonomy need not fall foul of this form of the objection.

However, the objection can be raised in a more nuanced and fundamental way. David Velleman writes:

> The agent's role cannot be played by any mental states or events whose behavioural influence might come up for review in practical thought at any level. And the reason why it cannot be played by anything that might undergo the process of critical review is precisely that it must be played by whatever directs that process. The agent, in his capacity as agent, is that party who

[39] This is the horn of the dilemma that Frankfurt grabbed in his later work, appealing to the concepts of decisiveness and satisfaction. See Frankfurt, *The Importance of What We Care About*, 21; Frankfurt, *Necessity, Volition, and Love*, 104.

[40] Christman, 'Autonomy and Personal History', 7. [41] Ibid. [42] Ibid.

[43] Frankfurt, 'Freedom of the Will and the Concept of a Person', 13, note 6.

[44] Watson, 'Free Agency', 208.

[45] For an early rationalist response to Frankfurt in this vein, see Watson, 'Free Agency'.

[46] Berofsky, *Liberation from Self*, 80. Berofsky's complaint here is most readily raised against rationalist theories that employ a Platonic conception of objective goods. See Watson, 'Free Agency'; Wolf, *Freedom within Reason*.

is always behind, and never in front of, the lens of critical reflection, no matter where in the hierarchy of motives it turns.[47]

In light of these remarks, Velleman posits that agency is not grounded in some collection of psychological elements that constitute a 'true self'; rather, it must be grounded by a motive that is never subject to critical reflection, and which is nonetheless functionally equivalent to the agent herself. Initially, he identifies this motive as the fundamental concern that all agents share to act in accordance with reasons, where reasons are 'considerations by which an action can be explained and in light of which it would therefore make sense to the agent'.[48] In more recent work, Velleman has further specified his understanding of the constitutive motive of agency in accordance with this understanding of reasons. On the further developed view, the constitutive inclination of agency is not merely the inclination to act for reasons, but rather the inclination to acquire self-understanding, that is, the inclination to render oneself 'intelligible' in the folk psychological sense.[49] I shall use the latter understanding in my discussion below.

Whilst Velleman offers an account for how the rationalist might respond to the problem of alienation, I shall not pursue it further here for two reasons. First, aspects of the view are in tension with objectivism about reasons that grounds the theory of rational autonomy that I am developing here. On Velleman's understanding, our reasons for action only apply if we have the higher order inclination to render our actions intelligible. In making this claim, he is seeking to forge a middle ground between objectivism and subjectivism about reasons, insofar as our reasons still depend on a particular inclination, but one that is central to understanding ourselves as agents. However, the subjectivist element of this claim still seems open to Parfit's criticism of such theories; in particular, one might object that one's reason to avoid a period of agony is not merely contingent on whether one has the inclination to render one's actions intelligible. Moreover, Velleman's articulation of the nature of our reasons for actions also incorporates subjectivist commitments. On Velleman's view, holding a particular lower order desire for some outcome, in conjunction with a higher order desire for my actions to be intelligible, is sufficient for having a reason to act to bring about this outcome; the two desires can explain the action in the required sense. However, for reasons I explored in Chapter 1, the objectivist will find this claim and the absence of evaluation in this model problematic; for the objectivist, it is crucial that our practical reasons *justify* our actions, rather than merely explain them.

However, the second more fundamental issue with this approach is that we may doubt the underlying premise that motivates it, namely that the only mental state that can have the authority to speak for the agent is one that is itself not subject to critical review. This assumption motivates Velleman's claim that agency requires an inclination towards self-understanding. This is not only a considerable theoretical commitment about the nature of agency, it is also empirically dubious that the individuals that we would typically categorize as agents all share this inclination. Yet, rather than making this assumption, one might instead claim that the relevant psychological

[47] Velleman, 'What Happens When Someone Acts?', 477. [48] Ibid.

[49] Velleman, *How We Get Along*.

elements can plausibly receive agential grounding, even if they themselves can be subject to critical review. Instead of being grounded by some fundamental and 'pure' inclination as Velleman claims, it seems plausible that certain psychological elements could be mutually reinforcing and justificatory. Not only that, but these mutually reinforcing psychological elements can plausibly have agential authority just because they constitute our practical identities.[50] This is the thrust of Laura Waddell Ekstrom's coherence approach, a modified version of which I shall defend in the remainder of this chapter.[51]

4. Defending a Modified Coherence Approach to Rationalist Authenticity

On the coherence approach, an agent is autonomous when they act on a first-order desire if they have a 'personally authorized preference' for that desire to be effective. This terminology requires some explanation. First, a 'preference' in this context is understood to be a desire for a certain first-order level desire to be effective in moving the agent to act. However, this understanding of a preference moves away from a Frankfurtian picture of second-order volitions, since a preference on this account is formed in accordance with the agent's subjective conception of the good. Crucially, although this evaluation need not occur at the conscious level, it must actually be performed at some point.[52] Notice then that this understanding of 'preferences' is compatible with objectivism about reasons; the point is the agent forms her preferences on the basis of her beliefs about what is valuable. Such preferences are thus grounded by reasons of the sort that objectivists champion and subjectivists deny.

Second, a preference is *personally authorized* if it 'coheres' with the agent's 'character system',[53] that is, the agent's set of preferences at time *t*, in conjunction

[50] Michael Bratman adopts a similar approach in Bratman, 'Planning Agency, Autonomous Agency'. However, like Velleman, Bratman's approach incorporates a number of important subjectivist assumptions. In particular, he is quite clear that planning attitudes that underlie autonomous agency do not need to be grounded by an evaluative judgement. For Bratman's own understanding of valuing, see Bratman, 'Valuing and The Will' and Bratman, 'Identification, Decision, and Treating as a Reason'.

[51] Although I am choosing to explicate autonomy in terms of authenticity conditions, an alternative approach from the moral responsibility literature that is amenable to my rationalist approach claims that moral responsibility requires some form of reasons responsiveness. See Fischer and Ravizza, *Responsibility and Control*; Haji, *Moral Appraisability*. In turn, reasons responsiveness requires that agents are both receptive and reactive to a broad set of reasons. An agent is *receptive* to reasons if they are able to identify and process good reasons. An agent is *reactive* to reasons if their decision-making mechanism would give rise to different action in some hypothetical cases where different reasons obtained. Although I am sympathetic to the claim that autonomy requires reasons receptivity, I am less certain that it requires reasons reactivity. For discussion, see Mele, 'Fischer and Ravizza on Moral Responsibility', 288–94. For other objections to the claim that autonomy (as opposed to responsibility) requires reasons reactivity, see Christman, *The Politics of Persons*, 141.

[52] Ekstrom, 'A Coherence Theory of Autonomy', 603.The criterion of unconscious reflection is presumably a pre-emptive defence against the charge that people do not typically reflect on their motivational states at the time of action. In a similar vein, Savulescu appeals to the claim that autonomy is a dispositional property—evaluative reflection must occur at some point, although it need not be at the point of action. See Savulescu, 'Rational Desires and the Limitation of Life Sustaining Treatment', 199–200.

[53] Ekstrom, 'A Coherence Theory of Autonomy', 606.

with the set of propositions that the agent accepts at *t*. The latter are termed the agent's 'acceptances', and are beliefs formed in accordance with the individual's subjective conception of the true.[54] Finally, a preference for a particular desire to be effective coheres with an agent's character system if it is either (i) more valuable for the agent to prefer that desire than it is for her to prefer a competing desire, on the basis of their character system, or (ii) as valuable for the agent to prefer the conjunction of that desire and another neutralizing desire *n*, as it is for her to prefer a competing desire.[55]

It is important to clarify an ambiguity here regarding Ekstrom's terminology of it being 'more valuable for an agent to prefer a *desire*'. It may be more valuable for an agent to prefer one thing to another for two different kinds of reason. The reason might be object-given in the sense I have been so far considering; that is, the object of one desire can be more valuable than another. Alternatively, it could be more valuable for an agent to prefer a desire because she has *state-given reasons* to hold a particular preference. To illustrate, suppose that someone threatened to torture you unless you held a particular desire. This would give you a state-given reason to be in the state of holding the desire in question, even if you had no object-given reason to want the object of the desire itself (suppose that you would be tortured unless you held a desire to do something you find repulsive). Whilst Ekstrom's choice of terminology might lead one to think that she is appealing to state-given reasons, I think it is most natural to understand her view as appealing to object-given reasons.[56]

There is much to be said in favour of the coherence theory. It can explain why those of an agent's preferences that cohere with her character system have agential authority, in so far as the agent's coherent preferences and acceptances may plausibly be understood as representing the agent's 'true self'. There is a strong case in favour of this view, since cohering elements of the self are likely to be 'particularly long lasting',[57] since they are 'well-supported with reasons'.[58] By virtue of this support, they will also be 'fully defensible against external challenges',[59] as well as being preferences that the agent feels 'comfortable owning'.[60] However, our characters are not thereby static; elements of our character systems can and do change. Crucially though, if new elements of our psychological economies are to cohere, then they must admit of rational justification in accordance with other elements of our characters. Accordingly, character change that is compatible with autonomy will be gradual, and akin to rebuilding Neurath's raft. New elements have to fit with the pre-existing structure; moreover, replacing the complete structure wholesale in one fell swoop would rupture the continuity of the agent's identity.

The coherence approach can thus offer a model for how our evaluative judgements about what we have reasons to do can be understood as the appropriate seat of self-governance. Practical rationality, understood as acting in accordance with our

[54] Ibid. [55] Ibid., 611.

[56] See Parfit, *On What Matters*, 50–2 and appendix A for further discussion of state-given reasons. Notably, he is sceptical about the import of such reasons, if they do in fact obtain in separation from object-given reasons.

[57] Ekstrom, 'A Coherence Theory of Autonomy', 608. [58] Ibid. [59] Ibid. [60] Ibid., 609.

rationally warranted preferences, has a positive role in autonomy because our preferences are abiding elements of our characters, and thus have agential authority. To conclude this chapter, I shall defend the coherence approach from three objections, and in doing so slightly refine the view. To be clear, in light of the distinction I drew in the introduction, the objections I consider here are objections to the claim that a rationalist coherentist condition should feature amongst the conditions of what *constitutes* decisional autonomy. I shall consider further objections to the implications of my theory for the *causal* conditions of autonomy (including objections grounded in concerns about demandingness and the role of emotions in rationalist autonomy), in Chapter 7.

(i) An Asymmetry of Theoretical and Practical Rationality?

On Ekstrom's description, the coherence theory allows for a possible asymmetry between theoretical and practical rationality. Preferences have to be rationally warranted in the objectivist sense that the agent must believe that they have reasons to have those preferences, reasons that are based upon their subjective beliefs concerning the good. Yet, acceptances need only be held in accordance with the agent's 'subjective conception of the true'; as such, the coherence theory denies that the autonomous agent's beliefs must be in any way rationally warranted. However, this asymmetry between practical and theoretical rationality is problematic. In section 1, I argued that autonomous decision-making plausibly requires a degree of theoretical rationality. Towards the end of section 2, I also mentioned that if one accepts this point, then consistency demands that we should claim that autonomous agents should be theoretically rational with respect to the evaluative beliefs about the good. Crucially, these evaluative beliefs significantly ground our practical rationality. This point comes to fore in cases where agents might plausibly lack autonomy with regards to their motivating desire, not because the motivating desire itself is incongruous with their subjective conception of the good, but rather because the agent's *beliefs* about the good are theoretically irrational. For instance, as Fulford explains, delusions that threaten autonomy can be evaluative and not simply factual.[61]

To illustrate this point, consider a sufferer of clinical depression. In some cases of this psychiatric disorder, the sufferer may have a suicidal desire that they personally authorize; but this authorization may stem from a belief about the disvalue of their own life that they hold irrationally.[62] In saying that the belief is irrational in this sense, I do not mean to say anything about whether the content of the belief is objectively true or false. As I observed in the previous chapter, it is a mistake to assume that delusions are necessarily false; so accepting that evaluative delusions are possible does not entail the claim that they involve *false* evaluative judgements. Moreover, as I shall clarify in Chapter 8, I am not denying that a desire to end one's own life can never be practically rational, nor grounded by theoretically rational evaluative beliefs. The point here is rather that in some cases agents are not themselves able to offer any cogent reasons as to *why* they hold certain dubious evaluative

[61] Fulford, 'Evaluative Delusions'. [62] See Beck, *Depression*, 3.

beliefs (perhaps about their own self-worth), or to respond to any epistemic reasons with which they are presented against holding such beliefs (for instance, evidence that other people care about them, contrary to their own impression). Instead, they may simply adopt these beliefs unshakeably in a manner that bespeaks a delusional state.

There are important questions about how we should delimit the scope of the concept of an 'evaluative delusion' to which I shall return in Chapter 8. Moreover, we should of course take care not to automatically assume that sufferers of psychiatric disorder always lack autonomy with respect to desires that constitute a significant diagnostic criterion of their condition (again, a point to which I shall return). Yet, it seems plausible to claim that the agent in the particular case under consideration plausibly does lack autonomy with respect to their suicidal desire given the nature of the evaluative belief upon which it is based; I suggest that just as we believe that an agent can lack autonomy if they are compelled by a motivating desire from which they feel alienated, so too can an agent lack autonomy if their endorsement of their motivating desire is based upon an irrational belief about the good. In cases such as the one I am considering here, it seems possible that an agent's decisional autonomy can be undermined by delusional evaluative beliefs, as well as compulsive first-order desires.[63]

Whilst the coherence theory's appeal to a purely subjective understanding of the truth with respect to the agent's acceptances is problematic for this reason, the problem is easily remedied. Like rationalist theories of autonomy in bioethics, the coherence approach should adopt a condition of theoretical rationality with respect to acceptances.

(ii) Competing Desires and Coherence

The second objection pertains to the criteria of what it is for an agent's preferences to cohere. On Ekstrom's view, when agents have to decide which of two competing preferences should win out and cohere with their other central preferences, the autonomous agent will decide that one preference defeats another on the basis that it is *more valuable* for her to prefer the object of desire *d* to the object of desire *g*, or at least as valuable to prefer the object of desire *d* and some neutralizing desire *n*.

A problem with this view is that it is unable to account for the possibility that an agent could be autonomous with respect to a desire to act in manner that they believe to be sub-optimal. Consider the following example. Suppose that Jim values having a career in medicine, but also values spending more time with his family. Following a great deal of consideration, let us suppose that Jim forms the judgement that it would be slightly more valuable for him to prefer that his desire to spend more time with his

[63] Radoilska argues that depression can undermine decisional autonomy because it involves paradoxical identification, in which one identifies with what one loathes, in this case, oneself. See Radoilska, 'Depression, Decisional Capacity, and Personal Autonomy'. I am sympathetic to this view, and acknowledge that this is a related way in which depression can serve to undermine decisional autonomy.

family be effective in moving him to act.[64] Would it really be the case that, having made this assessment about what is more valuable (and sticking to it), Jim would no longer be autonomous with respect to his decision if he became motivated to instead pursue a career in medicine? Admittedly, he would be doing so in the knowledge that he could be doing something else that he believed to be slightly more valuable; however, it still seems plausible to claim that Jim could nonetheless still be autonomous with respect to this decision.[65] Notice that this is compatible with the claim that Jim would have been *more* autonomous if he had chosen to act in accordance with what he believed to be his strongest reasons. The point that I am making here is that it is more plausible to make these two claims, rather than to rule out the possibility of Jim's autonomy here.

Indeed, as I have stressed throughout this chapter, truths regarding the relative strength of our different competing self-interested reasons can be highly imprecise, and there may just be no clear way of deciding which of two competing preferences *A* and *B* it would be more valuable for one to prefer. Paul Hughes has argued that when a person acts from volitional ambivalence like this:

> ...she is not autonomous either with respect to the desire that prompts her action or the action itself...[since]...in cases of volitional ambivalence there is no single conative 'self' directing the agent's actions.[66]

Hughes seems to be making a similar assumption to Velleman here in appealing to the need for a single conative self directing critical evaluation. As I have explained, the coherence approach can explain why this is not necessary; cohering elements of our character systems admit of both rational justification, and mutually reinforcing justifications. Moreover, *pace* Hughes, it is not clear why an agent in this situation would not be autonomous with respect to their action once they had elected to act in accordance with, say, preference A rather than preference B. Once the agent has plumped for A, it seems plausible to claim that they will be autonomous with respect to acting in pursuit of A *in so far as preference A is itself still rationally warranted.* In plumping this way, otherwise ambivalent agents simply act in a manner that serves to constitute their will.[67] Although A is no better or worse than B, this only means that the agent may lack a rational basis for their choice of A over B; but this does not mean that they lack autonomy with respect to their acting in pursuit of A, since that act itself is still rationally warranted.[68] The choice of A over B is thus a choice to prioritize a certain set of reasons over another, and to emphasize the corresponding

[64] For simplicity, I am assuming here that the beliefs that Jim knows he has at the time of deliberation prior to this judgement exhaust all of the beliefs he has relevant to this decision. However, as Arpaly points out, this need not be the case. See Arpaly, 'On Acting Rationally against One's Best Judgment'.

[65] Sher discusses a similar example. Sher, 'Liberal Neutrality and the Value of Autonomy', 143. See also Raz, *The Morality of Freedom*, 304.

[66] Hughes, 'Ambivalence, Autonomy, and Organ Sales', 238–9. Bratman also raises this sort of underdetermination case as raising a concern for theories of autonomy that appeal to rationalist considerations. See Bratman, 'Reflection, Planning, and Temporally Extended Agency'.

[67] Ruth Chang defends a similar view, and a detailed account of the nature of what she calls 'hard choices' in Chang, 'Hard Choices'.

[68] Sher, 'Liberal Neutrality and the Value of Autonomy', 144 makes a similar point.

aspects of one's character system, even whilst acknowledging that the alternative choice also represents elements of one's character system that one would not otherwise repudiate.[69] An agent's chosen preference can still cohere with her other central preferences and acceptances, and ground an autonomous choice in such circumstances. Indeed, in light of this discussion, it is notable that in medical contexts, a patient's demonstrable ambivalence in the face of difficult choices in an end of life decision-making context is not understood to readily undermine decision-making competence.[70]

In light of the above, the coherence approach should adopt the weaker claim that autonomous agents should choose in accordance with preferences that they have a sufficient reason to adopt. On this understanding, coherence is incompatible with irrationality in Parfit's sense, but not with choosing in a less than fully rational manner. With this amendment, the coherence approach can accommodate the plausible claim that autonomous agents can make sub-optimal choices, which may still reflect central elements of the agent's characters, particularly in the light of the imprecise truths governing the strength of our competing practical reasons.

(iii) Authentic Alienation?

Suzy Killmister has recently raised an important challenge for rationalist theories of autonomy that is apposite here.[71] She asks us to consider a case in which an agent accepts that a motivational attitude they hold is irrational, but which they nonetheless regard as providing them with sufficient justificatory reasons to act, because it reflects what they take to be their true self. Most theories of autonomy, she claims, cannot account for the thought that such an agent seems to be autonomous along some dimensions, but less autonomous along others.

To give a concrete bioethical example, an anorexic patient might regard her desire to refrain from eating as irrational, and yet also regard it as providing her with sufficient justificatory reason to refrain from eating. The justificatory reason arises from the fact that the patient understands this irrational desire to partly constitute her real self.[72] Killmister claims that in order to account for this sort of case, we need to split what I am calling the reflective element of autonomy into two components, which she terms 'self-definition' and 'self-realization'. Self-definition pertains to the reasonableness of an agent's attitudes, whilst self-realization pertains to the extent to which the agent's intentions track what she takes herself to have most reasons to do.

However, the rationalist theory developed here can also provide a theoretical basis for those who are ambivalent with regards to such an agent's autonomy, providing certain assumptions are met. The theory can also provide a basis for critiquing the intuition that the autonomy of such an agent is in some way 'mixed'. To see why, we need to think more deeply about both the nature of the reasons and the conceptions of rationality in play in Killmister's example. Recall that the patient in this example

69 Joesph Raz argues that such choices play a particularly important role in shaping our character. See Raz, *Engaging Reason*, 242.

70 Gavaghan, 'In Word, or Sigh, or Tear', 248.

71 Killmister, 'The Woody Allen Puzzle'.

72 For some empirical support for the plausibility of such an example, see Tan et al., 'Competence to Make Treatment Decisions in Anorexia Nervosa'.

regards her desire to refrain from eating as irrational. Nonetheless, she takes that desire as providing her with reasons for action, in so far as she regards that desire as partly constitutive of her authentic self. On Killmister's model, such a patient would lack autonomy in one sense, that is, with respect to her self-definition (in so far as her authentic self incorporates elements that she herself takes to be irrational). Yet she would also, in some sense, be autonomous with respect to her self-realization, in so far as she is acting in accordance with what she believes she has most reason to do, that is, act in accordance with her authentic self.

On the framework that I have presented here, the plausibility of such a patient being 'mixed' with respect to their autonomy in this way relies on two assumptions. First, that an agent's authentic self could incorporate attitudes that she herself takes to be irrational. Second, that acting in accordance with one's authentic self *for its own* sake can be regarded as good in a reason-implying sense. I shall consider each in turn.

Our views regarding the plausibility of these assumptions are likely to be complicated by different interpretations of the 'true self'. On some understandings of authenticity that are implicit in philosophical theories of autonomy, the true self is understood as being perpetually created; living authentically is a matter of consciously shaping one's own character in accordance with one's desires and values.[73] In contrast though, one might endorse an alternative essentialist understanding of authenticity, according to which the true self is an extant and largely static essence that we need to discover rather than create.[74]

The claim that the above anorexic patient is partly autonomous in the way that Killmister understands her to be seems to rely on an essentialist conception of authenticity.[75] The reason for this is that many existentialist understandings of authenticity would most likely reject the first assumption outlined above: If, as existentialist approaches maintain, it is the agent herself who decides how to shape her authentic self on the basis of her own values and conception of the good, then it is not clear how the authentic self could be understood to incorporate elements that the agent *herself* takes to be irrational. Notice though that this claim is compatible with the thought that an existentialist conception of the true self might plausibly incorporate elements that one believes others will deem to be irrational. Indeed, some anorexic patients might claim that their true selves incorporate irrational elements in this normative sense, in so far as they might admit that it would be more rational to prioritize their health over a low weight, from a third-party perspective. Crucially though, this need not commit such patients to regarding their desire to maintain a low weight as irrational; they may yet believe that they are acting in accordance with what *they* have strongest reason to do.

[73] For a discussion of the existentialist approach and autonomy, see DeGrazia, *Human Identity and Bioethics*, ch. 3.

[74] For discussions of this distinction, see Levy, 'Enhancing Authenticity'; Pugh, Maslen, and Savulescu, 'Deep Brain Stimulation, Authenticity and Value'.

[75] Interestingly, Killmister's interpretation of the anorexic case here runs contrary to an essentialist tradition in bioethics that claims that the 'anorexic self' must be *inauthentic*, on the basis that it is grounded by pathological or self-destructive values. See Tan et al., 'Competence to Make Treatment Decisions in Anorexia Nervosa'; Nordenfelt, *Rationality and Compulsion*. I shall discuss such accounts in greater detail in Chapter 8.

The rationalist theory that I have developed here can accommodate the thought that such individuals can be autonomous with respect to desires that are rationally endorsed in this sense, as long as the beliefs about the good upon which they are based are not held in a theoretically irrational manner. Yet, if this is the correct interpretation of Killmister's view, then the agent is not mixed with regard to her autonomy; she is acting in accordance with a desire that she rationally endorses, even though she acknowledges its apparent irrationality. Yet this just means that she disagrees about the strength that we ought to attribute to different reasons; this alone is not sufficient for practical irrationality as I have described it in this chapter.

The authentic self cannot incorporate irrational elements in this motivational sense on a number of plausible existentialist understandings of authenticity. However, this is not a problem for the essentialist understanding; one's static essence may incorporate attitudes that one now takes to be irrational on the basis of one's own beliefs about value, or one's beliefs about what one *should* value according to impersonal criteria. So Killmister's suggestion that the agent in her case partly lacks autonomy seems to rely on an implicit essentialist conception of authenticity.

The second question is whether this essentialist conception of authenticity can provide a sufficient justificatory reason for action, as Killmister's second assumption requires. Naturally, the first potential problem with this claim is that the essentialist conception of authenticity is somewhat contentious, in so far as it seems to rely on the assumption that we have a deep, immutable, hidden essence that is immune to our own evaluative stance.[76] Notwithstanding this issue, the essentialist understanding also owes us an account of why living authentically on this conception should be regarded as good in a reason-implying sense. Even assuming that an essential self exists, to claim that this essence must be good and that it ought to be promoted without further argument seems to come close to making the naturalistic fallacy.

Suppose, though, that such an account can be provided;[77] if living in accordance with an essentialist conception of the self can be construed as good in a reason-implying sense, and that conception of the self incorporates elements that the agent herself takes to be irrational, then it seems that Killmister's ambivalent intuition about the agent's autonomy in this case can be compatible with the rationalist account that I have developed here. However, we may notice that the strength of one's reason to live in accordance with this essence on such an account would also have to be particularly strong. After all, the reasons associated with living authentically would need to be sufficient to compete with the agent's reasons to pursue other goods, perhaps even including survival in the case of severe anorexia.

The rationalist framework I have outlined here can not only account for Killmister's own ambivalent intuition in such cases, but it can also account for the possibility that we may not find the intuition about ambivalence compelling. Whether we share Killmister's intuition will depend on our credence in essentialist conceptions of authenticity, their value, and the possibility that an agent could

[76] Strohminger, Knobe, and Newman, 'The True Self'; DeGrazia, *Human Identity and Bioethics*, 233–4.

[77] For a classic defence of essentialist authenticity as a normative ideal in this respect, see Taylor, 'The Ethics of Authenticity'. For some considerations that speak in favour of this approach in the context of mental disorders, see Erler and Hope, 'Mental Disorder and the Concept of Authenticity'.

rationally prioritize this value over other goods that may be in play in her decision-making.

In contrast to the essentialist conception of authenticity upon which Killmister's case seems to rely, the coherence approach I have outlined in this chapter draws on both essentialist and existentialist themes in the conception of authenticity that it invokes. From the essentialist tradition, it takes the claim that we may have certain more or less fixed elements that partly constitute our character system. From the existentialist tradition, it takes the claim that we may be able to choose which of these more or less fixed elements to bring to the fore in a coherent nexus, and which to downplay on the basis of the web of values that we come to develop. On this approach, if the individual herself believes that a certain element of her character system is not valuable, as Killmister's anorexic patient does, then this element of her character system is inauthentic, and cannot be understood as a suitable ground of autonomous decision-making. However, as I shall explore in Chapter 8, the theory is also compatible with the thought that some anorexic patients may coherently experience their disorder as a part of their authentic self. In this part of the book, I shall also return to Craigie's concern that such patients may also later regret the values that previously informed their decision-making, and the implications that this should be understood to have for their autonomy.

Conclusion

The assumption that there is a close relationship between autonomy and rationality in bioethics is well-grounded. Whilst previous theories of rationalist autonomy have made important progress in outlining the kind of role that rationality might play in autonomy, they have been somewhat hampered by certain misunderstandings about the nature of rationality. Furthermore, they have not adequately engaged with the deeper question of why our evaluative judgements should be understood to serve as an appropriate seat of self-government. By drawing on an objectivist account of reasons and the broader literature on philosophy of action in this chapter, I am now in a position to offer the following rationalist minimal conditions of autonomy:

Theoretical Rationality: Decisional autonomy is precluded by theoretically irrational beliefs about information that is material to one's decisions.
Practical Rationality: The autonomous agent's motivating desires must be rational in the following sense:
They must:

(a) Be endorsed by preferences that are sustained on the basis of the agent's holding (rational) beliefs that, if true, would give the agent reason to pursue the object of the desire.
And
(b) These preferences must cohere with other elements of the agent's character system.

In turn, a preference coheres with other elements of an agent's character system if there is a sufficient reason for the agent to maintain that preference in the light of other competing preferences and theoretically rational acceptances. Coherence is thus incompatible with irrationality, but it is compatible with being less than fully rational.

As I mentioned above, Rebecca Walker claims that a negative rationality condition should replace the standard account's condition concerning the absence of internal control. I agree with this sentiment, but I have made the stronger claim that considerations of practical rationality should feature in a positive condition on autonomy, one that requires that autonomous decisions be grounded by authentic preferences. This account can offer a deeper justification for why practical rationality matters for autonomy.

We may also notice that the positive condition of practical rationality is stronger than the negative criterion of theoretical rationality. One reason for this is that in the case of practical rationality it is possible to draw a meaningful distinction between irrationality and arationality, and both are incompatible with the approach that I am advocating here. The explanation for this is that the positive contribution that practical rationality makes to autonomy is to facilitate our ability to decide in accordance with elements of our character that should be understood to have agential authority. Our decisions can clearly lack that authority if they are irrational, but they also lack it if they are arational. Furthermore, they also lack this authority if they are not endorsed by cohering elements of the agent's character system.

Yet, even if these conditions are necessary they may not be sufficient. It still seems that a suitable theory of autonomy should follow the standard account in maintaining a condition excluding controlling forms of influence such as manipulation, deception, and coercion. It is to these forms of influence that I shall now turn. In particular, in the next chapter, I shall argue that the rationalist conditions that I have set out here can provide a plausible foundation for understanding why manipulation and deception undermine autonomy, and the bearing that this should have on our understanding of authenticity.

3

Controlling Influences

Recall that the standard account of autonomy states that autonomy requires the absence of both internal and external controlling forces that determine the agent's decision. As I suggested in the introductory chapter, the claim that autonomy requires the absence of *internal* controlling forces is too strong if it is understood to foreclose the possibility of compatibilist approaches to autonomy. Accordingly, I have argued that we should replace the condition concerning the absence of internal control with a rationalist authenticity condition. In this chapter, I now want to consider the implications of this account for the *external* forms of controlling influence to which the standard account appeals: manipulation, deception, and coercion.[1]

Although it is all but universally agreed that manipulation, deception, and coercion can undermine an agent's decisional autonomy, it is less clear how we ought to distinguish these forms of influence from those that are compatible with decisional autonomy. After all, our decisions are continually and (as relational theorists of autonomy stress) unavoidably influenced in a number of ways that are not aptly construed as undermining decisional autonomy.

To illustrate, suppose I tell you that you ought to buy a novel, telling you that it incorporates beautiful prose and cutting social commentary. *Ceteris paribus*, it does not seem that this way of attempting to influence your decision is aptly construed as undermining your autonomy with regards to your decision about which book to buy. Even at a pre-theoretic stage, this clearly stands in stark contrast to a case in which I threaten to significantly harm you if you do not read the book. Consider also a case in which I maliciously deceive you into reading a book that I know you will dislike, or, even more fantastically, hypnotizing you into doing so.

Accordingly, the challenge that we face in understanding controlling influence is to explain how we are to distinguish those forms of influence that serve to undermine an individual's decisional autonomy from those that do not. Although the standard account stipulates a condition regarding the absence of controlling interference, the

[1] 'Undue influence' is arguably a more natural term for what I am referring to as controlling influence. However, I have avoided this term due to the fact that, in some circles it is taken to have a rather more specific meaning than I intend. For example, the Belmont Report defines undue influence as follows: 'Undue influence . . . occurs through an offer of an excessive, unwarranted, inappropriate or improper reward or other overture in order to obtain compliance.' See Largent et al., 'Misconceptions about Coercion and Undue Influence' for discussion. I shall discuss the implications of incentives for autonomy in the next chapter.

Autonomy, Rationality, and Contemporary Bioethics. Jonathan Pugh, Oxford University Press (2020). © Jonathan Pugh.
DOI: 10.1093/oso/9780198858584.001.0001

account itself provides us with few clues about how to draw these distinctions; it simply stipulates by fiat that coercion, psychological manipulation, and deception are examples of interventions that undermine autonomy. It relies on the intuitive plausibility of these judgements in order to justify partially defining autonomous decisions as those that are made in the absence of these influences. This seems somewhat theoretically unsatisfactory.

The rationalist approach that I developed in the previous chapter can offer a deeper account of the relationship between autonomy and these different forms of influence. On this approach, an individual's decisional autonomy can be undermined if either the cognitive or reflective elements of decisional autonomy are disrupted as follows:

(i) The individual is led to either (a) sustain theoretically irrational beliefs or (b) fail to hold decisionally necessary true beliefs.
(ii) The individual is led to sustain a motivating desire in a manner that bypasses the cognitive element of autonomy, such that they either (a) do not endorse the desire, or (b) they endorse it with a preference that fails to cohere with other cohering elements of their character system

In accordance with this framework, we may categorize deception as amounting to (i)[b] but not necessarily (i)[a]. It can be theoretically rational to believe others who are lying to us. However, informational manipulation more broadly may involve either (i)[a] or [b]. I shall consider these forms of controlling influence in sections 4 and 5.

In contrast, *psychological* manipulation involves the manipulation of motivational states rather than beliefs, and may be said to amount to forms of influence that are involved in either (ii)[a] or [b]. One might argue that psychological manipulation could also operate at a more global level, such that an agent is brainwashed into holding an entirely new character system as follows:

(ii)[c] An individual is led to radically change the overall coherent nexus of preferences and acceptances by which she endorses her motivating desires.

Whilst the theory of autonomy that I outlined in the previous chapter can explain why (ii)[a] and [b] undermine autonomy, it is not clear that it can explain why global manipulation of the sort identified in (ii)[c] would. As I shall explain, this has led some philosophers to argue that an adequate theory of autonomy should certain incorporate historical conditions.

I shall reject this view in section 3. Prior to doing so though, I shall in the first two sections begin by outlining more mundane forms of psychological manipulation that may more plausibly be employed in biomedical contexts, and explaining how they differ from forms of rational persuasion that are compatible with decisional autonomy. I shall delay consideration of coercion until the next chapter, and explain why it does not fit naturally within the framework I have just outlined.

To conclude these introductory remarks, it is important to be clear that I am only interested here in the implications of these forms of influence for the *autonomy* of the targeted individuals. I do not mean to deny that these influences can have other important moral implications that can and should factor into an all things considered moral analysis of them.[2] For instance, there has been a great deal of recent debate regarding the extent to which instances of psychological manipulation might violate a putative right to mental integrity, even if they do not constitute threats to autonomy per se.[3] Although my autonomy-based analysis of manipulation is not entirely unrelated to these other questions, we should not assume that the conclusions I draw here translate straightforwardly to how we should understand other important moral properties of manipulation and deception.

Finally, the terminology of 'controlling influence' is perhaps somewhat unfortunate, since it seems to imply that these forms of influence must be exerted intentionally, in a manner that connotes that the one who influences is actively *controlling* the target of their influence. However, as I shall explain in this chapter, non-intentional and indeed non-agential forces can cause the phenomena indicated in (i) and (ii) above. Despite this unfortunate implication, I shall retain this terminology in the interests of consistency with the literature.

1. Rational Persuasion

On the standard account, rational persuasion is understood to be compatible with autonomy on the basis that it enhances understanding; persuasion is thus broadly similar to simply informing.[4] However, on the approach that I outlined in the previous chapter, we can understand persuasion in a broader sense to involve attempting to change an agent's beliefs by drawing their attention to reasons. Rational persuasion on this approach thus involves attempting to change an individual's desires indirectly, by actively engaging with the cognitive element of their practical decision-making process. This can include interacting with both the target's descriptive beliefs about the world (as the standard account implies), but also their evaluative beliefs about the good. Desires that are formed following rational persuasion are thus likely to accord with the cohering elements of the agent's character system in a manner that betokens autonomy, because they will have been explicitly developed in light of the individual's acceptances. When successful, persuasion must appeal to the values we hold, or convince us to change our values in response to reasons.

Typically, rational persuasion will involve highlighting descriptive facts about another's options; for example, you might persuade a friend not to cross a bridge by drawing their attention to the large hole in the middle of it. We may call this factual persuasion. In factual persuasion, the persuader presumes that both they and the subject of their persuasion share an understanding of the target's preferred outcomes. One explanation for why factual persuasion can fail is that the persuader has made an incorrect assumption about the target's preferred outcome.

[2] For a comprehensive discussion, see Blumenthal-Barby, 'A Framework for Assessing the Moral Status of "Manipulation"'.

[3] Bublitz and Merkel, 'Crimes Against Minds'; Douglas, 'Neural and Environmental Modulation of Motivation'.

[4] Faden and Beauchamp, *A History and Theory of Informed Consent*, 354–68; Beauchamp and Childress, *Principles of Biomedical Ethics*, 137–9.

Alternatively, the two parties may agree on all the relevant descriptive facts of the matter but disagree about the outcome that ought to be pursued in a particular context. In such cases, simply bringing further relevant descriptive facts to the target's attention is unlikely to be successful. Rather, if persuasion is to succeed in such a context, it must involve what I shall call 'evaluative persuasion'; that is, the persuader must bring reason-giving facts about other outcomes to the target's attention, in an attempt to change their assessment of the relative strength of their reasons to pursue different courses of action.

Evaluative persuasion might involve advocating the value of goods that the target will forgo if they follow through on their planned course of action; for example, we might seek to persuade a suicidal person against their planned course of action by drawing their attention to various good things in their life that are worth living for. Alternatively, evaluative persuasion might involve questioning the value of the agent's preferred outcome, asking her to explain the grounding of her belief that the outcome in question is good in a reason-implying sense. For example, one might attempt to persuade a person to stop smoking by asking her to reflect on whether she actually enjoys the experience of smoking, or whether she simply reaches for her cigarettes on a habitual, non-rational basis.

In the context of medical ethics, evaluative persuasion is often viewed with suspicion, particularly by those who endorse the so-called shared decision-making model of the doctor–patient relationship.[5] On strong versions of this view, it is assumed that:

> The physician should objectively answer questions but should avoid influencing the patient to take one path or another, even if the physician has strong opinions or if the patient asks for advice.[6]

On this model, it is usually assumed that physicians would be exerting controlling influence if they were to encroach on the evaluative domain of the decision-making process. The General Medical Council (GMC) adopts a weaker version of this position, stating that:

> The doctor may recommend a particular option which they believe to be best for the patient, but they must not put pressure on the patient to accept their advice.[7]

Whilst there are different ways of understanding the shared decision-making model, we should reject versions of the model that construe the doctor–patient relationship in a manner that demands that doctors should adopt a wholly value-neutral approach in their dealings with patients.[8] First, it is highly questionable to assume that it is even possible for doctors to provide medical information in a value-neutral manner. After all, medical concepts such as health and disease are themselves value-laden, in so far as they are commonly understood to imply certain value judgements

[5] Veatch, 'Abandoning Informed Consent'.

[6] Quill and Brody, 'Physician Recommendations and Patient Autonomy', 764.

[7] General Medical Council, 'Ethical Guidance for Doctors, Part 1'.

[8] Veatch, 'Abandoning Informed Consent'. For an understanding of the doctor–patient relationship that corresponds to the rationalist approach that I am defending here, see Savulescu, 'Liberal Rationalism and Medical Decision-Making'.

(particularly in the conversational context of a treatment discussion).[9] Second, physicians must make certain evaluative judgements in deciding upon what information to disclose to patients (such as information about risks associated with treatment) and deciding what treatment options to propose to their patient. In both cases, it seems that the physician's evaluative judgements will inevitably bear upon what is (and is not) disclosed.

However, the theory of autonomy that I am outlining also gives us reasons to reject even the weaker version of this value-neutral approach adopted by the GMC. The strategies of evaluative persuasion noted above should not be understood to constitute controlling influence of the sort that undermines decisional autonomy, because evaluative, as well as factual, persuasion can facilitate autonomous decision-making. Evaluative persuasion does not involve seeking to impose values on the target; rather, it involves seeking to elicit the rational justification underlying the values that are now guiding the agent's conduct, and alerting them to other reasons that are at stake in a particular choice context. In so far as this mode of persuasion causes the subject to reflect on these reasons, it can be construed as enhancing the agent's autonomy with respect to their decisions, even if it is not successful.[10] Indeed, part of the physician's role can be to advocate the import of certain sorts or reasons, reasons that reflect the values that shape the profession of medicine.[11] Moreover, in an era in which physicians have to battle with the widespread distribution of misinformation about medicine proliferating in the online world, it may be a mistake to assume that the dispassionate provision of medical facts alone can be enough to allow them to adequately compete in this environment, and to ensure that their patients are appropriately informed about their treatment options.[12]

Of course, a decision to engage in evaluative persuasion must be sensitive to the particular vulnerabilities of specific patients. In particular, it is important to be clear that the physician is engaging in evaluative persuasion rather than simply aiming to elicit the patient's capitulation to their view. Whilst this is an important danger, we should not simply assume that the best way to avoid it is to require that doctors say nothing in the face of patient decisions that seem to be grounded by badly skewed evaluative judgements. To illustrate, a physician would be quite warranted in engaging in evaluative persuasion to persuade a patient that she really ought to receive a life-saving shot to prevent an anaphylactic shock, if her reason for refusing it is that she wants to avoid the small pain involved in the injection. A physician can go beyond merely recommending the injection in this sort of case without unduly encroaching on the patient's autonomy.

Having outlined forms of persuasion that are compatible with autonomous decision-making, I now want to turn to forms of influence that are not, starting with psychological manipulation.

[9] For a classic account of conversational implicature, see Grice, *Studies in the Way of Words*.

[10] For defence of similar views, see Savulescu, 'Liberal Rationalism and Medical Decision-Making'; Widdershoven and Abma, 'Autonomy, Dialogue, and Practical Rationality'.

[11] Brock, *Life and Death*, ch. 2, especially 69.

[12] For a sobering editorial on this point, see Ranjana Srivastava 'My Patient Swapped Chemotherapy for Essential Oils. Arguing Is a Fool's Errand'.

2. Psychological Manipulation

In rational persuasion, one attempts to alter the target's motivational states indirectly by engaging with the cognitive element of their decisional autonomy, including their beliefs about the world and the good. Psychological manipulation involves attempting to directly alter the motivational states themselves, in a manner that bypasses the cognitive element of the target's decisional autonomy.

As Anne Barnhill notes, one of the difficulties in theorizing about manipulation is that ethicists often fail to provide a working definition of what they are talking about, or they offer definitions that are either over-inclusive or under-inclusive.[13] Indeed, one over-inclusive theory that Barnhill adverts to is an account of psychological manipulation that Tom Beauchamp and Ruth Faden develop in outlining a detailed version of the standard account of autonomy in bioethics. According to Beauchamp and Faden, psychological manipulation can be defined as:

> any intentional act that successfully influences a person to belief or behavior by causing changes in mental processes other than those involved in understanding.[14]

This account of psychological manipulation is theoretically incomplete because the link between this type of manipulation and the explanation for why it undermines autonomy is left unclear. This is particularly problematic because there are ways in which the definition is *both* over- and under-inclusive. One way in which the theory may be under-inclusive is that it rules out the possibility that manipulative influence could be non-intentional. However, one reason for questioning Beauchamp and Faden's claim to the contrary is that they (and other advocates of the standard account of autonomy) readily accept that *some* non-intentional forces can amount to controlling influence that undermines decisional autonomy. This is due to the fact that advocates of the standard account accept the possibility of internal controlling forces (such as psychiatric disease) that may undermine decisional autonomy.

There are of course some pragmatic reasons for understanding manipulation to require intentional agency. First, one might want to stress the semantic point that the term 'manipulation' itself seems to connote intentional agency, in the same way that the term 'controlling' influence does. Furthermore, there may be a range of morally relevant features of intentional manipulation that are not applicable to non-intentional forms of the same sort of phenomenon. For my purposes here though, these points are somewhat moot. As I stipulated in the introduction to this chapter, I am solely interested in the effects of manipulation on the target's autonomy. Crucially, that non-intentional forces can exert forms of influence that have relevantly similar effects on the target's autonomy as intentional psychological manipulation follows straightforwardly from the account of autonomy that I have defended. If authenticity of a certain sort is required for decisional autonomy, and if authenticity as I have spelled it out can be threatened by non-intentional and non-agential forces (as well as agential forces), then we should deny the claim that autonomy-

[13] Barnhill, 'What Is Manipulation?', 51.

[14] Faden and Beauchamp, *A History and Theory of Informed Consent*, 366.

undermining psychological manipulation is necessarily intentional.[15] What matters for decisional autonomy is that we endorse our motivating desires with certain kinds of rationally endorsed preferences, namely, ones that fit in with other cohering elements of our characters. Now, it is true that we might fail to act on the basis of such a desire because another agent has intentionally induced a different motivating desire. However, it is also possible that our failure in this regard may not be due to the machinations of another intentional agent. 'Internal' forms of controlling influence of the sort I considered in the previous chapter can lead individuals to form and sustain desires in this way, and undermine autonomy for the same reason.

I shall consider some further arguments regarding the necessity of intention that have been made specifically with respect to deception in section 5. To return to psychological manipulation though, one might worry that my theory of autonomy will lead to too broad an understanding of manipulation. For instance, Barnhill argues a theory of manipulation ought to exclude drugs and brainwashing as examples of interference that undermine autonomy, on the basis that they evince *global* changes to the target's psychology. Such global changes mean that these interventions do not directly target particular elements of the target's psychological economy in the manner that manipulation arguably requires.[16] It seems plausible that psychiatric diseases could also constitute another example of what Barnhill has in mind here.

I am sympathetic to Barnhill's claim here; indeed, in the next section, I shall explain why forms of interference that evince global changes to a person's psychology do not threaten autonomy per se. However, I do not believe that these examples are problematic for the conception of manipulation that can be grounded by my rationalist approach. First, I am sceptical of the claim that drugs or psychiatric disorders must *always* involve such global changes. Indeed, some drugs have direct effects on a limited set of motivational states. Consider, for example, the use of chemical castration in the punishment of individuals who have been convicted of sexual offences. Contrary to Barnhill's analysis, this seems a paradigm case of psychological manipulation; these individuals are compelled to take a drug that has a direct effect on their libido, but which may nonetheless leave large swathes of their character systems intact. Indeed, they may lament their lack of sexual drive whilst experiencing the effects of the drug, in accordance with preferences that they have sustained from a point in time prior to the intervention. Furthermore, with respect to psychiatric diseases, we may also note that the standard account of autonomy explicitly accepts the claim that psychiatric disease can undermine decisional autonomy.

As I mentioned above, Barnhill also claims that Beauchamp and Faden's account of manipulation is over-inclusive. According to Beauchamp and Faden's approach, methods of changing beliefs and desires that do not qualify as rational persuasion will constitute psychological manipulation. Yet as Barnhill argues, it appears that intentional expressions of emotions may serve to change another's beliefs or behaviour,

[15] Mele makes a similar point with respect to his theory in Mele, *Autonomous Agents*, ch. 6, section 2 and Mele, *Free Will and Luck*, 177–90.

[16] Barnhill, 'What Is Manipulation?', 65.

but this does not entail that such expressions must be manipulative.[17] It might be argued that my approach will fall foul of a similar complaint, given the emphasis I place on the fact that psychological manipulation involves inducing desires directly by bypassing the cognitive element of autonomy. However, my approach can accommodate the thought that emotional influences can be compatible with autonomy, as I shall now explain.

One explanation for this is that emotional influences need not lead us to develop motivational states in a manner that bypasses the cognitive element of decisional autonomy. To illustrate, consider Barnhill's own example of a woman deciding to hand back some embezzled money after her father tells her that 'he didn't raise her to be a thief'.[18] I agree with Barnhill that this is plausibly an example of a non-manipulative, yet emotional form of influence (via shame) that is compatible with autonomy.

However, I deny that it involves inducing a desire in a manner that entirely bypasses the cognitive element of the agent's autonomy. It is a mistake to assume that decisions substantially grounded by affective experiences are wholly divorced from our beliefs about what is valuable. Whilst it is true that emotional experiences of fear and anger (amongst others) can involve us becoming divorced from our evaluative judgements or theoretically rational beliefs about the nature of the world, some affective attitudes and emotional experiences can instead give rise to values, ground certain kinds of reasons for choice, and even reveal the presence of certain reasons that were previously obscure to us. Indeed, an increased understanding of our reasons can sometimes also be facilitated by emotional engagement, as well as simpler forms of information disclosure. In this particular case, my claim is that the emotional influence of the woman's father enabled her to perceive a powerful set of reasons not to steal.

Of course this may not be true of all forms of emotional influence; when it is not, I suggest that emotional influence can be manipulative. However, we should also acknowledge the point that the fact that one has been initially manipulated into holding a desire (by emotional means or otherwise) does not entail that one must thereby *forever* lack autonomy with respect to it. One can come to critically reflect on the content of the manipulated desire, and to decide for oneself whether or not to *sustain* it in the light of one's preferences.

To illustrate, suppose that you were brainwashed by subliminal advertising to form the desire to give money to charity. Even if you later came to reject the causal history of this desire (having been made aware of it), it still seems plausible to claim that you could autonomously hold the desire, just because you endorse the *content* of the desire itself. As Bernard Berofsky points out, one may reasonably have objections to the causal process that led one to develop a desire, without having any qualms about the results.[19] By reflecting on a desire that one has been manipulated to develop, one can come to take ownership of the desire itself in a manner that betokens autonomy; call this 'post-factum reflection'.

[17] Ibid., 62. [18] Ibid. [19] Berofsky, *Liberation from Self*, 212.

Post-factum reflection on changes to our motivational states following emotional influence may often lead to their endorsement, because our emotions can plausibly serve as a source of reasons that may not be immediately accessible at the time of deliberation, but which may nonetheless ground rational behaviour.[20] More broadly though, we are of course more likely to engage in post-factum reflection on manipulated desires if they represent either a striking departure from our characteristic motivations, or if the manipulative process itself was particularly overt. The problem is that many manipulative processes, including many forms of emotional influence, subvert this sort of post-factum reflection because their effects are covert and subtle. Accordingly, they do not give us cause to reflect on, or indeed even recognize, the changes that they have evinced.

On a related point, we may note that on the approach that I am defending here is that psychological manipulation need not be covert.[21] In light of the above remarks though, my account is compatible with the claim that covert manipulation is likely to be more successful in sustaining a lack of autonomy with respect to a desire; after all, if the target of manipulation is aware of the existence of a manipulative influence they are more likely to be able to both employ mechanisms to resist its influence, and to engage in post-factum reflection that will allow them to repudiate or take ownership of the desire itself. However, it is also compatible with the claim that overt influences can still involve psychological manipulation. This seems to me a benefit of the account. To see why, reconsider the use of mandatory chemical castration in the criminal justice system.[22] Now, whatever we think of the permissibility of this sort of policy, it seems quite clear that intervention can be understood to be a form of psychological manipulation, despite the fact that it is not covert, if the target repudiates their lack of sexual desires following the intervention.

With this in mind, what might plausible forms of psychological manipulation look like in the biomedical context? Philosophers who discuss manipulation typically appeal to extraordinary cases of manipulation involving nefarious neurosurgeons and hypnotists. However, the justification for appealing to such examples is the theoretical clarity that they permit, rather than the fact that they represent common cases of manipulation. Yet, there are a number of common ways in which we might be subjected to this form of interference in the biomedical sphere. For instance, physicians may exert control in these sorts of ways through subliminal suggestion, and by appealing to irrationally grounded emotional attitudes such as guilt.[23] To illustrate, a physician could psychologically manipulate a patient who refuses a treatment by telling them that they are just 'being awkward', or by telling the patient that all of their other patients just 'do what their doctor says'. In such cases, the physician is attempting to influence the patient, not by appealing to reason-giving facts about the nature of the treatment that could give the patient reasons to change their decision, or by making an emotional appeal that serves to reveal the strength of

[20] Arpaly, 'On Acting Rationally against One's Best Judgment'.

[21] For accounts that claim that manipulation must necessarily be covert, see Goodin, *Manipulatory Politics*, 9; Ware, 'The Concept of Manipulation', 165.

[22] Forsberg and Douglas, 'Anti-Libidinal Interventions in Sex Offenders'.

[23] Faden and Beauchamp, *A History and Theory of Informed Consent*, 366–7.

the patient's reasons (such as an injunction to 'think of your family' in making a treatment decision). Instead, this is an appeal to a non-rational bias that the patient may have to conform to a 'norm' of 'the good patient' perpetuated by a medical authority.

Over the latter half of the twentieth century, psychologists and behavioural economists have also highlighted ways in which environmental cues can be strategically used to influence our practical decision-making in ways that might be deemed manipulative in various ways. Following Thaler and Sunstein, such strategies are commonly referred to as 'Nudges'. According to Thaler and Sunstein's own definition, a nudge can be constituted by:

> Any aspect of a person's choice architecture that alters people's behaviour in a predictable way without forbidding any options or significantly changing their economic incentives.[24]

The debate in the bioethical literature about whether nudges are compatible with autonomous choice has been somewhat impeded by the exceedingly broad nature of this definition of nudges. The problem with the definition is that it can be understood to incorporate both strategies that influence decision-making by facilitating the involvement of the cognitive element of our decision-making, and also those that subvert this. In doing so, it conflates two morally distinct categories of influence.[25] For instance, rational persuasion as I have described it above could qualify as a nudge on this definition; so too could the use of incentives.[26]

However, I suggest that there are some cases in which nudges are psychologically manipulative, by virtue of the fact that they entirely bypass the cognitive element of our decision-making (as well as subverting post-factum reflection). Consider for example the use of priming. In one famous example of priming, criminal justice authorities found that if they exposed prison inmates to a particular shade of pink, violent behaviour amongst those inmates dramatically reduced. It is not as if the colour prompted the inmates to engage in reflection about their reasons to engage in violent behaviour. Rather, their exposure to this environmental factor seemed to somehow serve to diminish their violent impulses without engaging with the offenders' rational processing.[27] Moreover, the covert and subtle nature of this influence makes it less likely that the targets will be aware of the changes evinced, and to critically reflect on the question of whether to endorse or reject them (assuming that the effects themselves could indeed be wilfully resisted).

Despite the breadth of the commonly invoked definition, discussions of the effects of nudging on autonomy do not always attend to the particular significance of nudges that bypass (and subvert) the rational processes alluded to above.[28] A number of commonly discussed nudge strategies, such as priming, would fall into this category

[24] Thaler and Sunstein, *Nudge*, 6.

[25] For other defences of the claim that not all nudges need pervert our decision-making processes, see Wilkinson, 'Nudging and Manipulation'; Cohen, 'Nudging and Informed Consent'.

[26] Blumenthal-Barby and Burroughs, 'Seeking Better Health Care Outcomes'.

[27] For discussion, see Pugh, 'Moral Bio-Enhancement, Freedom, Value and the Parity Principle'; Douglas, 'Neural and Environmental Modulation of Motivation'.

[28] Some authors employ a narrower definition of nudging, according to which nudges by definition take advantage of non-rational processes. For example, see Hausman and Welch, 'To Nudge or Not to Nudge'.

quite uncontroversially. However, in the case of some strategies the matter is not so straightforward. One reason for this is that some nudges involve forms of informational manipulation, rather than psychological manipulation as I have defined it here, and the distinction between informational manipulation and enhancing understanding through information disclosure can be somewhat blurred. I shall consider this form of influence in section 4.

Prior to doing so, to complete my analysis of psychological manipulation, I shall in the next section consider forms of global psychological manipulation outlined in (ii) [c] in the introduction to this chapter. Such instances of psychological manipulation have prompted some philosophers to argue that we ought to understand authenticity in a strictly historical sense. I shall defend my account from this objection, and in doing so outline how my theory can accommodate the pervasive relational influences on our values within a framework of decisional autonomy.

3. Global Manipulation and Autonomy

One might be sceptical that there is a practical need for a theory of autonomy to accommodate the prospect of global manipulation. For instance, Marilyn Friedman has argued that philosophers should refrain from engaging with bizarre counter-examples to autonomy, and that we should only refine such concepts in 'helpful practical ways'.[29] I am sympathetic to Friedman's frustration in this regard. Nonetheless, some comments on global manipulation are necessary. One reason for this is that critics of the kind of rationalist approach that I have endorsed here might contend that it is ill-equipped to accommodate the pervasive relational influences that we are all subject to as members of society. This is important because these influences arguably represent a very real way in which external forces can substantially mould and shape our character systems as a whole. As I shall explain, this sort of observation has led some relational theorists to abandon the idea that autonomy requires authenticity conditions (since authenticity would inevitably be tainted by this social influence). Second, cases of global manipulation have led other theorists to argue that authenticity should be understood in an explicitly historical sense. I shall consider each point in turn.

(i) The Pervasiveness of Relational Influence and Autonomy

It is undeniable that relational autonomy theorists have captured a number of important insights about autonomy. We are social beings, and our decisions are both guided and enabled by societal influences in a pervasive fashion.[30] Yet, these insights are compatible with a wide range of theories of decisional autonomy, including the one developed in the previous chapter.[31]

[29] Friedman, *Autonomy, Gender, Politics*, 28.

[30] For detailed discussion of the forms that relational influence can take, see the entries in the seminal Mackenzie and Stoljar, *Relational Autonomy*. See also Christman, *The Politics of Persons*, ch. 8; Oshana, 'Personal Autonomy and Society'; Nedelsky, 'Reconceiving Autonomy'.

[31] Foster suggests that relational theorists who have supposed otherwise are largely attacking a straw man. See Foster, *Choosing Life, Choosing Death*, 14–15.

In particular, most theories are compatible with the claim that certain relational conditions are *causally* necessary for autonomy.[32] This is significant, as the key claim of relational autonomy theory is sometimes understood as a claim about the *causal* conditions of autonomy. Consider for example, Anderson and Honneth's claim that:

> The key initial insight of social or relational accounts of autonomy is that full autonomy... is only achievable under socially supportive conditions.[33]

This is an important claim, but it is also one that can (and should) be accommodated straightforwardly by procedural theories of decisional autonomy that outline *constitutive* conditions of autonomy. In the terms of the theory that I have developed, one may maintain that decisional autonomy requires both theoretical and practical rationality whilst accepting both (i) that these capacities themselves may be socially mediated and (ii) the more fundamental point that one can only exercise these capacities in a social environment that furnishes one with the opportunities and abilities to make one's decisions in this way.[34]

The more challenging question arising from relational theory concerns whether the constitutive conditions of decisional autonomy adequately accommodate the pervasiveness of relational influences.[35] Indeed, a widespread criticism of the kinds of procedural theories of autonomy that I discussed in the previous chapter is that they focus on an unduly individualistic conception of autonomy and the self.[36]

I believe that this criticism is somewhat misplaced with regards to the rationalist theory that I have developed, since the theory is compatible with relational influence on the self and autonomy in a number of ways.[37] First, many of our practical reasons can be other-regarding. Our practical reasons are often self-interested reasons; but they can also include the reasons we might have to promote the interests of others, or reasons grounded by the value that our relationships instantiate. Accordingly, the theory is well-placed to accommodate the fact that our relationships can be of the utmost importance to us as autonomous agents.[38]

Furthermore, the claim that decisional autonomy requires practical and theoretical rationality is quite compatible with the claim that many of the values, desires, and beliefs that ground our rationality will often have been formed as a result of our relationships and social forces. Accordingly, I wholeheartedly agree with John

[32] John Christman makes a similar point. See Christman, *The Politics of Persons*, 177–82.

[33] Anderson and Honneth, 'Autonomy, Vulnerability, Recognition, and Justice', 130. For further discussions of relational causal conditions of autonomy, see also Nedelsky, 'Reconceiving Autonomy'; Mackenzie and Stoljar, 'Autonomy Reconfigured'; Oshana, 'Personal Autonomy and Society'.

[34] Nedelsky particularly stresses this point in Nedelsky, 'Reconceiving Autonomy'.

[35] Oshana similarly identifies this as the most significant challenge posed by relational influences. See Oshana, 'Personal Autonomy and Society', 97.

[36] For example, see Oshana, 'Personal Autonomy and Society'; Mackenzie and Stoljar, 'Autonomy Reconfigured'; Meyers, *Self, Society, and Personal Choice*; Anderson and Honneth, 'Autonomy, Vulnerability, Recognition, and Justice'.

[37] Christman's theory, which I criticize below, is also compatible with these claims. See Christman, *The Politics of Persons*, chs. 7 and 8. For discussions of this trend more broadly with regards to liberal conceptions of autonomy, see Friedman, *Autonomy, Gender, Politics*, 81–97.

[38] Christman, 'Relational Autonomy, Liberal Individualism, and the Social Constitution of Selves'.

Christman when he writes that there are a number of ways that any plausible theory of autonomy must:

> ...take into account the various ways in which humans are socially embedded, intimately related to other people, groups, institutions and histories, and that they are motivated by interests and reasons that can only be fully defined with reference to other people and things.[39]

The theory of autonomy I have outlined readily accepts these claims; the important point is whether individuals are able to reflect upon these socially mediated values in the process of cultivating their characters. It does not require that these values were developed in a social vacuum. However, the agent must take ownership of these values by ensuring that they hold their evaluative beliefs in a theoretically rational sense, and incorporate them into a coherent character system.

As I mentioned in the introductory chapter, some feminist philosophers have argued that the fact that our values have a social source is a damaging criticism of theories of autonomy that incorporate considerations of authenticity. If our 'true selves' have been uncritically forged in the crucible of a society that ensures that individuals simply internalize socially oppressive norms, then perhaps we should be sceptical of the claim that these selves are the locus of autonomous agency.[40] Instead, perhaps we ought to appeal to substantive conceptions of autonomy, or to develop non-authenticity based procedural accounts that appeal to social conditions, or competency conditions.[41]

I have already noted that relational competency conditions can be compatible with a wide range of procedural theories of decisional autonomy. However, procedural and substantive relational accounts of autonomy face a deeper conflict. The crux of the issue here is captured in the example of cosmetic surgery that I alluded to in the introduction. If one holds the view that a woman's desire for a beautifying cosmetic procedure is merely an artefact of the influence of the patriarchal society in which she lives, then one might deny that a woman can be autonomous with respect to that desire, no matter how much she personally endorses it. In this sort of example, procedural and substantive relational accounts come into irreconcilable conflict.

It would be impossible to significantly advance the debate between substantive and procedural theories on this point in the space available here. I must make do with adverting to existing work that extensively defends the procedural approach in this regard,[42] and reiterating my own concern (outlined in the introduction) that substantive accounts could legitimize paternalistic interference under the rubric of autonomy. Further, I suspect that part of the reason that this conflict appears irreconcilable is that at least some substantive theorists conceive of autonomy as something akin to a socialized ideal of what it would be live a life of independence and equal standing, rather than to live one's life in accordance with one's own

[39] Christman, *The Politics of Persons*, 165.

[40] Stoljar, 'Autonomy and the Feminist Intuition'.

[41] Mackenzie, 'Three Dimensions of Autonomy', 31. See Westlund, 'Rethinking Relational Autonomy'; Meyers, *Self, Society, and Personal Choice*; Benson, 'Autonomy and Oppressive Socialization'; Benson, 'Feminist Intuitions and the Normative Substance of Autonomy'; Stoljar, 'Autonomy and the Feminist Intuition'.

[42] Christman, *The Politics of Persons*, ch. 8; Friedman, *Autonomy, Gender, Politics*, ch. 1.

values.[43] It may be that autonomy theorists in this context are simply interested in different things that nonetheless get lumped together under the umbrella term of autonomy.

(ii) A Need for Historical Conditions?

Rather than attend further to the debate between procedural and substantive theorists, I shall instead consider whether these considerations of pervasive relational influence suggest a need to incorporate historical conditions into our understanding of what it is for a motivating desire to be authentic.

Advocates of historical theories claim that the theories of decisional autonomy that I considered in the previous chapter are *ahistorical*.[44] These theories are ahistorical in the sense that they claim that an agent's subjecting their motivating desire to a certain sort of psychological scrutiny at a particular point in time is sufficient for their being autonomous with respect to it. They are not particularly concerned about *how* the agent came to form the desire (or indeed the components of their psychology that might critically reflect on the desire). The motivation for claiming that an adequate theory of decisional autonomy should incorporate historical conditions is that agents may have been caused to have either their motivating desires, or other elements of their psychological economies in ways that appear to undermine their autonomy.

In the previous section, I explained how the account I have developed can explain why certain forms of influence constitute psychological manipulation that undermines autonomy. However, I noted that the mere fact that a desire was elicited via manipulative means does not entail that the agent must forever lack autonomy with respect to it. As I shall explain, this is a point that historical theories can also accommodate (although at some cost). However, the main point of disagreement between the theory of autonomy that I have outlined and historical approaches is that my theory cannot account for why global forms of manipulation (as outlined in (ii) [c] in the introduction to this chapter) would undermine autonomy.

One of the most widely discussed cases of global manipulation is Alfred Mele's case of Beth and Ann, in which Beth, an unproductive philosopher, is covertly brainwashed to become psychologically identical to Ann, a very productive philosopher. The brainwashers instil the same hierarchies of value that Ann has into Beth, while eradicating all of Beth's other competing values; she embraces her newfound passion for philosophy following critical reflection.[45]

Historical theorists typically use this case to object to ahistorical theories on the basis that the latter cannot account for the plausible intuition that Ann is autonomous with respect to her future philosophical behaviour in a way that Beth is not; *ex hypothesi*, both Ann and Beth (following the intervention) have identical

[43] Christman identifies this implicit conception of autonomy in some feminist discussions of autonomy in Christman, *The Politics of Persons*, 175.

[44] Mele distinguishes between internalist and externalist forms of psychological autonomy rather than ahistorical and historical forms. Mele, *Autonomous Agents*, 146–56. I have avoided the former terminology to avoid confusion with the way in which internalism and externalism have featured in debates about practical reason.

[45] Mele, *Autonomous Agents*, 145.

psychologies and thus reflectively endorse their love of hard philosophical work (a new passion in Beth's case).[46]

In contrast, one might accommodate the intuition that Beth lacks autonomy by claiming that there is either an objective or subjective historical condition of authenticity. I shall first briefly consider Mele's own approach, before turning to consider Christman's historical approach in more detail, given its recent influence in bioethical discussions.

According to Mele, a necessary condition of an agent's possessing an authentic desire is that she was not 'compelled' to have that desire, such that she is practically unable to shed it.[47] To be compelled is not merely to be *caused* to have some desire; rather it is to be caused to have a desire in a manner that bypasses the subject's capacities for control over their mental life.[48] Notice here that Mele appeals to objective facts about how the agent came to hold the desire in question; it can thus be construed as an objective historical account. Notice also that the account is framed negatively; authenticity requires the *absence* of certain types of causes. A further necessary condition is that the agent neither performed nor arranged for the bypassing that led her to develop the psychological characteristic in question.[49]

I shall have cause to refer to a further necessary condition that Mele specifies in the course of refining his view below. However, the first two conditions specified here are enough to see that Mele's account can offer a way of explaining how Beth might lack autonomy in a way that Ann does not. She is compelled to now value the life of a productive philosopher in a manner that bypasses her control over her mental life. The main challenge facing Mele's account as I have so far specified it is that it sets a seemingly high bar for autonomy. As those who espouse relational views of autonomy point out, we are all, at least in part, an outcome of social and environmental forces that determine many of our values and desires at a pre-critical stage of our development. There is '... no self before the socialization that creates it'[50] in pre-critical childhood development. In a sense then, by Mele's lights, we are all victims of manipulative processes that serve to undermine our autonomy, in so far as we have all had certain values and desires imputed to us during the pre-critical stages of our development, some of which we are now practically unable to shed. Accordingly, it seems plausible that autonomy is compatible with the fact that many of our desires were caused in ways that bypassed our mental control.[51]

Consider now John Christman's alternative subjective historical account. Rather than appealing to objective facts about how a desire was caused, subjective accounts instead ask '... if the person would have, or did resist the adoption of a value or desire, and for what reasons'.[52] In the early iteration of the view, Christman argued that the relevant question for autonomy is whether the agent would have resisted *the process* by which she came to have a particular desire (in a minimally rational, and self-aware manner). One obvious problem with this initial iteration of the view is a phenomenon I explored in the previous section. One can reject the process by which

[46] Ibid., 145. [47] Ibid., 166. [48] Ibid., 171. [49] Ibid., 166.

[50] Noggle, 'Autonomy and the Paradox of Self-Creation', 104.

[51] Christman raises a similar criticism at Christman, *The Politics of Persons*, 141.

[52] Christman, 'Autonomy and Personal History', 10.

one acquired a desire, and yet still hold that desire autonomously if one endorses it on other grounds. Partly in view of this objection, Christman has recently revised his subjectivist view by defending the following three necessary[53] authenticity conditions of an agent's being autonomous with respect to some basic evaluative characteristic C:

1. Were the person to engage in sustained critical reflection on C over a variety of conditions in the light of the historical processes (adequately described) that gave rise to C;
2. She would not be alienated from C in the sense of feeling and judging that C cannot be sustained as part of an acceptable autobiographical narrative organized by her diachronic practical identity;
3. The reflection being imagined is not constrained by reflection-distorting factors.[54]

Notice that condition 1 shifts the focus of the relevant reflection from the *causal history* of a particular desire, to the desire itself, *in light of* its causal history. This move circumvents a significant part of the above criticism. However, it does so at the cost of considerably weakening the relevance of history per se to authenticity. The relevant reflection now concerns the nature of the psychological characteristics themselves, rather than the manner in which one came to acquire them. Indeed, I suggest that the need for historical theories to make this move suggests that historical views of autonomy are in fact focusing on the wrong aspect of our desires, since these revised versions maintain that it is not the causal history of our desires that really matters with regards to our autonomy; what really matters is whether the agent *now* believes that they ought to endorse their desires. The history of the desire is one thing that may contribute to that decision, but it is not the only consideration.

This latter point emphasizes the fact that it is uncharitable to characterize the rationalist view that I have defended as entirely ahistorical. The rationalist view rejects what David Zimmerman refers to as source historicism; that is, it rejects the thesis that our autonomy with respect to a particular psychological property depends on the manner in which it is acquired. However, it is perfectly compatible with what Zimmerman calls process-historicism, that is, the thesis that 'autonomy grounding psychological states and processes are temporally extended'.[55] As I explained in the previous chapter, the constituents of our character systems have authority to speak for the 'true self' because they are diachronically extended, and relatively stable features of our psychological economies.[56] Process-historicism matters for autonomy, but it is not at all clear that source-historicism does.

We may also note that the objective historical account can also make a similar move to the one discussed above to circumvent Berofsky's concern. That is, the

[53] Necessary but not sufficient. These authenticity conditions are supplemented with three conditions concerning the competencies that are causally necessary for autonomy. See Christman, *The Politics of Persons*, 155.

[54] Ibid., 155.

[55] Zimmerman, 'That Was Then, This Is Now', 642.

[56] Indeed, what I refer to as the agent's character system shares a number of salient similarities with what Christman refers to as the agent's diachronic practical identity in Christman, *The Politics of Persons*.

objectivist can (and should) claim that an agent can initially acquire a desire in a manner that bypasses her mental control, and yet still be autonomous with respect to it, as long as she later exerts mental control by deciding to sustain that desire once she is made aware of its dubious causal history.[57] Indeed, Mele supplements his theory with the following necessary condition that responds to this kind of problem: S will only fail to be autonomous with respect to a particular value P which she was compelled to have in a manner she did not arrange if it is also true that:

> *S* neither presently possesses nor earlier possessed pro-attitudes that would support his identifying with *P*, with the exception of pro-attitudes that are themselves practically unsheddable products of unsolicited bypassing; then *S* is compelled* to possess *P*.[58]

With this condition, Mele's account moves closer to the view of manipulation that I defended in the previous section. In typical cases of manipulation where the agent endorses the changes evinced, it seems plausible that they do so by virtue of the fact that the new characteristic coheres with *pre-existing* elements of their character system. Such agents can be autonomous because they do not meet the above necessary condition of compulsion. Mele and I are in agreement on this point.

However, our approaches come apart when we consider cases in which the agent's endorsement of a manipulated psychological characteristic is *itself* a product of elements of one's character system that one has also been compelled to have. Crucially, Beth endorses her manipulated values in this kind of way. For Mele, endorsement of a manipulated value by *other* compelled values would meet the further necessary condition just outlined, and so such an agent would fail to be autonomous because they would meet all the necessary conditions of having been compelled to have the relevant values in a manner that she did not arrange. This is an important point, because it is here where the relational objection to the objectivist externalist account shows its teeth. Why does Beth lack autonomy in a way that most people do not, if their character systems as a whole are unsheddable in a relevantly similar way, by virtue of their formation in pre-critical periods of their lives?

One response to this problem is to appeal to the subjectivist approach, and claim that Beth lacks autonomy because she would hypothetically feel alienated from her new values were she to reflect on them in light of their causal history. I am not convinced by the subjectivist explanation of why Beth lacks autonomy, but we can put that point to one side.[59] Instead of attacking this explanation, I believe that we should adopt the revisionist view that *both* Beth and Ann are autonomous in an important sense, even if Beth meets all of Mele's conditions of compulsion in a way

[57] Mele, *Autonomous Agents*, 165. [58] Ibid., 172.

[59] Briefly, my concern is that Beth could plausibly have been manipulated in such a manner that she would *not* feel so alienated. Christman's third condition outlined above is intended to block off this kind of example. Yet, it is not clear that it can be successful; for it to be so, we would need a good theory of what it is for a factor to be reflection-distorting in the relevant sense. In his discussion, Christman relies on our 'independent knowledge' of such factors. Yet, in borderline cases, this is precisely what seems to be missing. Consider for example a young woman who prioritizes the avoidance of weight-gain over all other values including her own survival; alone, the mere fact that we might diagnose such an individual as having a psychiatric disease tells us little about whether we should understand her mode of reflection to be distorted in the relevant sense.

that Ann does not. On this revisionist view, Mele's example is still powerful because it raises a plausible question about whether we should employ historical conditions on Beth's prospective *morally responsibility* following global manipulation. However, the point is that we should be wary of assuming that these intuitions translate straightforwardly to the claim that Beth is not autonomous.[60]

This is particularly true when we think about the way in which we understand autonomy in the biomedical sphere. To illustrate, suppose that following the manipulation, Beth is told that she has a medical condition that will result in paralysis unless she undergoes a neurosurgical procedure that is likely to cause a mild cognitive impairment (equivalent let us say to her losing 5 IQ points). Prior to her global manipulation, it may be that Beth would have prioritized her motor capacities far above a small reduction in her cognitive capacities. Following the manipulation though, let us suppose that her priorities have changed; she no longer cares for non-philosophical pursuits, and even a small reduction in her cognitive capacities would be hugely damaging. Here is the key point: all other things being equal, 'post-manipulation' Beth can clearly autonomously decide to refuse to consent to the procedure, even though she did not arrange for the global change in values that manipulation evinced, and which now grounds the autonomy of her decision. We may also note that a significant benefit of claiming that Beth is autonomous is that it obviates the problem facing Mele's theory, of how to explain the way in which we can generally be autonomous in a way that Beth is not, if all of our characters are grounded by values that appear to be unsheddable by his lights.

However, why should we think that the intuitive appeal of Mele's example is grounded in the fact that our judgements regarding Beth's autonomy and moral responsibility can diverge?[61] In defending a similar view, Nomy Arpaly alludes to the way in which our judgements about moral responsibility may be muddied by conflicting understandings of the notion of personal identity. However, for this argument to succeed, one would need to explain why these intuitions do not similarly affect our judgements about autonomy. An alternative explanation for why our judgements about autonomy and responsibility might differ can be sourced in Gary Watson's distinction between accountability and attributability. According to Watson, it can be possible for conduct to be *attributable* to an individual, where the conduct itself admits of appraisal and when it make sense to appraise the individual herself as an adopter of ends. Yet, the attributability of conduct does not entail that the agent is also accountable for that conduct, in the sense of her deserving sanction for it. One way in which we can cash out the conflicting claims about the responsibility and autonomy in the Beth/Ann case is to make the following two claims:[62] (i) these agents' conduct is attributable to them following global manipulation, but they

[60] Nomy Arpaly defends this revisionist view in Arpaly, *Unprincipled Virtue*, 126–30.

[61] Mele has offered a response to Arpaly's critique. However, he is mainly concerned with demonstrating that certain counterexamples raised by Arpaly to the bypassing condition (not provided here) fail. Crucially, he does not engage with the point regarding the putative differences between autonomy and moral responsibility, which are fundamental to Arplay's argument and my own criticism. See Mele, *Free Will and Luck*, 179–84.

[62] Watson, 'Two Faces of Responsibility', 263.

are not accountable for that behaviour and (ii) autonomy only requires that our conduct is attributable to us, whilst accountability may be necessary for some conceptions of moral responsibility.[63,64]

On the view that I am proposing here then, cases of global manipulation epitomized in the Beth/Ann case and identified in (ii)[c] in my schema above are primarily relevant to questions of personal identity and moral responsibility rather than autonomy, at least with regards to the sort of autonomy that is of practical interest in bioethics. Notably, although I have suggested Christman's subjective approach would imply that Beth lacks autonomy, it seems that the view could be amended to endorse the same conclusion on the Beth/Ann case that I have suggested here. To conclude my analysis of the role of history in decisional autonomy, I shall highlight two ways in which the theory I presented in the last chapter further departs from a subjective account that might be amended in this way.

As I discussed above, although considerations of history are no longer the primary consideration on Christman's revised theory, they still play a significant role; the agent must not (hypothetically) feel alienated from a given psychological characteristic *in light of its causal history*. However, whilst I agree that the dubious causal history of a desire may mean that we ought to critically assess the content of those desires to ensure that we endorse them, I remain sceptical of the claim that the agent's own attitude towards that causal history itself should matter with respect to the authenticity of their psychological characteristics themselves.

Indeed, an agent's own attitude towards the causal history of a characteristic can be irrelevant to their autonomy with respect to it. Suppose Alex loathes Ben and detests his world-view. Ben is giving a detailed, well-researched speech about why the government ought to adopt policy A rather than policy B. Although Alex previously endorsed policy B, he finds that he is rationally persuaded by the arguments in Ben's speech to now endorse policy A. Nonetheless, he feels alienated from this new preference, simply by virtue of the fact that it was Ben, his fiercely detested enemy, who succeeded in persuading him. By Christman's lights, it seems that Ben is not autonomous with respect to this new preference, but this seems implausible. The mere fact that Alex feels alienated from his preference because of Ben's role in it is not sufficient to show that Ben's rational persuasion is a form of controlling influence that serves to undermine Alex's autonomy.

Furthermore, Christman's theory can only provide practical guidance if we assume that we have an adequate grasp of the causal history of our psychological characteristics. However, the causal histories of some of our desires may remain opaque to us,[65] and we may even hold false beliefs about them. Indeed, this represents a considerable challenge in the psychiatric context, where clinicians may face the challenge of distinguishing between those forms of apparently psychotic phenomena

[63] For a defence of the claim that Beth/Ann are in fact both morally responsible, see Talbert, 'Implanted Desires, Self-Formation and Blame'.

[64] Of course, there may be other differences between the two concepts. For instance, we may lack autonomy due to reasons of ignorance without thereby lacking moral responsibility on the basis that our ignorance was culpable.

[65] Levy, *Hard Luck*, 105.

that constitute pathological but benign delusional states, from eccentric beliefs and values that are deeply embedded within an individual's character system.[66] In some cases, there may be little clear difference in the causal history of the cognitive states in question. Christman denies that his theory is problematic in this sort of way, because his account requires that the agent's conception of the relevant causal history need only be 'minimally adequate . . . in the sense that it be consistent with accepted evidence and known causal sequences'.[67] Yet, a recent application of Christman's theory in neuroethics reveals that the opacity of the causal histories of our psychological characteristic still affects the practical application of his theory.

In a recent paper, Daniel Sharp and David Wasserman have argued that Christman's theory can provide much needed illumination about questions of moral responsibility that are arising in problematic real-life cases in which patients who have undergone neurosurgical treatment (Deep Brain Stimulation) exhibit uncharacteristic behaviours following the intervention.[68] In considering a hypothetical example of an individual who develops a gambling addiction following neurosurgical treatment, and who endorses this new behaviour, the authors write:

> Many (ourselves included) have the intuition that the gambler is not fully responsible for his conduct because his endorsement itself *appears to be caused by personality-altering effects of DBS.*[69]

Setting aside the important point that Christman's theory is primarily intended as a theory of autonomy rather than responsibility, I want to focus on the emphasized phrase here. Philosophers and neuroethicists generally assume that changes to behavioural traits or personality that are sometimes observed following Deep Brain Stimulation are directly caused by the treatment itself. However, as Frederic Gilbert and colleagues have forcefully argued, we have very little evidence to suggest that this is the case; the phenomenon could also be adequately explained by a host of other mechanisms. It could be the result of the treatment unmasking extant psychiatric symptoms or of the patient experiencing difficulties with social integration following the amelioration of a chronic medical condition.[70]

The problem here is that the very context that the historical theory is apparently required to illuminate is one in which we lack even a minimally adequate understanding of the causal history of the relevant psychological characteristics. It is one thing to assume that an individual would hypothetically be alienated from a desire that has been induced by brain stimulation. It is another to assume that they would be alienated from a desire that they have formed as a result of their recovering from a chronic medical condition.

[66] For discussion of some enlightening case studies in this regard, and an argument for basing a distinction between spiritual and pathological forms of psychotic phenomena in considerations of their role in what I have called the agent's character system (and not the causal history of these cognitive states), see Fulford and Jackson, 'Spiritual Experience and Psychopathology'.

[67] Christman, *The Politics of Persons*, 154.

[68] Sharp and Wasserman, 'Deep Brain Stimulation, Historicism, and Moral Responsibility'.

[69] Ibid., 179, my emphasis.

[70] Gilbert, Viaña, and Ineichen, 'Deflating the "DBS Causes Personality Changes" Bubble'.

Finally, Christman stipulates that the reflection that his theory demands is only hypothetical, and that it can thus accommodate the thought that many central aspects of our lives have never been reflectively endorsed.[71] In contrast, rationalist theories tend to stipulate that critical reflection must be carried out at some point, even if only unconsciously, or in a dispositional sense.[72] The virtue of Christman's hypothetical approach is that it makes his account of autonomy significantly less demanding; however, in the biomedical context it also comes at a cost, since it renders the view difficult to operationalize. In assessing an agent's autonomy with respect to a decision, rather than simply enquiring about their general values, we not only have to know the causal history of the agent's desires, we have to make a judgement about what that agent would hypothetically feel about that causal history if it was brought to their attention.

This feature of the view raises the bar for third-party assessments of autonomy. However, in other ways the view also lowers the bar too far for the standards of decisional autonomy itself (rather than its third-party assessment); if it is true that an agent has *never* evaluated some central element of their psychological economy in any way, be it implicitly or unconsciously, then I do not hasten to conclude that the agent lacks autonomy with respect to that aspect of her psychology. Whilst this may seem a hard bullet to bite, we may note that those who endorse the hypothetical reflection condition have to bite the bullet of accepting that an agent qualifies as self-governing without ever actually attending to any element of his practical identity, no matter how minimally. I struggle to agree that this would be indicative of an agent engaged in any sort of active self-governance.

4. Informational Manipulation

At the beginning of this chapter, I distinguished psychological manipulation from informational manipulation, and deception. The latter two forms of influence affect the agent's beliefs, albeit in somewhat different ways. Beauchamp and Childress classify deception as a form of informational manipulation in outlining the standard view of autonomy. However, I believe that the clarity of the discussion will be best served by separating the two. One reason for this is that it can often be theoretically rational to believe *x* when one has been deceived into believing *x*, since we can be rationally justified in believing the testimony of others, even when it is false. In contrast, whilst informational manipulation may also involve leading another to develop false beliefs, it more typically involves leading an agent to adopt theoretically *irrational* beliefs.

We humans are subject to a considerable number of cognitive biases when it comes to forming our beliefs, and these biases can compromise our autonomy in a number of ways. Some biases may lead individuals to misapply their values, either by

[71] Christman, *The Politics of Persons*, 145.

[72] Ekstrom, 'A Coherence Theory of Autonomy'; Savulescu, 'Rational Desires and the Limitation of Life Sustaining Treatment'.

causing them to form a false belief about the world or to make basic logical errors; others can cause a patient to act in a way that does not reflect her values.[73]

Cognitive biases that can compromise autonomy in the first way include the phenomenon of motivated reasoning, in which agents regard an argument as fallacious simply because they are already predisposed to reject its conclusion.[74] Consider also the framing effect. Evidence from behavioural psychology suggests that if information provided to a patient is framed positively, then agents deciding on the basis of that information are more likely to be risk averse than if the information is framed negatively. Savulescu uses the following example to illustrate the importance of the framing effect in medical consultations:

> ...(l)ung cancer can be treated by surgery or radiotherapy. Surgery is associated with greater immediate mortality (10 per cent v 0 per cent mortality), but better long-term prospects (66 per cent v 78 per cent five-year mortality). The attractiveness of surgery to patients is substantially greater when the choice between surgery and radiotherapy is framed in terms of the probability of living rather than the probability of dying.[75]

The framing effect engenders a form of theoretical irrationality because it involves logical incoherence; in the above example, it would be contradictory for a patient to prefer surgery when the comparative risk/benefit profiles are framed positively, but to also prefer radiotherapy when the (very same) comparative risk/benefit profiles are framed negatively.

Cognitive biases that can compromise autonomy in the second way include the bias that agents exhibit towards the present, and their reluctance to consider the possibility of future harms when they weigh their reasons for pursuing different outcomes.[76] For example, a patient may reject their physician's recommendation that they stop smoking, not because they believe that the pleasure they get from smoking is more valuable than increasing the probability of a longer lifespan, but rather because they fail to attend to the disvalue of the later consequences of smoking.

The evidence regarding cognitive biases suggests a further reason to reject value-neutral approaches to the shared decision-making model that I considered in section 1. It is a mistake to assume that the information we might need to give to individuals to ensure they adequately understand their options can be provided in a value-neutral way. Although the *content* of the information we provide can enable autonomy by ensuring adequate understanding, the *manner* in which it is presented can covertly influence individuals to develop irrational beliefs, or to act in practically irrational ways. Indeed, it seems that some nudge techniques are designed to capitalize on the forms of theoretical irrationality to which our propensity to cognitive biases makes us particularly vulnerable.

However, it is not always clear how we should demarcate kinds of informational manipulation from forms of influence that enhance the understanding that is necessary for decisional autonomy. To illustrate, Blumenthal-Barby and Burroughs suggest that the use of vivid examples and explanations can constitute a nudge,

[73] Levy draws this distinction in Levy, 'Forced to Be Free?', 298. [74] Ibid., 298.

[75] Savulscu, 'Rational Non-Interventional Paternalism,' 328–9. See also Brock, *Life and Death*, 88.

[76] Levy, 'Forced to Be Free?', 6. See also Brock, *Life and Death*, 84.

noting that these items can elicit strong emotional responses that powerfully shape decisions and behaviours. By way of example, they describe the following study by Volandes et al.:

> A group of elderly adults was shown a 2-minute video about what life with advanced dementia was like along with a written description, while the other group was just given the written description. The group that saw the video had 86% of its members indicate that they would want 'comfort care only' in such a state, whereas in the control group that number was only 64%.[77]

Blumenthal-Barby and Burroughs' discussion suggests that they understand this to be an instance of the use of affect to influence decision-making, and that such use of affect will typically amount to a manipulative interference.[78] However, it seems that more needs to be said in favour of this interpretation, particularly in light of my discussion of emotions and persuasion in section 2. In particular, it seems plausible that the video in question may simply have made reason-giving facts about the badness of life with dementia more vivid to the viewers; if so, it seems that the strategy should be construed as facilitating rather than impeding rational decision-making.[79]

In light of my discussion of the kinds of psychological and informational manipulation that nudge techniques can employ, what should we say about the implications of these techniques for decisional autonomy? Advocates of these techniques often argue that they are compatible with individual autonomy by appealing to the fact that they do not limit the agent's choice set (unlike bans) or involve significantly altering incentives.[80] Whilst true, such observations miss what is primarily at stake in the debate about nudging and autonomy. The fact that nudges do not undermine autonomy in some ways (by restricting freedom or coercing) does nothing to answer the fact that they may yet pose other threats to our decisional autonomy by inducing forms of theoretical and/or practical irrationality.[81]

Proponents of nudges alternatively might advert to the fact that normal human decision-making is plagued by non-rational influences.[82] Here, it might be claimed that nudges can do little to undermine decisional autonomy if we *already* lack such autonomy. Of course, the fact that non-rational influence of some sort is inevitable in a given choice domain does not imply that steps should not be taken to mitigate these non-rational effects. Recall the example of the framing effect above. In this circumstance, even though the physician has to make a choice about whether to frame the

[77] Blumenthal-Barby and Burroughs, 'Seeking Better Health Care Outcomes'. [78] Ibid., 5.

[79] Indeed, these videos might prompt the sort of 'vivid imagination of alternatives' that Savulescu argues is a requirement of autonomous decision-making. See Savulescu, 'Rational Desires and the Limitation of Life Sustaining Treatment'.

[80] Thaler and Sunstein, *Nudge*.

[81] Saghai has developed a philosophically robust defence of a closely related argument that nudges are compatible with autonomy, by invoking considerations of freedom of choice and resistibility. See Saghai, 'Salvaging the Concept of Nudge'. See Ploug and Holm, 'Doctors, Patients, and Nudging in the Clinical Context—Four Views on Nudging and Informed Consent' for a rebuttal of this argument drawing on rationalist themes.

[82] Thaler and Sunstein, *Nudge*; Blumenthal-Barby and Naik, 'In Defense of Nudge–Autonomy Compatibility'.

information positively or negatively, this does not entail that he cannot seek to then mitigate the non-rational influence his framing might have on the patient's choice, by asking the patient to justify or explain their choice.[83]

Notwithstanding these claims, I shall suggest below that nudges may infringe an interpersonal form of voluntariness that standard non-rational decision-making does not. To conclude this part of the discussion though, we should, I believe, concede that some (but not all) of the nudge strategies that aim to influence individual behaviour are manipulative in a manner that serves to undermine autonomous decision-making. Despite the powerful, and potentially beneficial effects of such strategies, we should not labour under the illusion that interventions are always compatible with local autonomous choice. As I argued in section 2, they may fail to be so if they bypass and subvert the cognitive element of our practical rationality. However, they will also fail to be so if they engender forms of theoretical irrationality.

Again, it is important to be clear that this is a point about the implications of nudges for decisional autonomy, and not an all things considered moral judgement on their use. One might argue that broadly beneficence-based concerns could outweigh these considerations of local autonomy; however, such a strategy will naturally require that one is able to respond to the (justified) allegation of paternalism that would be weighed against it.[84] An alternative, and I believe more promising strategy, might seek to justify these strategies of influencing behaviour by appealing to the value of the agent's global, rather than local autonomy. I shall explore this point when I consider the value of different kinds of autonomy in Chapter 9.

5. Deception

On one prominent understanding, deception involves imparting false beliefs to another person.[85] If it is the case that decisional autonomy requires that agents hold certain decisionally necessary true beliefs, then deception (so-construed) will serve to undermine autonomy just in so far as it leads individuals to hold false beliefs about features of their choice domain that are subjects of what I am terming 'decisionally necessary' beliefs. However, the account of autonomy and true beliefs that I have been sketching so far (and which I shall flesh out further in Chapter 5) points towards a broader account of deception. I have suggested that decisional autonomy can require that agents hold certain true beliefs about features of the decision in question; crucially, it seems that there can be cases in which one causes another to fail to hold the relevant true beliefs by *omitting* key information. If this is

[83] Ploug and Holm, 'Doctors, Patients, and Nudging in the Clinical Context—Four Views on Nudging and Informed Consent'. See also Miller and Fagley, 'The Effects of Framing, Problem Variations, and Providing Rationale on Choice'. In their discussion, Ploug and Holm imply that the framing effect undermines autonomy in so far as it undermines the understanding required for autonomous decision-making. I agree with Blumenthal-Barby and Naik's criticism of this claim. Blumenthal-Barby and Naik, 'In Defense of Nudge–Autonomy Compatibility'.

[84] This strategy corresponds to what Ploug and Holm describe as the 'priority view'. See Ploug and Holm, 'Doctors, Patients, and Nudging in the Clinical Context—Four Views on Nudging and Informed Consent', 36 for discussion.

[85] Shiffrin, *Speech Matters*, 19.

so, then it is also possible to undermine autonomy by deception via omission on the theory that I am outlining here.[86] Accordingly, in the following discussion, I shall seek to defend a broader conception of deception as involving either causing another to hold false beliefs, or causing them to fail to hold decisionally necessary true beliefs.

This is a controversial way of broadening the scope of deception. Another controversial implication of the view that I have so far defended is that deception need not be intentional. In discussing psychological manipulation I noted that the claim that manipulation need not be intentional follows straightforwardly from the claim that rational authenticity is a necessary condition of decisional autonomy. Strikingly, an analogous claim can be made with regard to deception if one holds that sufficient understanding is a necessary condition of autonomy. Deception need not be intentional in order to undermine decisional autonomy as long as it serves to lead agents to fail to hold decisionally necessary beliefs.

The clarity of the following discussion will be aided by making some distinctions between possible forms of deception. Of course, one of the most common methods of deception is lying. However, lying is not co-extensive with deception, in so far as a lie does not entail that a liar successfully imparts a false belief in the manner that deception connotes.[87] We may say that an agent lies, when she intentionally provides her target with information that she believes to be incorrect, and her doing so manifests her intention to get her target to treat the information as an accurate representation of what she (the liar) believes.[88] A lie will also deceive if this has the effect of imparting a false belief to the target. In contrast, unintentional deception can occur when one provides an agent with information that they believe to be true, but which is in fact false. Deception via omission occurs when the target is led to develop a false belief, or to fail to hold a decisionally necessary true belief because of the omission of certain key information.

Of course, a great deal here turns on the feasibility of decisionally necessary beliefs. I briefly defended this view in the previous chapter, and I shall offer a more principled defence in Chapter 5. Here though, to illustrate deception via omission in a medical context, a physician may so deceive their patient by providing them with only a partial disclosure about their condition, or employing euphemisms to obscure the true nature of the condition. In such a case, deception via omission may lead the patient to explicitly hold false beliefs, or to fail to hold true beliefs of the sort that are crucial for making certain future decisions with the kind of understanding that autonomy requires. Suppose that tests revealed that Maurice has motor neurone disease; however, instead of explicitly informing Maurice of this particular diagnosis, the physician tells him that he has a condition that will cause him increasing weakness, but that he will be made 'as comfortable as possible'. On the basis of the

[86] For another detailed defence of this view, see Cox and Fritz, 'Should Non-Disclosures Be Considered as Morally Equivalent to Lies within the Doctor–Patient Relationship?'

[87] Shiffrin, *Speech Matters*, 19–21.

[88] Ibid., 13. Notice that on this account, it is possible to lie without deception in the sense that '... a lie does not depend on its recipient being deceived'. In such cases, I suggest that the lie may not undermine the voluntariness of the recipient's decision, but that there may nonetheless be reasons to sanction the liar. Another interesting feature of Shiffrin's account is that lying must be intentional in the sense indicated above, but it need not involve the intention to deceive.

conjunction of this euphemism, and the partial disclosure about the effects of the increasing weakness caused by motor neurone disease, Maurice forms the false belief that his condition is not all that serious. If so, on the definition that I am employing here, the physician would have deceived Maurice via omission, even if this were not his intention; Maurice fails to understand his situation in a manner that allows him to draw accurate connections between his values and his available options.

There is a significant philosophical debate as to whether lying is morally on a par with deception via omission.[89] However, as I mentioned at the outset of this chapter, I am interested only in the question of the effects of different sorts of influence on autonomy. Insofar as lying and omission can lead individuals to either form the same false beliefs or to fail to have decisionally necessary true ones, I claim that both can undermine autonomy. However, there are some important distinctions between the two. First, there is often a straightforward causal connection between the telling of a lie, and the target holding a false belief, such that the target can straightforwardly blame the liar for the fact that they hold a false belief. However, in the case of deception via omission, this causal relationship is far less straightforward, particularly when the deception is non-intentional. The explanation for this is that it seems plausible that autonomous agents have *some* degree of doxastic responsibility to obtain their own true beliefs about the world. If so, the fact that others omit to provide one with information cannot be said to be the only causal factor in one's ignorance. Just as we can distinguish between culpable and non-culpable ignorance in discussions of moral responsibility and blame, it also seems possible to distinguish between autonomy-undermining ignorance that is the fault of a third party, and that which is the fault of the agent herself.[90]

Accordingly, in some cases an individual's failure to hold a decisionally necessary belief is not best attributed to the fact that *others* have omitted to provide certain information. In everyday life, individuals plausibly have some responsibility to make attempts to understand the situations in which they find themselves, and the reasons that obtain for them in those situations. However, in biomedical decision-making, patients place a great deal of trust in their physician due to the considerable knowledge gap that exists between them with regards to salient medical facts. An upshot of this is that patients may transfer much of their everyday responsibility to cultivate decisionally necessary beliefs onto the physician in this context, in the form of a presumed duty of the physician to disclose information that is necessary for the patient to make an autonomous treatment decision. This represents an important way in which individuals in the biomedical context are more vulnerable to deception (broadly conceived) than they are in everyday life.

The understanding of deception I am employing here also runs contrary to the claim that only *intentional* deception undermines autonomy.[91] Interestingly,

[89] Pugh et al., 'Lay Attitudes toward Deception in Medicine'; Benn, 'Medicine, Lies and Deceptions'; Gillon, 'Is There an Important Moral Distinction for Medical Ethics between Lying and Other Forms of Deception?'; Jackson, 'Telling the Truth'; Bakhurst, 'On Lying and Deceiving'.

[90] For discussions of the doxastic responsibilities of patients, see Kukla, 'How Do Patients Know?'; Foster, *Choosing Life, Choosing Death*, 104.

[91] See Wilkinson, 'Nudging and Manipulation'.

Beauchamp and Childress claim that only intentional deception undermines autonomy. This is somewhat perplexing given their view that substantial understanding is a necessary condition of autonomy; why suppose that only intentional forms of deception can subvert substantial understanding? The claim that *only* intentional deception undermines autonomy is on more solid ground when it is held in conjunction with the claim that autonomy does not require certain true beliefs. Wilkinson, for instance, adopts this strategy.[92] He writes:

> A person may have false beliefs about his or her options without his or her autonomy being affected; who has true beliefs about all their options? But if those beliefs came about through deceit, his or her autonomy has been harmed.[93]

However, the fact that holding *some* false beliefs is compatible with decisional autonomy does not entail that *any* particular false belief about one's options is compatible with decisional autonomy. To illustrate, an individual can autonomously decide to undergo a medical procedure on the basis of a belief that it will be successful in ameliorating their condition, even if their belief turns out to be false. This reflects the fact that not all sorts of information about our choices are decisionally necessary, a point I raised in Chapter 2. However, this is quite compatible with the claim that some information is. To repeat an example from earlier in the book, an individual cannot be said to have autonomously decided to undergo a vasectomy if they fail to understand that it will lead them to be infertile.

More generally, simply showing that autonomy is compatible with individuals holding some false beliefs is not sufficient to demonstrate that decisional autonomy does not require that individuals must hold any true beliefs. To appeal to the compatibility of autonomy with certain false beliefs in order to deny the existence of *any* decisionally necessary beliefs is rather like pointing to a white swan in order to disprove the possibility of a black one. Following the Aristotelian claim that we can sometimes fail to be autonomous due to reasons of ignorance, and in accordance with the standard account's criterion of understanding, we should, I believe, acknowledge the possibility of decisionally necessary beliefs, and their implications for our understanding of deception. I shall offer a principled approach to identifying decisionally necessary beliefs in Chapter 5.

There are of course important non-autonomy based moral reasons to separate out the different forms that deception can take. Intentional deception plausibly involves wrongs that non-intentional deception does not, and intentional deceivers will often be culpable in a manner that may not be the case if deception was unintentional. Indeed, from a legal perspective, the question of whether a physician intentionally lied to their patient or unintentionally omitted vital information in obtaining consent to a medical intervention might make the difference between the procedure being an instance of battery rather than negligence. However, from the perspective of the

[92] For other examples of theorists who claim that false beliefs do not undermine autonomy, see McKenna, 'The Relationship between Autonomous and Morally Responsible Agency', 208–9; Arpaly, 'Responsibility, Applied Ethics, and Complex Autonomy Theories', 175.

[93] Wilkinson, 'Nudging and Manipulation'. Note that Wilkinson uses this observation to defend the view that only intentional manipulation undermines autonomy.

individual's autonomy *alone*, my claim is that failing to hold decisionally necessary true beliefs undermines an individual's ability to make an autonomous decision, no matter how they were influenced to fail in this way.

There are various ways in which a physician can either intentionally or unintentionally deceive a patient. Lying, of course is the most obvious method. However, there are also more subtle means of deception. For instance, as I illustrated with the example of Maurice above, the physician may not provide the patient with any false information, but simply be selective about the information that they choose to divulge to a patient, so that the latter forms an inaccurate impression of their condition, an impression that means that they do not fully understand the salience of the choices they face. These observations about deception via omission raise important questions about how we should understand the standards of information disclosure that valid consent requires in a medical context. I shall postpone this discussion until Chapter 6. To conclude this chapter though, I want to reconsider the role of intentionality in controlling influence, and the further interpersonal sense of voluntariness it connotes.

6. The Role of Intentions and Interpersonal Voluntariness

I have so far defended a view of controlling influences that downplays the necessity of third-party intentional agency in determining whether a particular form of influence undermines decisional autonomy. As I mentioned above, my approach in this regard is a corollary of the fact that I have endorsed (i) a rationalist authenticity condition on decisional autonomy and (ii) the possibility of decisionally necessary beliefs. However, I do not mean to claim that the interference of intentional agents on another's autonomous decision-making is therefore morally equivalent to non-intentional or non-agential interference. There are clearly some important differences between the two that are not primarily grounded in their implications for the sense of autonomy that I am outlining here. First, in the former case, the interfering agent violates the Kantian imperative that enjoins one to act in such a way that one treats other rational agents never merely as a means, whilst the same need not be true in the latter. Second, whether or not one agent intentionally interfered with another may be significant with regards to assessments of culpability for the harm caused through one's interference. In many cases, I believe that our concern with the intentions of those who exert influence over us is primarily grounded in moral concerns that are largely orthogonal to the question of the target's autonomy per se. Moreover, the ambivalence that some authors claim to have about whether a certain form of influence (such as manipulation)[94] necessarily requires intentional agency, may be attributable to the fact that we may be invoking the concept of the influence at stake to answer quite different moral questions.

Nonetheless, there does seem to be some intuitive plausibility to the claim that intentional interference is somehow worse from the point of view of the agent's

[94] Barnhill, 'What Is Manipulation?'

autonomy. The agent who is intentionally deceived seems to have experienced a greater affront to her autonomy than the agent who is unintentionally deceived. Despite the claims that I have so far advanced in this chapter, I believe that this intuition captures an important truth. Crucially though, and contrary to what some theorists have implicitly claimed, it is not the *only* truth about autonomy.

The Aristotelian distinction between two types of non-voluntary action (those performed from reasons of ignorance and those that take place by force) captures aspects that are central to our understanding of decisional autonomy, at least in the biomedical sphere. In this concluding section though, I want to consider the possibility that when an agent's deficit in decisional autonomy is attributable to intentional third-party agency, this can be understood to undermine a separate kind of 'freedom from domination' that undergirds a sense of voluntariness that the Aristotelian distinction fails to acknowledge. I also suspect that this further form of voluntariness also adds further fuel to the fire regarding our ambivalence about the necessity of intention to our concepts of different forms of controlling influence.

The conception of freedom I have in mind here might be understood to denote a particular kind of negative freedom, namely the absence of positive constraints that have been intentionally imposed *by another agent*. This freedom is a specific kind of the broadly libertarian type of freedom that stresses the importance of the absence of constraints. However, freedom from domination has historically been understood in a broader sense within the republican tradition.[95] In this tradition, it is noted that dominance over another can be exerted even if it does not involve the *actual* imposition of constraints. For example, if another agent has the mere *capacity* to arbitrarily interfere with another's choices, they may be said to dominate the other in a sense that undermines the latter's freedom from domination.[96]

Accordingly, on the republican understanding, this freedom is violated if another has the mere capacity to interfere with one's choices. In contrast, on the libertarian understanding of freedom from domination as a particular kind of positive constraint, this freedom is only undermined if the dominating party does *in fact* exercise that capacity and actively interferes with the agent's decision. The sense that I mean to invoke here is the libertarian conception, although this is not the place to try and settle the debate as to whether it is more plausible than the republican conception. Although very little of what I shall claim turns on the fact that I endorse the libertarian rather than republican understanding of this freedom, it is important to acknowledge that the libertarian conception of this freedom is more robust. In order to undermine it, one must actually interfere with another's choices; it is not sufficient to merely have the capacity to do so.

[95] Pettit, *Republicanism*; Pettit, 'Freedom as Antipower'; Skinner, *Liberty before Liberalism*. For a discussion of the concept of domination itself, see Lovett, 'Domination'.

[96] This republican understanding of freedom can thus be invoked by those who claim that Savulescu and Persson's famous God Machine example involves the violation of individual freedom, even for those law-abiding individuals whom the machine does not directly act upon. See Savulescu and Persson, 'Moral Enhancement, Freedom, and the God Machine'; Sparrow, 'Better Living Through Chemistry?' for a republican response.

The key element of freedom from domination for my purpose here is that it is an *interpersonal* form of freedom; a lack of this freedom amounts to the subjugation of one's own will to another's authority. It may thus plausibly be construed as referring to a different sense of voluntariness than the one that is captured by the cognitive or reflective elements of decisional autonomy. The sense of voluntariness that reflective autonomy captures is the sense that is grounded by the thought that voluntary choices must reflect the agent's own character. The sense of voluntariness that the cognitive element captures is the sense that is grounded by the thought that ignorance can preclude us from acting effectively in pursuit of our ends, by rupturing the connection between our beliefs about our choices and our values. In contrast, the sense of voluntariness that freedom from domination captures is the sense that is grounded by the claim that it must be the agent *herself*, rather than other parties, who is in control of her decision-making if she is to be autonomous. This is the thought that Robert Wolff seeks to capture in his claim that 'The autonomous man, insofar as he is autonomous, is not subject to the will of another'.[97]

Why should we suppose that freedom from domination matters? Part of the explanation might be phenomenological; perhaps it is simply the case that third-party interference feels like more of an affront to our autonomy.[98] Elinor Mason, however, goes deeper than this phenomenological point in her discussion of this difference:

> What agents do to us is different to what non-agents do to us ... when there is another agent, that agent takes the place of 'self' in self-determination. Other agents are qualified to do that because they themselves have wills and are self-determining – the blind forces of nature cannot take over in the same way.[99]

A claim that seems implicit in Mason's comment here is that there is a difference in *the nature* of the lack of control of an agent whose decision-making is subjected to intentional interference, and an agent whose decisional autonomy is undermined by forces of hazard.

The difference can be helpfully illustrated by way of analogy. The sense of voluntariness captured by the two elements of decisional autonomy I have discussed prior to this point may be understood as pertaining to the strength of a ship captain's grip on her vessel's helm, and her ability to navigate to her destination. The captain has the relevant control to the extent that she (i) has true beliefs about where to go, and (ii) is able to dictate the ship's movements through her own influence on the helm. She may lack control because she is lost, or because the wheel is simply left spinning, and the course of the ship is left to the uncontrolled dictates of the sea and wind. In contrast, the interpersonal sense of voluntariness may be understood as pertaining to whether it is the captain, or a usurper who has taken control of the helm; there is an important difference between the course of one's ship being left to the vagaries of the elements, which have little interest in your destination, and your

[97] Wolff, *In Defense of Anarchism.* [98] Wertheimer, 'Voluntary Consent', 244–5.

[99] Mason, 'Coercion and Integrity', 196. Jennifer Blumenthal-Barby similarly denies the moral equivalence of environmental and agential influences on autonomy in Blumenthal-Barby, 'A Framework for Assessing the Moral Status of "Manipulation"', 125–6.

course being decided upon by an intentional agent who takes great interest in where you end up.

As I mentioned in the introductory chapter, some theorists claim that only intentional forms of controlling influence undermine autonomy. Such theorists place a great deal of stock in the sense of voluntariness that I am outlining here. In contrast, on the account of autonomy and controlling influence that I am outlining here, this sense of voluntariness supplements those outlined in the Aristotelian distinction. Decisional autonomy can be undermined by either non-agential processes (such as psychiatric disease) or the intentional interference of third parties. However, in the latter case, the influence exerted may serve to nullify an additional interpersonal sense of voluntariness. Crucially though, on the account of decisional autonomy that I have developed, one can lack decisional autonomy even if one's freedom from domination has not been violated. This distinguishes my account from those theories that claim that *only* intentional agents can undermine another's autonomy.[100] Indeed, I suggest that in order for one's will to have been dominated by intentional manipulation or deception, it must be the case that the interference in question has undermined the reflective or cognitive element of one's decisional autonomy. If the intentional deception or manipulation does not succeed in undermining one's decisional autonomy in a particular instance, it is difficult to make sense of the claim that one's will has been dominated in any significant sense by those exerting the influence.

One of the trends in the philosophical literature has been to understand the senses of voluntariness incorporated into decisional autonomy as being a matter of *solely* reflective autonomy, or *solely* freedom from domination. Both of these views, however, are mistaken. Our beliefs matter for decisional autonomy, and *both* agential and non-agential influences on our behaviour can undermine our autonomy. To return to the above analogy, one can fail to be in control of one's ship either because one does not have a strong enough grip on the helm, or because another has usurped one's position at the helm. Yet the former, which we may term *non-autonomy*, is not equivalent to the latter, which we may term *heteronomy*; this is not just so from the perspective of morality all things considered. It is also true from the perspective of interpersonal voluntariness.

Conclusion

In this chapter, I have outlined an approach to understanding different forms of manipulation and deception in light of the rationalist conception of autonomy that I developed in Chapter 2. In doing so, I also highlighted the significance of an interpersonal form of voluntariness not captured by the Aristotelian distinction.

I did not, however, address a salient form of controlling interference in this chapter, namely coercion. The reason for this is that coercion admits of greater

[100] Bublitz and Merkel, 'Autonomy and Authenticity of Enhanced Personality Traits'; Taylor, *Practical Autonomy and Bioethics*.

theoretical complexity than deception and manipulation. Moreover, as I shall explore in the next chapter, acknowledging the sense of freedom from domination that I explored in the second half of this chapter is crucial to providing a plausible theoretical basis for the ambiguous effects that coercion seems to have with respect to the voluntariness of the choices made in coercive situations.

4

Coercion

Consider the following as a paradigm case of coercion:

> Terry is targeted by an armed thief. The thief tells Terry to hand over his wallet. Terry refuses to cooperate. The thief then tells Terry that he will shoot him unless he cooperates. Terry agrees to hand over his wallet.

In accordance with the standard account of autonomy in bioethics, I assume that it is uncontroversial to claim that Terry is not autonomous with respect to his decision to hand over his wallet. Yet, despite the strength of our intuitions in this regard, coercion raises a number of puzzles, two of which in particular shall be my focus in this chapter. First, in what sense does coercion undermine voluntariness, and second, can offers as well as threats be coercive?

I shall begin this chapter by explaining my motivation for exploring these particular questions in more detail, before going on to explore two prominent streams in the literature on coercion that seeks to address these questions. I shall go on to argue for an account of coercion that accommodates the possibility of some coercive offers, and suggest that the answers to the two questions are interrelated. That is, I shall suggest that the way in which we should distinguish threats from offers (in responding to the second question) should draw on considerations that are closely linked to one's understanding of the way in which coercion undermines the interpersonal sense of voluntariness that I introduced in the previous chapter.

First though, since coercion is a term that is subject to a number of different interpretations in bioethical contexts, it is prudent to begin by delimiting the understanding that I shall invoke in my discussion. Although coercion is most often associated with the use of threats, some theorists adopt a broader understanding of the concept, according to which physically forcing an agent to do something (or to have something done to them) against their will can also amount to coercion.[1] For example, the term 'coerced treatment' is sometimes used in psychiatry to refer to treatment that has been forced in this sense. However, this use of the term conflates an important moral distinction between interventions in which an agent is forced to act, and interventions in which an agent is *acted upon*, potentially in the absence of their assent and even despite their dissent.[2]

[1] For instance, Wood claims that an agent can be said to be coerced when they do not choose to perform some action. Wood, 'Coercion, Manipulation, Exploitation', 21.

[2] See Bayles, 'A Concept of Coercion'; Lamond, 'Coercion, Threats, and the Puzzle of Blackmail'.

Autonomy, Rationality, and Contemporary Bioethics. Jonathan Pugh, Oxford University Press (2020). © Jonathan Pugh.
DOI: 10.1093/oso/9780198858584.001.0001

In order to avoid this conflation, I shall understand coercion to refer to a form of interference that necessarily involves the use of conditional proposals that render certain options ineligible for rational choice.[3] However, unlike the standard account of autonomy's approach to understanding coercion I shall *not* assume at the outset that the kinds of conditional proposals involved in coercion must, *by necessity*, be threats.[4]

1. Two Questions Facing an Adequate Account of Coercion in Bioethics

With this in mind, I can now turn to the two broadly interrelated questions with which I shall be concerned in this chapter. The first is why we should understand coercion to amount to a form of controlling interference of the sort that undermines voluntariness *at all*.

Coercion represents something of a problem for authenticity-based approaches to decisional autonomy because, although we want to be able to say that victims of coercion do not decide autonomously, these individuals will often meet the authenticity conditions set out by the accounts I have so far considered in this book. As Irving Thalberg notes, most persons who are subjected to coercion '... would, at the time and later, give second-order endorsement to their cautious [and compliant] motives'.[5] With regards to the theory that I have defended in the previous chapters, the motivating desire that an individual forms following a coercive threat could very plausibly be one that they rationally endorse with a preference that coheres with their character system. For instance, in the above example, Terry may endorse his desire to hand over his wallet, because the content of his motivating desire can be understood to include the outcome of staying alive, and he understands this to be a more valuable outcome than safeguarding his money. We may also note that victims of coercion also normally have adequate understanding of their situation.

Explaining how and why coercion undermines the voluntariness of the victim's decision is a considerable challenge for any authenticity-based conception of autonomy. However, in view of my claims in the previous chapter, it is perhaps a particularly acute challenge for the view that I am developing here. Recall that in the previous chapter, I claimed that deception and manipulation are forms of controlling influence that can undermine decisional autonomy without being intentional. This raises an important question for my theory because it appears that the same is not true of coercion; coercion must be intentional if it is to undermine decisional autonomy of the sort that undergirds the doctrine of informed consent. To see why, consider the following two cases:

> Alan is told by his doctor that if he refuses to start taking painkillers that will cause him to suffer from alopecia as a side-effect, he will start to experience significant pain as a result of an underlying medical condition. Although Alan agrees to take the pills, he would strongly prefer to be in a situation in which his

[3] Feinberg, *The Moral Limits of the Criminal Law*, 191.

[4] Beauchamp and Childress, *Principles of Biomedical Ethics*, 138.

[5] Thalberg, 'Hierarchical Analyses of Unfree Action', 126.

not experiencing pain was not also attended by the consequence of losing his hair.

Bernie is in fine health, but someone threatens to cause him similarly significant pain if he does not agree to take a drug that causes alopecia. Although Bernie agrees to take the pills, he would strongly prefer to be in a situation in which he does not experience pain, and where his not experiencing pain is not also attended by the consequence of losing his hair.

It seems that Alan can be autonomous with respect to his decision to take the drug, despite the limited choices available to him: Valid consent must be possible in the light of limited treatment options.[6] On the other hand, it is highly counter-intuitive to claim that Bernie is autonomous with respect to his decision to take the drug; like Terry, it seems that Bernie has plausibly been subjected to controlling influence of the sort that might be said to undermine the voluntariness of his decision. However, the only difference between the two cases is that Bernie's available options have been influenced by an intentional agent, whilst Alan's have been engineered by forces of hazard. The question is why should this matter for coercion, but not for deception or manipulation?

Aristotle recognized the nature of the theoretical challenge that coercion raises in his discussion of voluntariness, when he suggests that our actions following such threats are 'mixed' with regards to voluntariness. He writes:

> If a tyrant, for example, had one's parents and children in his power and ordered one to do something shameful, on the condition that one's doing it would save them, while one's not doing it would result in their death – there is some dispute about whether they are involuntary or voluntary. The same sort of thing happens also in the case of people throwing cargo overboard in storms at sea. Without qualification, no one jettisons cargo voluntarily; but for his own safety and that of others any sensible person will do it. Such actions, then, are mixed, though they seem more like voluntary ones, because at the time they are done they are worthy of choice, and the end of an action depends on the circumstances. So both voluntariness and involuntariness are to be ascribed at the time of the action.[7]

Despite claiming that these kinds of action are 'mixed' with regards to voluntariness, Aristotle himself eventually concludes that coerced actions should in fact be understood to be voluntary, in so far as the moving principle of the coerced agent's action lies in the agent herself.[8] Notice though that Aristotle here does not draw a moral distinction between coercion manufactured by an intentional agent (i.e. the

[6] A number of authors have raised this sort of counterexample to accounts of coercion discussed in the bioethics literature. See Wertheimer, 'Voluntary Consent'; Richards, *The Ethics of Transplants*; Pugh, 'Coercion and the Neurocorrective Offer'.

[7] Aristotle, *Nicomachean Ethics*, 1110a 4–12.

[8] Ibid., 11110b 5–7. Notably, in her discussion, Meyer suggests that Aristotle believes such acts are mixed with regards to voluntariness because they are voluntary with respect to the sense pertaining to ignorance, but involuntary with respect to the sense pertaining to choice. See Meyer, 'Aristotle on the Voluntary', 141–2. However, this interpretation seems to miss out on the nuance of Aristotle's discussion quoted above, since the mixed nature of voluntaries here makes no reference to understanding; instead, the belief that coerced acts could be voluntary is grounded by the claim that no one would perform the act in question without the qualifications provided by the context of the choice.

tyrant example) and coercion manufactured by forces of hazard (i.e. the cargo example). Similarly, one could adopt an Aristotelian approach and simply claim that both Alan and Bernie make voluntary decisions in the above example, in so far as the moving principle of action in both cases is in some sense 'internal' to the agent. However, such an interpretation would run contrary to the widely held view in bioethics that coercion does undermine the voluntariness of the victim's decision to comply.[9] As such, I suggest that we instead need an account of why this is so, which is compatible both with an authenticity-based understanding of autonomy, and the claim that neither deception nor manipulation need be intentional to undermine decisional autonomy.

The second question I shall consider in this chapter is whether offers as well as threats can be coercive. For some, this question might seem misguided—it has been claimed that offers are just categorically different from threats for reasons that I shall consider below. Moreover, the view that only threats can be coercive is commonly assumed in bioethics; it is endorsed by advocates of the standard view in their discussion of coercion,[10] and it is also enshrined in the Belmont Report, which states that 'coercion occurs when an overt threat of harm is intentionally presented by one person to another to obtain compliance'.[11] However, although this position has been highly influential we should be careful not to simply assume that it is true, particularly when invoking the concept of coercion in the context of contemporary bioethics. The reason that we should take particular care in this context is that coercion-related concerns are commonly raised not with respect to the use of explicit threats, but rather by the use of incentives.

To further illustrate this, consider the following three cases in which bioethicists have argued that offers can be coercive. To be clear, the charge of coercion is not the only moral criticism that has been raised in the debates surrounding the issues outlined below. However, this moral criticism is particularly significant. Given the salient value that we attribute to personal autonomy in contemporary bioethics, establishing that a practice amounts to controlling interference that invalidates consent is a particularly powerful moral criticism.

(i) Paying Research Subjects

In 2006, eight healthy subjects were offered £2000 to participate in a phase I trial of a novel monoclonal antibody agent, TGN1412. As part of the informed consent form, participants were told that they were free to leave the trial at any time without giving a reason. However, they were also told that if they chose to withdraw and exercise their right not to give a reason, or if they were required to leave the study for non-compliance, then they would forfeit their entitlement to payment.[12] Having

[9] Interestingly, drawing on some comments in Arthur Caplan's *Am I My Brother's Keeper?* Wertheimer notes (but does not endorse) the possibility that one could adopt the complete opposite view and claim that examples like Alan and Bernie above suggests that terminally ill patients cannot provide valid consent to treatment. Wertheimer, 'Voluntary Consent'.

[10] Beauchamp and Childress, *Principles of Biomedical Ethics*, 138. See also Nelson et al., 'The Concept of Voluntary Consent', 7.

[11] The Belmont Report.

[12] 'TGN1412 Trial Consent Form'.

previously tested the drug in animals, researchers gave six of the subjects in this first in-human trial 1/500th of the highest dose used in animal testing (the remaining subjects received a placebo). However, the six who received a dose of the drug quickly developed serious adverse reactions to the experimental agent, as result of a cytokine storm.[13]

Although regulatory reports on the trial suggested that it fulfilled all ethical requirements for clinical research (including the criteria of social value, scientific validity, favourable risk/benefit ration, informed consent, independent review, and respect for participants),[14] some bioethicists raised concerns about the quality of the participants' consent, with one commentator arguing that the language used in the consent process was 'very coercive'.[15] This sparked a number of commentaries on the trial discussing whether the payment offered for participation in the trial amounted to coercion.[16]

(ii) Reduced Sentences for Sexual Offenders Who Agree to Undergo Chemical Castration

Chemical castration refers to the use of an anti-libidinal agent to significantly reduce the recipient's sex drive. Although the anti-libidinal effects of the drugs that are typically used for this purpose are generally reversible, there are concerns about the long-term safety of chemical castration.[17] Despite both this and the scarcity of robust data about the effectiveness of chemical castration in preventing recidivism,[18] the procedure is sometimes performed on convicted sex offenders. Whilst chemical castration is compulsory for sex offenders in some jurisdictions, in others, sex offenders who would otherwise face a long prison sentence may be offered a significantly reduced sentence on the condition that they agree to undergo chemical castration.[19] Supporters of this 'offer' model argue that this benefits the offenders by giving them the chance to avoid a long prison sentence, whilst also respecting their autonomy by leaving the choice in the offender's hands. However, opponents have objected that the offer is inherently coercive. Here is a typical example:

The convicted rapist is faced with two options – a lengthy prison sentence or even death on the one hand and... castration on the other. Freedom of choice is impossible because the convict's

[13] Suntharalingam et al., 'Cytokine Storm in a Phase 1 Trial of the Anti-CD28 Monoclonal Antibody TGN1412'.

[14] For an overview of such principles, see World Medical Association Declaration of Helsinki.

[15] Evans, 'Parexel Misled Subjects Sickened in London Study, Ethicists Say'.

[16] Wertheimer and Miller, 'Payment for Research Participation'; Emanuel and Miller, 'Money and Distorted Ethical Judgments about Research'; Schonfeld et al., 'Money Matters'.

[17] Garcia and Thibaut, 'Current Concepts in the Pharmacotherapy of Paraphilias'.

[18] Thibaut et al., 'The World Federation of Societies of Biological Psychiatry (WFSBP) Guidelines for the Biological Treatment of Paraphilias'.

[19] Forsberg and Douglas, 'Anti-Libidinal Interventions in Sex Offenders'; Douglas et al., 'Coercion, Incarceration, and Chemical Castration'. For discussion of the neurocorrective offer and coercion, see Pugh, 'Coercion and the Neurocorrective Offer'.

loss of liberty constitutes a deprivation of such a magnitude that he cannot choose freely and voluntarily, but he is forced to give consent to an alternative he would not otherwise have chosen.[20]

(iii) *Markets for Organs*

In light of the global shortage of kidneys for transplantation, a number of bioethicists have suggested that we ought to permit a regulated market in which individuals are free to sell one of their kidneys.[21] Effectively, on such a model, individuals would be offered a sum of money in return for their kidney. A common objection to such a market is that it would coerce the poorest members of the global community into selling their kidney. Michael Jaycox captures this objection as follows:

> From the perspective of the poorest and most vulnerable persons in this world, the market of human organs is not something in which all persons choose to participate as equally free and self-determining individuals. For the poorest and most vulnerable members of the world community effectively have no or little choice but to participate in this market as vendors.[22]

In order to ascertain whether the charge of coercion may appropriately be raised in these three examples, we need to have a sound understanding of the nature of coercion, how it undermines voluntariness, and how offers differ from threats. In short, we need to provide an answer to the two questions that I have raised in this section; however, as I shall now explain, our responses to these questions are likely to be importantly interrelated, since the way in which one might distinguish threats from offers (in responding to the second question) might plausibly draw on considerations that are closely linked to one's understanding of how coercion undermines voluntariness.

With these framing remarks in mind, I shall proceed as follows. In the next section, I shall introduce a highly influential 'content-based' view of the distinction between threats and offers, and the normative and non-normative accounts of coercion that are grounded by this view. Having outlined problems facing normative accounts, I shall, in section 3 consider non-normative accounts in more detail. Although I shall suggest that these accounts get closer to the truth about coercion, I shall argue that they offer inadequate accounts of why coercion undermines voluntariness. The reason for this is that they do not adequately emphasize the importance of interpersonal voluntariness in this context. In section 4, I shall argue that the significance of this sense of voluntariness can be better captured if we adopt a structural rather than content-based understanding of the distinction between threats and offers. This understanding accommodates the possibility of some coercive offers. In the final section, I shall consider the practical implications of my approach for the cases delineated above.

[20] Green, 'Depo-Provera, Castration, and the Probation of Rape Offenders'. More recently, Wood has defended an account of coercion according to which an agent is coerced to do something when they have no acceptable alternative. Wood, 'Coercion, Manipulation, Exploitation'.

[21] Richards, *The Ethics of Transplants*; Taylor, *Stakes and Kidneys*; Wilkinson, *Bodies for Sale*.

[22] Jaycox, 'Coercion, Autonomy, and the Preferential Option for the Poor in the Ethics of Organ Transplantation'. See also Rippon, 'Imposing Options on People in Poverty'; Annas, 'Life, Liberty, and the Pursuit of Organ Sales'.

2. The Content-Based View of Threats: Normative and Non-Normative Accounts of Coercion

On one prominent approach to coercion, one that is endorsed by the standard account of autonomy in bioethics, it is claimed that coercion necessarily involves the use of threats. Of course, the appeal of this understanding of coercion depends in large part on our understanding of threats. Although I shall refine this terminology over the course of this section, we may say, at this stage roughly, that a proposal constitutes a threat if it announces a conditional intention to make the recipient worse off if she does not perform some action that the coercer wants her to perform.

The first thing to acknowledge with regards to the 'threat-based' understanding of coercion is that even if *only* threats can be coercive, clearly not *all* threats are. For instance, suppose the thief from my previous example had instead threatened to verbally insult Terry if he refused to hand over his wallet. It does not seem plausible to describe this as an instance of coercion. Accordingly, advocates of the threat-based understanding of coercion must offer an account of why some threats are coercive and some are not.

I shall not be concerned primarily with such conditions here; my interest in this section is rather to explore the way in which the threat-based understanding of coercion seeks to distinguish threats and offers, and the implications of this view for our understanding of the implications for voluntariness in each case. Nonetheless it will be useful to have a broad understanding of some commonly accepted necessary conditions of coercive threats for my discussion below. Broadly, we may say that in order for P's threat to have coerced Q into doing A, it must, *inter alia*, be the case that:

(1) Prior to the threat being made, Q believes he has a decisive reason to not A.
(2) Q has sufficient reason to believe that P's threat is credible.
(3) The fact that the non-performance of A will lead to the consequence that P threatens to bring about if Q does not A is the operative reason in Q's decision to A; the consequences render the non-performance of A for Q 'ineligible' for rational choice.[23]
And
(4) Q does A.

These conditions essentially state that for P's threat to be coercive, it must not only be successful in getting Q to A, it must also be the case that Q came to be motivated to do A because she believed P's threat, and wanted to avoid the consequences that P has credibly threatened to bring about.[24]

I do not mean to claim that these conditions are *sufficient* for a threat to be coercive; one might wish to add further conditions in order to distinguish coercive

[23] I have adopted the terminology of eligibility for rational choice from Feinberg's useful discussion. See Feinberg, *The Moral Limits of the Criminal Law*, 192. However, this terminology (and this condition generally) is compatible with the various accounts of coercion that I shall consider here.

[24] Feinberg, *The Moral Limits of the Criminal Law*, 198; Raz, *The Morality of Freedom*, 149; Nozick, 'Coercion'.

threats from warnings, for example.[25] Moreover, as I suggested above, the example of Alan and Bernie might be taken to suggest that we should incorporate a condition of intentionality here, according to which, the coercing party must intend to coerce their victim if their threat is to be truly coercive.[26] Nonetheless, such a condition has been contested, as I shall discuss. In the interests of brevity, and to focus my discussion, I shall simply accept the above four conditions as broadly accepted necessary conditions of coercive threats without further discussion.

With this in mind, why should we accept the claim that coercion necessarily involves the use of threats? Arguably, our intuitions may speak in favour of this view. In addition to the fact that paradigmatic cases of coercion (such as Terry above) pre-theoretically seem to involve threats, we also commonly get people to do things that they would otherwise not do by offering them inducements, and it seems clear that this does not usually involve coercion. If Terry had been offered a million pounds to hand over his wallet to an eccentric collector (rather than being threatened with death), it perhaps seems more plausible that he could have been autonomous with respect to his decision to hand over his wallet (assuming it contained far less than a million pounds).

However, one problem with relying on these sorts of intuitions to ground the threat-based understanding of autonomy is that it is not at all clear how we should philosophically distinguish threats and offers. As Scott Anderson points out in his introduction to the concept of coercion:

> ... offers may also be made with the same general intention as coercive threats: that is, to make some actions more attractive, others less so.[27]

Anderson goes on to point out that both threats and offers share the same basic structure; in both cases, the proposing agent, P, claims that she will bring about consequence C if and only if (*iff*) the proposed-to agent, Q, does some action A.[28] I shall suggest below that Anderson's structural analysis here is subtly incorrect. However, the claim that threats and offers are structurally similar has led both defenders and opponents of the threat-based understanding of coercion to adopt what I shall call a 'content-based' view of the difference between the two types of proposal.

The content-based view claims that threats can be distinguished from offers by appealing to the difference in the nature of the consequences that the proposer announces a conditional intention to bring about in each case. Advocating such a view in his seminal account of coercion, Robert Nozick claims that threats announce a conditional intention to bring about a consequence that would make the recipient *worse off* in comparison to the baseline of the 'normally expected course of events'.[29] Recall the original example of Terry. On this account, the thief's proposal amounts to a threat because it announces a conditional intention to bring about a consequence that would make Terry worse off than he might normally expect to be if he refrained from handing over his wallet to a stranger. In contrast, on this approach, offers announce a conditional intention to bring about a consequence that would make the

[25] Nozick, 'Coercion', 453–8. [26] Ibid. [27] Anderson, 'Coercion'. [28] Ibid.
[29] Nozick, 'Coercion', 447.

recipient *better off* in comparison to the baseline of the 'normally expected course of events'.

The ambiguity of the concept of 'the normally expected course of events' has led to two different accounts of coercion grounded by this way of distinguishing threats and offers, one non-normative, one normative. The ambiguity of the concept is attributable to the fact that there are different norms of expectability that might govern our understanding of the baseline 'normal expected course of events'.[30] More specifically, the 'normal' expected course of events can be understood in a merely descriptive sense, to refer to what one might reasonably expect to happen, given one's prior knowledge concerning descriptive facts about the world. However, it is also possible to understand the baseline in a normatively laden sense, to refer to how the world *ought* to be. To illustrate this point, consider the following example from Nozick's discussion:

> Suppose that usually a slave owner beats his slave each morning, for no reason connected with the slave's behaviour. Today he says to his slave, 'Tomorrow I will not beat you if and only if you now do A.[31]

In relation to a descriptive understanding of the normal course of events, the slave-owner's proposal qualifies as an offer, since the slave-owner proposes to make the slave better off than he could normally expect to be (given his previous experience of being a slave of this owner) if he performs the task that the slave-owner asks him to perform.

This raises something of a problem, because it seems highly plausible to claim that the slave is nonetheless coerced in this case. Accordingly, theorists who claim that *only* threats can be coercive must argue that it is possible to recast the slave-owner's proposal as a threat if they are to accommodate this intuition. One way in which it is possible to do this is to consider the proposal against a normative baseline that incorporates what the agent might *morally* expect:

> *Morally Expected Course of Events*: The baseline comparison course of events that incorporates what is minimally morally required of others in their actions towards the recipient in the pre-proposal situation.

In comparison to this normative baseline, the slave-owner's proposal can be understood as a threat, since the proposal does not make the slave better off in comparison to the course of events in which others meet their moral obligations towards the slave. After all, in this course of events, the agent would not be a slave who is beaten every day, but rather a free man.[32] Other normative accounts of coercion parse the normative baseline in terms of circumstances in which the individual's *rights* are respected, and in which others meet their obligations towards the individual.[33] Rights-based normative accounts also claim that we should *always* invoke a normative baseline when distinguishing coercive proposals from non-coercive proposals. In contrast, in his original theory, Nozick suggests that when the normative and

[30] Feinberg, *The Moral Limits of the Criminal Law*, 219–27. [31] Nozick, 'Coercion', 450.
[32] Ibid. [33] Wertheimer, *Coercion*, 217–21.

non-normative baselines diverge, it should be up to the agent which baseline should be invoked.[34]

This normative approach is also understood to provide a theoretical foundation for an account of why coercion undermines voluntariness. Due to the different content of threats and offers on this approach, Nozick suggests that a rational agent would be willing to move from their pre-proposal 'baseline' situation to the post-proposal choice situation. With respect to offers, they would be willing to do this because the nature of the consequence that the third party announces an intention to bring about is such that it would make the recipient better off than they would have been in comparison to the baseline of the normal expected course of events. The same cannot be said in the case of threats; after all, in the case of a threat, the recipient is in a position in which their rights will be violated if they fail to comply, or they will not be treated in the manner that morality demands.[35] Accordingly, the reason that coercive threats undermine voluntariness on this account is that they involve moving the recipient into a post-proposal choice situation unwillingly.

This normative account of coercion captures the Aristotelian insight that a coerced act is 'mixed' with regards to voluntariness. Even though the coerced agent may willingly comply with the coercer's demands, they have unwillingly been placed into the post-proposal choice situation. Nonetheless, there are significant problems with this understanding of coercion. Some of these problems pertain to the content-based view of the distinction between threats and offers that partly grounds the account. Naturally, these problems are also shared by other (non-normative) accounts of coercion that are also based on this distinction; I shall consider such accounts in the following sections. However, to conclude my discussion of normative accounts, I shall outline those problems that are uniquely faced by normative accounts of coercion.

First, if coercion only occurs when one agent proposes to violate another's rights, or if they fail to meet some other sort of moral obligation, it makes the definition of coercion, and more importantly its moral wrongness, parasitic on these prior moral wrongs.[36] Yet this is to divorce the moral wrongness of coercion from the implications that it has on the voluntariness of the target's choice. This is problematic because it seems that these implications are fundamental to our understanding of why coercion is wrong, particularly in a bioethical context. Indeed, the normative account of coercion seems to jar with our intuitions in this regard. For instance, consider the following case:

S is a justly imprisoned prisoner who would strongly prefer not to be imprisoned. The warden tells S that if he is caught attempting to escape, he will be liable to have his entertainment privileges withdrawn. Assume that S does not have any right to leave prison, and that prison authorities would not be violating S' rights if they withdrew certain entertainment privileges from him following an escape attempt. Suppose that these privileges are highly valuable for S in

[34] Nozick, 'Coercion', 451. Notably though, Nozick himself came to endorse a rights-based understanding of the normative baseline in later work .See Nozick, *Anarchy, State and Utopia*.

[35] Nozick, 'Coercion', 459–60.

[36] Zimmerman, 'Coercive Wage Offers', 123.

prison, and, because he believes that he cannot risk losing them, he decides not to try and escape.[37]

On the normative account, S's deciding not to escape because of the warden's threat of withdrawing these privileges would not qualify as coerced, and we would have no reason to claim that his decision to not try and escape here was non-voluntary. After all, the warden has not threatened to violate S's rights in any way. Yet this seems implausible; given that S takes himself to have very strong reasons to escape, but even stronger reasons to avoid the threatened consequence, it is not clear why the mere fact that the latter consequence would not violate S's rights should have any bearing on the effect of these threatened consequences on the voluntariness of S's choice.

More broadly, it is not clear that the normative account can make sense of morally legitimate instances of coercion that plausibly serve to undermine voluntariness, despite the fact that they are morally legitimate. In addition to the above example, we might also note the quite common example of parents legitimately shaping their children's behaviour through the use of coercive threats. It seems that we might want to say that parents can coerce their children (perhaps by telling them to eat their vegetables or they will not get dessert) without necessarily threatening to treat them in ways that violate their rights, or failing to treat them as morality demands.

Another reason that the normative account of threats and offers is jarring is that it is somewhat unnatural to describe the slave-owner's proposal in Nozick's case as a threat rather than an offer. In section 4, I shall provide a structural explanation of the proposal in question that explains why the normative interpretation is counter-intuitive. Of course, the point that the normative account of coercion can jar with our common understanding of threats and offers is not, by itself, a knock-down objection. Philosophers commonly invoke conceptions of everyday terms that do not map neatly on to our common usage of those terms. However, this point at least speaks against the normative account, particularly if there is an understanding of coercion that incorporates a construal of threats and offers that is congruous with the common understanding of these terms, and which can accommodate morally legitimate coercion that nonetheless undermines voluntariness.

3. Non-Normative Approaches, Coercive Offers, and Interpersonal Voluntariness

As I explained in the previous section, non-normative accounts of coercion can also be grounded by a content-based understanding of the distinction between threats and offers. Unlike normative theories, non-normative accounts appeal to a *descriptive* baseline of the normal expected course of events in drawing this distinction. This allows non-normative approaches to classify the slave-owner's proposal in Nozick's example as an offer, rather than a threat.

I believe that non-normative theories reach the right conclusion in this regard, although I shall argue that they do so for the wrong reasons. Notwithstanding this point though, presuming that a plausible theory of coercion ought to claim that the

[37] This is a modified version of an example given by Olsaretti, 'Freedom, Force and Choice', 59.

slave-owner's proposal is coercive, then plausible non-normative accounts must deny that only threats can be coercive. They must allow for the conceptual possibility of coercive offers. Accordingly, a key challenge that such accounts face is explicating which offers should qualify as coercive. In this section, I shall delineate what we might term the 'preference-based' view of coercive offers.[38]

Recall that on a non-normative approach, offers will announce a conditional intention to make the recipient better off than they would normally expect to be given descriptive facts about the world. According to the preference-based view, this feature of offers is significant because it means that recipients will typically prefer to receive offers. The reason for this is that they would strongly prefer to move from the normally expected course of events (in their pre-proposal situation) to the post-proposal situation (laid out in the terms of the offer).

However, an offer may nonetheless qualify as coercive on the preference-based view if two conditions are met. First, it must be the case that the recipient would *even more* strongly prefer to move from their actual pre-proposal situation to some alternative feasible pre-proposal situation. Second, the proposer must be *actively preventing* the recipient from being in this alternative feasible pre-proposal situation.[39] On this view, the slave-owner's offer is coercive because he can be understood as actively preventing the slave from being in a feasible alternative pre-proposal situation that he would strongly prefer to be in; namely one in which he is not a slave who receives daily beatings.

In the case of coercive offers, the preference-based view holds that an offer will be coercive if the offering party is frustrating the recipient's desire to be in some other feasible alternative pre-proposal situation. In turn, this feature of coercion is central to its prima facie moral wrongness on the preference-based view; coercion renders the victim unfree by frustrating their preference to be in some other pre-proposal situation. The preference view can further cash out the wrongness of frustrating an agent's desire in this way in both broadly utilitarian and broadly Kantian terms. On the utilitarian approach, rendering another unfree in this manner is wrong because desire frustration per se is prima facie wrong, whilst on the Kantian approach, frustrating another's desires is wrong because it fails to acknowledge the victim's full status as a rational being.[40]

I shall return to the utilitarian and Kantian approaches to the wrongness of coercion on the non-normative preference-based account below. Prior to doing so though, we may notice that both the normative account of coercion and the non-normative preference-based account answer the first question outlined at the beginning of this chapter in broadly the same way. They both endorse the general picture that coercion undermines voluntariness because coercive proposals serve to frustrate a certain set of the victims' preferences (namely, to be in a different set of

[38] Zimmerman, 'Coercive Wage Offers'. Notice that Zimmerman's use of the term 'preferences' differs from Ekstom's understanding (which I have been invoking), since Zimmerman does not claim that preferences presuppose the existence of higher order mental states in the way that Ekstrom does.

[39] Zimmerman, 'Coercive Wage Offers', 132. [40] Ibid., 129.

circumstances).[41] They simply disagree on their understanding of how we ought to define and correspondingly distinguish threats and offers.

There are three reasons for thinking that the non-normative approach is at least more plausible than the normative approach. First, on the former approach, the wrongness of coercion is not parasitic on other normative violations. Second, it is more compatible with our intuitions regarding the effect of morally legitimate threats on voluntariness; the prisoner's decision not to escape in the example in the previous section qualifies as having been coerced, even if the warden is not threatening to violate his rights in any way. Third, the non-normative account classifies the slave-owner's proposal in Nozick's case as an offer rather than a threat in a manner that corresponds with natural use of the term 'offer'.

However, I believe that that we ought to reject both the normative and non-normative approaches that I have so far outlined, due to their reliance on the content-based approach to the distinction between threats and offers. Their reliance on this view leads them to obscure a feature of coercion that is indispensable to an adequate understanding of its implications for voluntariness, namely the significance of intention.

To see why, recall the examples of Alan and Bernie from section 1. I suggested that it is plausible to claim that Alan can consent to treatment but that Bernie has been coerced in a manner that undermines the voluntariness of his decision. If this intuition is correct, it cannot simply be the case that coercion undermines voluntariness *just* because it frustrates a preference, or because it involves the recipient moving unwillingly from one choice circumstance to another less preferable one. The reason for this is that this occurs in *both* Alan and Bernie's cases.

It might be argued that I am being slightly uncharitable in suggesting that these cases raise problems for the normative and non-normative preference-based approaches to coercion. After all, at least some advocates from both camps explicitly stress that coercion is an interpersonal, intentional phenomenon.[42] Zimmerman, in particular stresses this by stipulating a prevention condition in his account of coercive offers. Recall that an offer will only qualify as coercive on his account if the proposer is *actively* preventing the recipient from being in a pre-proposal situation that they would strongly prefer to be in.

Whilst this is true, by cashing out the wrongness of coercion by appealing to the fact that it involves the frustration of preferences, these accounts obscure the role that intentional agency plays in the wrongness of coercion. This failure is clearest in the utilitarian approach to cashing out the wrongness of the frustration of preferences that coercion involves. According to the utilitarian interpretation, coercion is wrong because the frustration of desires per se is prima facie wrong. Yet, even if this is true,

[41] Zimmerman phrases the moral wrongness of coercion in terms of its effects on freedom rather than voluntariness. However, since Nozick (and others) believe that the effects of coercion on freedom have implications for voluntariness, and in so far as it seems plausible to claim that a desideratum of a theory of coercion is that it is able to capture the thought that coercion undermines voluntariness, I shall interpret Zimmerman's claims about the effects of coercion on freedom to have implications for our understanding of its implications for voluntariness.

[42] Nozick, *Anarchy, State and Utopia*, 272.

it is not clear why the fact that *the coercer*, rather than forces of hazard, is frustrating the individual's preferences is material to the wrongness of coercion on this approach. The problem with the utilitarian approach then is that it cannot account for the materiality of having one's desires frustrated by another agent to the way in which coercion undermines voluntariness.

In so far as intentional agency is a prerequisite of expressing an attitude of disrespect, the Kantian approach can claim that forces of hazard do not disrespect an individual's rational agency when they diminish her freedom. In this sense the Kantian interpretation is on stronger ground than the utilitarian approach to understanding the wrongness of coercion. I shall argue that the Kantian approach fails for other reasons that I shall detail in the next section. Here though, we need only acknowledge the point that the failure of the utilitarian approach in this regard suggests that in explicating the implications of coercion for decisional autonomy, we should focus less on the frustration of preferences it involves, and instead on its interpersonal features. That is, in order to adequately capture the effect of coercion on voluntariness in a way that is congruous with our intuitions in the Alan and Bernie cases, we have to focus not so much on the fact that the victim's preferences are frustrated, but rather on the fact that they are frustrated *by another agent*.

This echoes my discussion of the interpersonal sense of voluntariness that I highlighted at the end of the previous chapter. Coercion does not undermine voluntariness just because it frustrates the victim's preference; rather it does so because it subjugates the victim's will to the coercer's, violating the victim's freedom from domination.

However, the appeal to freedom from domination in the context of coercion raises a different problem, at least in view of the arguments I made in the previous chapter. There, I suggested that forces of hazard *can* manipulate or deceive an agent in ways that undermine their decisional autonomy. The question then is why intentional third-party influence should matter so much more in the case of coercion than it does in the case of manipulation—is there any relevant sense in which manipulation differs from coercion with respect to its implications for decisional autonomy?[43]

Gideon Yaffe has offered one account that denies this sort of difference, but which purports to explain why intentional third-party influence in particular might matter for freedom. Yaffe argues that intentional influence can undermine freedom in a way that forces of hazard do not, because those who exert intentional influence will track the compliance of their victims.[44] If an initial threat fails, an intentional coercer is likely to increase the severity of their threats until their victim agrees to comply. This matters for Yaffe, because tracking compliance in this manner involves a greater restriction of the target's freedom, and forces of hazard will not typically track compliance in this way.[45]

[43] Those who are sceptical of a plausible answer to this question have used this as motivation for accounts of autonomy that claim that only intentional interpersonal interference can undermine autonomy. Bublitz and Merkel, 'Autonomy and Authenticity of Enhanced Personality Traits'.

[44] Yaffe, 'Indoctrination, Coercion and Freedom of Will', 355–6.

[45] Yaffe acknowledges that there could be cases in which forces of hazard could track compliance, and that his conclusions would apply to such cases. Ibid., 354.

I believe that Yaffe is correct to highlight this feature to show how some forms of interpersonal influence infringe upon the victim's freedom in a manner that forces of hazard will typically not. However, I do not believe that this feature of interpersonal influence is *necessary* for undermining decisional autonomy. To see why, suppose the coercer in Bernie's case issued her initial threat, but privately resolved not to threaten anything worse if Bernie failed to comply with the issued threat. On Yaffe's analysis, the sort of coercion involved in this permutation of the case would be functionally equivalent to the restriction of choice by forces of hazard in Alan's case.[46] In contrast, it seems plausible to claim that Bernie may not be autonomous with respect to his decision, even if his coercer would hypothetically not track compliance in the way that Yaffe describes. To claim otherwise would be to adopt a highly revisionist understanding of the relationship between coercion and autonomy in bioethics.

However, discussion of Yaffe's position points towards a solution to the puzzle at hand. What actually seems to be important about a coercer's tracking compliance is that they are reducing another agent's freedom with the intention of affecting their victim's practical decision-making in a manner that will serve the coercer's *own purposes*. In contrast, when our freedoms are reduced by hazard, there is no rhyme or reason to it; as such, even though we might say that an agent's freedom can be diminished by hazard, it does not involve a *subjugation* of the coerced agent's will.

But why should this matter so much in the case of coercion? To begin to explain why, it is useful to compare how coercion and intentional manipulation violate the victim's freedom from domination. Compare the case of Terry with Simon. Suppose that prior to the thief's intervention, both Terry and Simon would harbour the following evaluative ranking of their available conjunctive options:

Best = Option A: (Don't hand over wallet) + (My money is safe).
Worst = Option B: (Hand over wallet) + (My money is stolen).

Psychological manipulaters might succeed in getting Simon to hand over his wallet by causing him to change his evaluative ranking of the available options (so that he now prefers option B to option A) without rationally engaging with his evaluative beliefs.[47] Let us suppose that this new preference ranking does not cohere with Simon's other core preferences and acceptances, those that led him to develop the initial preference ranking outlined above. Simon, nonetheless unreflectively acts on the manipulated preference, despite its conflict with his other preferences and acceptances; the preference is not responsive to his beliefs about the good.

My arguments in the previous chapter suggest that the violation of Simon's freedom from domination here is contingent on the fact that Simon lacks reflective autonomy with respect to this manipulated preference. Imagine now another thief targets someone with a different character system, Rupert. Rupert is somewhat repelled by his own wealth, and thinks that his life would be easier if he gave his money away; he acquired his wealth through complicity with things that he took to be immoral, and it deeply conflicts with his overall self-conception, and his positive

[46] Ibid., 354.
[47] Yaffe notes that indoctrination can evince a new pattern of taking facts to be reasons for acting in particular ways amongst its victims. Ibid., 342.

evaluation of helping others. Although he does not know what to do with his money, when faced with a would-be thief, he does not feel inclined to hand over his wallet.

Suppose that Rupert is similarly manipulated through hypnosis into changing his motivating desire. Unlike Simon though, Rupert comes to reflect on his changed motivation following his hypnosis, and comes to rationally endorse this ranking as being coherent with other core preferences and acceptances that have been in conflict with his initial preference not to hand over his wallet (for example, his belief that his money is morally tainted, that the thief is desperate, and his preference to help those in need). In Rupert's case, the account I have outlined in the previous chapters suggests that this psychological intervention does not violate Rupert's reflective autonomy; despite its causal history, his motivating desire is sensitive to his other pre-existing preferences and acceptances, in particular, his beliefs about the good. In view of my arguments in the previous chapter, this manipulation also does not violate his freedom from domination, insofar as it is Rupert *himself* who comes to rationally assimilate this manipulated preference into his own coherent self-conception.

In contrast to the cases of Simon and Rupert, when the thief *threatens* rather than manipulates Terry, his initial preference ranking is left intact; he still prefers option A to option B. However, the thief's coercive threat serves to take away option A from Terry's available choice set, and replaces it with option C which, for Terry, is less good than B:

Option C: (Don't hand over wallet) + (My money is safe) + (I am killed).

This analysis elucidates the following point. As Simon and Rupert's cases suggest, when manipulation *does* violate freedom from domination (i.e. in Simon's case), it does so by virtue of the fact that the third-party intervention undermines the reflective autonomy of another. When attempted manipulation fails to undermine reflective autonomy (i.e. in Rupert's case) it fails to amount to domination of the target's will. The third-party influence is immaterial to the individual's sustaining the desire following rational evaluation. Although the intervention caused Rupert to initially form the desire to hand over his wallet, it was Rupert himself who decided to rationally sustain the desire in the light of his other preferences and acceptances. In so far as Rupert sustained the desire on the basis of this sort of reflection, he can aptly be construed as the driving force underlying his decision to hand over his wallet to the thief; in hypnotizing Rupert to have this desire, the thief merely planted a seed in fertile ground.[48]

In contrast to manipulation, in coercion, the coercer must *rely* on their victim retaining their reflective autonomy if they are to dominate their victim's will. The control exerted in coercion does not function by undermining the victim's reflective autonomy; rather, it functions by influencing the practical parameters within which

[48] Such an interpretation does not commit me to claiming that the thief's intervention was therefore morally neutral. Even if it does not undermine Rupert's autonomy, we may still plausibly claim that the thief's intervention violated his right to mental integrity for example. For discussion, see Bublitz and Merkel, 'Crimes Against Minds'. See also McKenna, 'Responsibility and Globally Manipulated Agents'.

the victim's reflective autonomy will operate.[49] The coercer influences their victim to act in a certain way by taking away their most preferred conjunctive option from their choice set (option A above), and replacing it with an option (C) that is less preferable than the option that reflects the coercer's will (B). Accordingly, although coercion does not undermine reflective autonomy, it may still plausibly be understood to amount to a domination of its victim by virtue of this interference with the agent's practical freedoms, and the imposition on the agent's choice domain connoted by that interference.

This analysis is also compatible with the Aristotelian claim that coercion is 'mixed' with regards to voluntariness, without denying that we can draw a morally significant distinction between the cases of Alan and Bernie above (or Aristotle's own examples of the cargo and the tyrant). The reason that we believe that coercion is 'mixed' is that, on the one hand, we must concede that coerced agents would reflectively endorse their compliant motives; in fact, in order to formulate an effective threat of the sort that coercion requires, the coercing party must make an accurate assessment of the kinds of preferences and values that are central to their victim's character system. In this sense then, we can understand the victim as voluntarily performing the act, the non-performance of which would lead to consequences that he has strongly decisive reasons to avoid.

On the other hand though, in so far as it is a third party that is responsible for changing the parameters of the individual's choice situation in a manner that serves to further the coercer's own ends, coercion involves a subjugation of the victim's will, and violates his freedom from domination. Whilst this freedom pertains to a different sense of voluntariness from the sense related to reflective autonomy, it is nonetheless central to our assessment of ourselves as autonomous agents. Whilst in manipulation, the agent's reflective autonomy and their freedom from domination stand and fall together, in coercion they can be mixed in the way that Aristotle describes in his examples, and that I have explicated above.

I shall further support this point in the following section by offering a revised account of the distinction between threats and offers. To conclude this discussion though, one might object that my claims here contradict my assessment of the implications of global manipulation for autonomy in the previous chapter. Recall that I previously claimed that global manipulation does not undermine autonomy, but rather amounts to the creation of a psychologically 'new' person. I suggested that this new person could still be autonomous, despite the fact that her 'creation' was the result of another's agency. This might seem to be in tension with what I am claiming here, namely that the victim of coercion may lack decisional autonomy even though she meets the conditions of practical and theoretical rationality discussed in Chapter 2.

The key to reconciling these two contrasting claims about global manipulation and coercion is recognizing that in coercion, the central elements of the agent's character system are retained. We can sensibly say that the 'will' that is subjugated in coercion

49 In a similar vein, Yaffe suggests that coercion involves the manipulation of what reasons its victim has. Yaffe, 'Indoctrination, Coercion and Freedom of Will', 340.

existed both prior to the threat and following it. In contrast, in global manipulation, the will that exists following manipulation is, *ex hypothesi*, distinct from the will that existed prior to it. Global manipulation thus does not subjugate an extant will in a manner that undermines the autonomy of the agent following the intervention; rather it involves replacing the extant will with another of the manipulator's own design. This is an egregious harm; but it is, I suggest, a harm concerning identity, rather than autonomy. Coercion, in contrast, is a harm concerning autonomy that relies on the maintenance of the elements of identity that global manipulation destroys.

4. A Structural Account and Coercive Offers Revisited

In order to adequately understand why coercion undermines autonomy on my approach, we cannot merely appeal to the fact that coercion frustrates a certain kind of preference; we must also stress the fact that coercion violates the victim's freedom from domination. I shall now argue that we can better capture this aspect of coercion by abandoning the content-based view of the distinction between threats and offers, which is adopted by both the normative and non-normative accounts analysed above, instead adopting a structural account of the distinction between threats and offers. As well as capturing the moral significance of freedom from domination and interpersonal voluntariness, such an account is better placed to respond to Joel Feinberg's famous lecherous millionaire coercive offer example (outlined below), and the putative examples of coercive offers in bioethics that I delineated in section 1.

As I mentioned above, one reason that theorists have been attracted to the content-based view of the distinction between threats and offers is that these proposals seem to share the same sort of structure. Broadly, it might be claimed that it is true of both threats and offers that the proposing agent, P, claims that *she* will bring about consequences C if and only if the proposed-to agent, Q, does some action A.[50] If it were the case that offers and threats both had this precise structure, then it seems that the only way in which we could distinguish the proposals would be to appeal to the content of C, in the ways discussed above.

However, contrary to initial appearances, this analysis of the shared structure of threats and offers overlooks an important structural difference between the two types of proposal. In the case of offers, the proposer will bring about a certain consequence C that otherwise would not have occurred if and only if (*iff*) the proposed-to party *complies* with the proposer's demand to do A. In the case of offers, C is normally something that the proposer believes will make the recipient of the proposal better off; however, this is not a necessary feature, as the content-based view implies.[51] In contrast, in the case of threats, the proposer will bring about a certain consequence C that would not have otherwise occurred *iff* the proposed-to party *refuses* to comply with the proposer's demands to do A. Again, we might note that in the case of

[50] Anderson, 'Coercion'.

[51] For examples illustrating this point, see Sachs, 'Why Coercion Is Wrong When It's Wrong'.

threats, C is normally something that the proposer believes will make the recipient worse off, although this is not a necessary feature on the account that I am outlining here.

Accordingly, contrary to Anderson's analysis, there is a structural difference that we can appeal to in order to distinguish threats and offers. On this structural approach, the slave-owner's proposal in Nozick's example qualifies as an offer. As I illustrated above, non-normative approaches that endorse the content-based view of the distinction between threats and offers get the correct result here. However, they do so for the wrong reasons; the proposal is not an offer just because C is a 'good' consequence for the slave. Rather, the reason that the proposal is most appropriately understood as an offer is by virtue of the structural feature that the slave-owner will refrain from beating the slave *iff* the slave *complies* with his owner's demand to do A.

Compare this to a case in which the slave-owner will bring about a very *bad* consequence *iff* the slave complies with his demand to do A, say an even *worse* beating than usual. Such a proposal would be quite bizarre, and would be highly unlikely to be successful in motivating the slave to do A. Regardless of the bizarre nature of the proposal though, the badness of the consequence does not render the proposal a threat, as the content-based view would imply. Rather, such a proposal would most plausibly be understood to constitute a very unattractive offer, by virtue of its structural features.[52] By appealing to the nature of the consequences that the proposer announces a conditional intention to bring about in each case, the content-based account is focusing on something that is only *contingently* true of *most* threats and offers.

This structural understanding of threats and offers serves to elucidate the salience of interpersonal interference to the way in which coercion undermines voluntariness, as I began to describe at the end of the previous section. When P makes a threat, they make it the case that Q can no longer act in a way that is entirely independent of P's interference. Recall the options available to Terry (the original thief target), as I described them above, options B and C.

Option B: (Hand over wallet) + (My money is stolen).
Option C: (Don't hand over wallet) + (My money is safe) + (I am killed).

Notice that regardless of which option Terry chooses, the thief's influence will be apparent, either because Terry will suffer the consequences that the thief will bring about if he refuses to comply (in option C), or because he will comply with the thief's demands (in option B).

Contrast this with the case of an offer. On the structural account, an offer announces a conditional intention to bring about a certain consequence C if and only if Q *complies* with P's demands. In the case of an offer then, P's influence does not infect every option available to Q; P has only influenced Q's choice set by adding a further option of Q's performing some act for an inducement (i.e. consequence C). However, unlike the case of a threat, there will be no consequences for Q if she refuses

[52] Sachs calls such a proposal a 'ridiculously bad offer'.

to comply with the demand. As such, Q's pre-proposal status quo option remains intact in the post-proposal situation; in contrast, in the case of a threat, P's proposal takes away Q's freedom to maintain her pre-proposal status quo situation without further consequence.

Accordingly, we may say that in issuing an offer, the offering party influences the recipient's choice domain, but that this influence does not amount to the exertion of controlling influence. The reason for this is that offers leave open an option that is free from P's influence, namely Q's pre-proposal status quo option. If Q chooses to accept the offer, it is because she believes that compliance with what is demanded by the offering party in return for certain consequences is better than her extant circumstances, over which P will typically not exert influence.

However, the situation is different in the case of a threat. In issuing a threat, the threatening party exerts their influence through the terms of their proposal over *all* of their recipient's available options, in order to further their own ends. If Q refuses, P will intrude upon Q's sphere of autonomy by bringing about some consequence C that would otherwise not have occurred, and that P will typically not want to obtain (at least in most cases). If Q chooses to comply, it is only on the basis that acting in accordance with P's demands is better than this alternative way in which P would otherwise intrude into the sphere of Q's autonomy.

Whilst both successful offers and threats involve a third party creating the reason that is operative in the recipient's post-proposal decision about how to act, it is only in the case of a threat that the creation of this operative reason requires an intrusion into all of the recipient's available options in that context, robbing the recipient of the freedom to maintain their status quo situation. In so far as this is true, the terms of a threat involve the directed domination of one party's choice domain in the interests of another, in a way that offers do not.

To conclude this part of the discussion, recall that proponents of the content-based view explicate the moral wrongness of coercion and its effects on voluntariness by appealing to the fact that coercion involves a certain kind of preference frustration; furthermore, they note that individuals are willing to receive (non-coercive) offers, and that this represents the key difference between threats and offers with respect to voluntariness. The above discussion of the structural account illuminates the fact that there are in fact *two* dimensions underlying the rational agent's unwillingness to receive a coercive threat. On the one hand, such threats tend to (but need not) announce a conditional intention to bring about bad consequences. This is what the content-based view emphasizes. However, coercive threats also involve the frustration of a different kind of preference, one that is grounded by a desire to be free from domination. The reason for this is that threats involve the exertion of third-party influence over every available option in the recipient's choice set in a particular context. By emphasizing this supplementary feature of threats, the structural account makes salient the interpersonal aspect of coercion's moral wrongness.

Similarly, there is often a dual basis for why rational agents would be willing to receive offers. First, offers tend to (but need not) announce a conditional intention to bring about a consequence that would be good for the recipient if she complies with the demand. However, the recipient might also be willing to receive an offer insofar as it is often (though not always) advantageous to have more options available to one.[53]

This structural account of the distinction of threats and offers has important implications for our understanding of coercive offers. To see why, consider first the following example:

> *Lecherous millionaire*: *B* is in an otherwise hopeless condition from which *A* can rescue her if she gives him what he wants. He will pay for the expensive surgery that alone can save her child's life provided that she becomes for a period his mistress.[54]

On all of the accounts that I have surveyed in the first sections of this chapter, the proposal in this example uncontroversially qualifies as an offer. The key area of contention is whether we should understand it to constitute a *coercive* offer that undermines voluntariness. On the preference-based non-normative account, the question turns on whether we can construe the millionaire as preventing the woman from being in a feasible alternative pre-proposal situation. It might it be claimed that the millionaire is preventing the woman from being in this situation by omission. Yet, Zimmerman rules out this interpretation: he claims that an offer is only genuinely coercive if the offering party *actively* prevents the recipient from being in their preferred feasible alternative pre-proposal situation.[55] Merely omitting to provide Q with the means to be in an alternative preferable situation is not sufficient for genuine coercion. As such, the non-normative account denies that the lecherous millionaire's proposal is a coercive offer.

Joel Feinberg, who originally posed the example, claims that the offer *is* coercive. In contrast to the preference-based approach, Feinberg endorses what he terms a 'compatibilist approach', according to which offers can be coercive even if they *enhance* freedom overall. On the compatibilist approach, an offer is coercive if it meets three conditions. First, the offer must have been made with coercive *intent*; that is, the offering party P must have made the offer with the intention of getting the recipient Q to do what P wants her to do. Second, the offer must have a coercive *effect*; that is, the offer must succeed in getting Q to do what P wanted her to do.[56] Feinberg goes on to suggest that in order for an offer to be coercive in effect it must impose a sufficient degree of 'differential coercive pressure', where differential coercive pressure is understood to refer to 'the gap between the value tag of what is offered and the price tag of what is required';[57] the greater the gap, the more coercive the proposal.[58] Finally, in addition to imposing a sufficient degree of differential coercive pressure, in order to qualify as a coercive offer, the proposal in question

[53] This is not to say that this is *always* advantageous; see Dworkin, *The Theory and Practice of Autonomy*, ch. 6, and my discussion in Chapter 5.

[54] Feinberg, *The Moral Limits of the Criminal Law*, 229.

[55] Zimmerman, 'Coercive Wage Offers', 132.

[56] Feinberg, *The Moral Limits of the Criminal Law*, 233–5.

[57] Ibid., 234.

[58] Feinberg lists a number of other measurements of coercive pressure and their effects on voluntariness, including what he calls 'coercive force', 'total coercive burden', 'the coercive minimum'. However, in discussing coercive offers, he suggests that if our ultimate concern is to decide whether a recipient's consent was valid, the relevant measure is differential coercive pressure. Ibid., 254.

must offer a 'prospect that is not simply much preferred, but one which is an exclusive alternative to an intolerable evil'.[59]

The compatibilist approach adopts the broadly Aristotelian position, which claims that forces of hazard can exert coercive pressure just as intentional agents can; on the compatibilist approach, the woman in the lecherous millionaire case is understood to have essentially been coerced by her circumstances. I rejected this Aristotelian view of coercion above following my discussion of the examples of Alan and Bernie; it is highly revisionist to claim that non-agential forces can coerce in a way that invalidates consent in bioethics. Feinberg too seems to recognize this, and goes on to amend the compatibilist position in a manner that seems to bring it broadly into line with the preference-based view. He goes on to claim that on the compatibilist view, not all coercive offers undermine voluntariness to the extent of invalidating the recipient's consent: rather they will tend to do so if P's coercive offer is made after P has already *created Q's circumstances of vulnerability*. However, P's coercive offer frequently will not invalidate Q's consent when he was not responsible for creating those circumstances.[60]

The preference-based view and the amended compatibilist view are thus in broad agreement about a crucial necessary condition of what it is for an offer to be coercive in a manner that invalidates consent; the preference-based view's active prevention condition and the amended compatibilist's condition about the creation of the victim's circumstances of vulnerability seem to identify a very similar feature of coercive offers. The main difference between the two is that the compatibilist view holds that some offers can be coercive without diminishing voluntariness to the extent that is sufficient to invalidate consent.

In their defence of these accounts, Zimmerman and Feinberg both say little to defend their respective conditions, instead relying on their intuitive appeal. Yet, as I mentioned in the previous section, it is difficult to see how the utilitarian approach to cashing out the wrongness of coercion on the preference view can accommodate the significance of this. I am now also in a position to further explicate the problems with the Kantian approach. Recall that the Kantian approach claims that the wrongness of the way in which coercion frustrates the victim's desires lies in the fact that it fails to acknowledge the victim's full status as a rational being. The problem is that even if this claim is plausible, it does not explain why an offer will only *invalidate consent* if the offering party is actively preventing the recipient from being in their preferred feasible situation. The reason that this is problematic is that offers can plausibly fail to acknowledge the victim's status as a rational being without meeting the aforementioned necessary condition of coercive offers that invalidate consent. Indeed, the lecherous millionaire's proposal is a striking example of this. The proposal plausibly fails to acknowledge the recipient's full status as a rational being; however, as both the preference view and the amended compatibilist view hold, we may plausibly deny that the lecherous millionaire's offer invalidates the recipient's consent. The Kantian approach to understanding the wrongness of coercion on the preference view fails because it leaves us with the question of why

[59] Ibid., 234. [60] Ibid., 244.

offers that fail to acknowledge the recipient's full moral status only invalidate consent in some cases but not others.

In contrast, the new structural account of the distinction between offers and threats, and my discussion of freedom from domination, can help to elucidate the importance of the conditions that the preference view and the compatibilist view each adopt to accommodate valid consent in cases like the lecherous millionaire. To phrase this using the terminology of the compatibilist approach, when the offering party creates the recipient's circumstance of vulnerability, their proposal is similar to a coercive threat, insofar as the proposing party can then be said to have exerted influence over all of the options in the recipient's choice set in this context. In the case of normal non-coercive offers, I suggested that P's influence need not infect every option available to Q, since Q can simply choose to maintain her pre-proposal status quo situation, free from Q's influence, and without further consequence. This is not possible in the case of a threat. Moreover, it is also not possible in cases in which P makes an offer to Q having *already* placed Q into circumstances of vulnerability. In such a case, although the recipient may choose to remain in her pre-proposal status quo situation following the offer, this situation is one in which her will is *already* subjugated to her coercer's, by virtue of the fact that the coercer has created her current vulnerable circumstances. This is the situation in which the slave finds himself in Nozick's example.

One might object to the account that I have outlined here by suggesting that it gets the wrong conclusion in the lecherous millionaire case; contrary to the analysis that I have offered here, perhaps it might be claimed that the voluntariness of the victim in the lecherous millionaire case has been diminished in a manner that is sufficient to invalidate her consent. In support of this alternative interpretation, we might note that we would be reluctant to enforce a contract based on this kind of exploitative offer.

In response, the first thing to note is that there can be reasons for not enforcing a contract that have nothing to do with voluntariness of an individual's decision to accept its terms. My claim that the victim in the lecherous millionaire case provides valid consent thus does not commit me to the claim that we ought to enforce the terms of the contract. Morality might require that the millionaire simply saves the child without making any other demands. The woman might also claim that the contract is unduly exploitative. Yet this concerns a different set of issues about fairness that are distinct to those concerning whether the woman can autonomously agree to the terms of the millionaire's offer at the time that it was made.

More broadly, I am prepared to bite the bullet in maintaining this interpretation of Feinberg's example because of the importance of allowing for the possibility that people can make voluntary decisions in very poor circumstances. Indeed, to claim otherwise is to raise a grave threat to the autonomy of vulnerable individuals. Consider this permutation of the lecherous millionaire case: Suppose the woman is about to agree to the millionaire's offer in return for saving the life of her child. Suppose that we intervened and stopped this contract from being signed, citing the woman's lack of voluntariness. We surely could not congratulate ourselves for safeguarding the woman's autonomy as she now watches her child perish. The lesson here is that we should allow for the possibility that people can make autonomous decisions in desperate circumstances, and that our moral obligation in such cases is to alleviate these circumstances of vulnerability. If we fail in that obligation, this does not mean that we have the right to prevent the vulnerable individual from exercising a right to determine how to manage the terrible situation she finds herself in, and which we have failed to alleviate.

I suggest that we are now in a position to answer the questions delineated at the beginning of this chapter as follows: First, whilst acknowledging Aristotle's observation that coercion is mixed with regards to voluntariness, we can understand it to undermine decisional autonomy by virtue of the fact that the coercing party dominates their victim's will. The coerced agent may thus be understood to choose voluntarily in the sense that they retain reflective autonomy with respect to their choice, but they lack the sort of interpersonal voluntariness that is connoted by retaining freedom from domination. Second, on an adequate, structural understanding of the distinction between threats and offers, both kinds of proposal can be coercive. We should reject the claim that coercion necessarily involves the use of threats. Although offers typically enhance the recipient's freedom, some offers can be coercive if the offering party is actively preventing the recipient from being in a preferable alternative pre-proposal situation, or by creating their circumstances of vulnerability; this interference with the recipient's circumstances is necessary to ensure that the offer serves to dominate the recipient's will, even if it can be understood to enhance their freedoms in their post-interference circumstances. This conclusion echoes the conclusions of both the preference view and the compatibilist view; however, I have provided a new explanation of why this is the right conclusion to draw, that links our understanding of threats and offers to an account of the relationship between coercion and voluntariness that is absent in the preference and compatibilist views. In the final section, I shall explain how this theoretical analysis can help us in practical discussions of apparently coercive offers, with reference to the cases delineated in section 1.

5. Practical Applications

The first thing that should be clear from my above analysis is that the quoted justifications for claiming that the offers outlined in section 1 are coercive are unconvincing. Offers are not coercive just because they are made against the background of a substantial loss of freedom; to claim otherwise would jeopardize the possibility of informed consent in various medical contexts. However, there are a number of things we can learn from considering the practical application of theoretical accounts of coercion and autonomy.

First, the terminology of coercion in practical debates does not always follow the philosophical use, or map on to the kind of wrong that the philosophical use aims to capture. Consider for instance the case of the TGN1412 trial. On the philosophical analysis I have provided, the proposal to withhold the incentive of payment following withdrawal from the study can be understood as the negative expression of an offer. The initial offer amounted to a proposal to provide payment (which would otherwise not have been provided) *iff* the proposed-to party *complies* with the proposer's demand to fully participate in the study. Proposing to withhold the incentive if the proposed-to party does not comply is to restate the proposal in negative terms. Having established that the proposal in question is an offer, one can then ask whether it is coercive. On the account I have explored above, for this to be so, the body running the study would have had to have been responsible for ensuring that the participants were in a circumstance of vulnerability prior to the offer being made.

Some of the ethicists who made the claim that the participants of the trial were coerced focused on the large amount of money that had been offered to participants.[61] As my discussion of the nature of offers above should make clear, the problem with claiming that it is coercive to offer individuals large amounts of money in return for some service is that we often offer people inducements to perform tasks, and the recipients of these offers can clearly consent to these transactions. Indeed, in some cases, it may be irrational for them not to; I might plausibly be described as irrational if I refused the offer of £1million to give a lecture, say.[62] Naturally, the amount of money offered is relevant to our understanding of whether an offer is going to be sufficiently attractive to succeed in changing the recipient's beliefs about what they have most reason to do. However, such an offer can only be said to amount to a domination of the will of the sort that coercion entails if it is considered as part of a larger scheme in which the offering party has already placed the recipient in a circumstance of vulnerability.[63]

A plausible explanation of why ethicists might be concerned with the amount of money offered in these cases is that they are concerned about a different moral phenomenon. It might be suggested that being offered a large amount of money may lead the recipients of the offer to fail to adequately attend to other material information about the trial (such as the degree of risk to which they will be exposed); on this understanding, the offered amount may have overwhelmed the recipients into accepting the offer, no matter the cost.[64] Whether or not this was the case in the TGN1412 case is an empirical matter that I cannot address here. However, the point that I want to make is that this sort of interference with autonomous decision-making bears more resemblance to informational manipulation than the coercive interventions with which I have been concerned in this chapter. On this understanding, the offer serves to negatively affect the salience attributed to certain kinds of reasons, namely those associated with the risks of the trial. This may undermine autonomy; but it is, I suggest, obfuscatory to describe this intervention as coercive.[65]

Second, determining the involvement of third-party agency is central in claims regarding coercive offers, and this can be difficult to determine in practical contexts.

[61] Schonfeld et al., 'Money Matters'.

[62] On this point, see also Wilkinson, 'Biomedical Research and the Commercial Exploitation of Human Tissue'.

[63] Emanuel and Miller agree with this broad conclusion that the offer in the TGN1412 trial was not coercive, but do so by appealing to a normative approach to coercion. Emanuel and Miller, 'Money and Distorted Ethical Judgments about Research'.

[64] Wilkinson calls such cases 'enormous offer' cases. Wilkinson, *Bodies for Sale*. Both Macklin and Nelson et al. seem to implicitly support the view that such offers can be coercive. See Macklin, 'The Paradoxical Case of Payment as Benefit to Research Subjects'; Nelson et al., 'The Concept of Voluntary Consent'.

[65] On a similar point from a normative theorist of voluntariness generally, see Wertheimer, 'Voluntary Consent', 248–9. See also Largent et al., 'Misconceptions about Coercion and Undue Influence'.

Determining agency is central to claims regarding coercion because a key aspect of coercive offers (at least those that invalidate consent) on the account that I have developed in this chapter is that the offering party is actively preventing the recipient from being in a preferable pre-proposal situation, or has intentionally created their circumstances of vulnerability. Only then can such offers amount to the sort of domination that undermines interpersonal voluntariness. When the recipient's less preferable pre-proposal situation has been created by forces of hazard, offers made to them cannot coerce in a manner that would invalidate their consent.

In the philosophical thought experiments I have been considering, it is easy to ascertain whether the proposing party was engaged in such active prevention. However, coercive offers in practice raise far more difficult questions in this regard. To illustrate, it is easy to imagine a clean philosophical thought experiment in which Jones offers poverty-stricken Smith £10,000 for one of his kidneys; and we can say that this offer would only be coercive on the account I have developed if Jones had already somehow actively made it the case that Smith were financially destitute, and thus in a position in which refusing the offer was not eligible for choice given his circumstances. Part of the reason that this case seems so artificial is that it would rarely be the case that one individual would be responsible for another's poverty in this way. However, when we broaden the scope of our consideration in the context of real world markets for human organs, it might be claimed that structural injustices in the global economy mean that rich nations can appropriately be construed as actively preventing people in poor nations from escaping poverty.[66] Similarly, in the context of medical trials, even if the team organizing the study were themselves not responsible for creating the financial situation of those who signed up to the study, the research may have been funded by a governmental body that may at least be complicit in creating the circumstances of vulnerability that lead individuals to agree to participate in risky trials.

This of course is a far more complex question that I cannot hope to address here, and much will depend on the details of particular cases. However, in the light of my analysis of coercion, defining the scope of what constitutes the 'offering party' in these transactions (at an individual, organizational, or national level), and their role in intentionally creating the underlying circumstances of vulnerability amongst recipients of certain kinds of offers, is central to understanding whether we should construe these practices as coercive. It is also central to distinguishing the wrongs that coercion involves, from the wrongs involved in manipulation and exploitation. The less direct, and the less intentional the offering party's contribution to their target's underlying circumstances of vulnerability, the less appropriate the charge of coercion becomes, and the more likely it is that the wrong involved in making an offer does not primarily concern autonomy. Instead, if such offers are wrong, it is likely for the reason that by omitting to remedy their target's circumstances of vulnerability without further cost to themselves, the offering party fails to fulfil a

[66] See, for example Rippon, 'Imposing Options on People in Poverty'; Annas, 'Life, Liberty, and the Pursuit of Organ Sales'. For a response to arguments of this sort, see Wilkinson and Moore, 'Inducement in Research'.

moral duty of easy rescue.[67] In any case, contrary to what is widely claimed, it is these issues regarding the relationship between the offering party and their recipient's circumstances of vulnerability which are where the real questions about autonomy lie for coercive offers, rather than the size of the inducement per se.

We may also notice that those who endorse normative accounts of coercion have to answer a different question in this context. Rather than ascertaining whether such markets are coercive by asking whether rich nations are actively preventing individuals in poor countries from escaping poverty, they have to ask whether rich nations are *morally failing* these individuals by failing to alleviate their poverty. Although I have suggested that we ought to reject normative accounts, this shows how different theories of coercion can lead to different normative interpretations of pressing issues in practical ethics.

Similar issues concerning the role of the offering party in creating circumstances of vulnerability also arise in the context of offering incarcerated criminals chemical castration in return for a reduced sentence. Normative accounts can easily deny that the offer is coercive, presuming that the offender has been legitimately incarcerated in an establishment that respects the fundamental rights of prisoners; in such circumstances, the recipient's rights are not being illegitimately violated in his baseline state of affairs, against which the offer is made to him. However, on non-normative accounts, in order to determine whether the offer is coercive, we have to ascertain whether the proposing party created the prisoner's circumstances of vulnerability (or whether they are 'actively preventing the recipient from being in a preferable alternative situation' to use the framing of the preference view). This seems implausible when we understand the proposing party as the individual psychiatrist who makes the offer to the offender; however, it seems more plausible if we understand the criminal justice system as a collective to constitute the proposing party. Contrary to Green's analysis quoted at the beginning of the chapter, the key issue in considering the coerciveness of this sort of offer is thus not the offender's deprivation of liberty per se; the key issue is whether the proposing party should be construed as the same party that is actively preventing the prisoner from being released.

A further interesting aspect of this example that my account helps to elucidate is the relevance of the state's intentions. John McMillan has argued that the coerciveness of the chemical castration offer partly depends on the intention underlying it: Does the proposing party make the offer with the intention that the recipient will accept it? If not, then it is hard to see how the offer is coercive.[68] I agree that the proposing party's intentions are important here, since it seems plausible that intending one's offer to be accepted may be necessary for that offer to constitute domination of the recipient's will. As I have claimed, this is central to understanding the moral wrongness of coercion. If, on the other hand, the proposing party does not care whether or not their offer is accepted, it is difficult to see how they are dominating the recipient's will, in so far as domination implies directing another to a particular end.

[67] For more on this duty, see Rulli and Millum, 'Rescuing the Duty to Rescue'.
[68] McMillan, 'The Kindest Cut?' See also Shaw, 'Offering Castration to Sex Offenders'.

Conclusion

In this chapter, I have mapped out some of the theoretical complexity surrounding the concept of coercion and its relationship to voluntariness. In doing so, I have developed a structural account of threats and offers that accords with our common understanding of these kinds of proposal. Moreover, this account can naturally be incorporated into a plausible explanation of why coercion undermines decisional autonomy, in a manner that makes salient its implications for interpersonal voluntariness. In turn, this has important implications for our understanding of putative coercive offers, a concept that has been widely invoked in a number of bioethical debates. In order for such offers to be coercive in a manner that invalidates consent, they must involve a violation of the target's freedom from domination. I have suggested that offers can involve such a violation if they are made to an individual who has been placed into a circumstance of vulnerability by the offering party.

5

The Practical Dimension of Autonomy

So far in this book, I have been primarily concerned with the decisional dimension of autonomy. In this chapter though, I shall move away from considerations pertaining to the decisional dimension of autonomy, towards what I described in the introduction as the 'practical' dimension of autonomy. This dimension pertains to an agent's ability to act in pursuit of their chosen ends. My aim in this chapter is to explain both what it is for an agent to be practically autonomous in this way, and how this dimension of autonomy relates to the cognitive and reflective elements of the decisional dimension of autonomy (pertaining respectively to the kinds of beliefs and reflection on one's motivating desires that decisional autonomy requires). In particular, I shall suggest that the boundaries of the cognitive element of decisional autonomy, and of what it is for a belief to be decisionally necessary, are elucidated by considerations pertaining to the practical dimension of autonomy.

I shall begin by defending the claim that an adequate theory of autonomy should incorporate conditions pertaining to the practical dimension of autonomy. In section 2, I shall consider some prominent understandings of the nature of freedom, before going on to suggest, in section 3, how much freedom an agent must have in order to be minimally practically autonomous. In section 4, I shall argue that practical autonomy requires holding certain true beliefs; in doing so, I shall suggest that this informs how we should draw the boundaries of the cognitive element of decisional dimension of autonomy, a claim that that I shall consider further in my discussion of informed consent in Chapter 6. In section 5, I shall explain the relationship between the reflective and practical dimensions of autonomy, and argue that an agent's beliefs about what they are free to do importantly influences their decisions. Finally, in section 6, I shall consider the implications of my arguments for the enhancement and development of autonomy.

1. Introducing the Practical Dimension of Autonomy

The bioethical principle of respect for autonomy incorporates a negative obligation that enjoins us to not restrain the autonomous actions of others. As Dan Brock points out:

Autonomy, Rationality, and Contemporary Bioethics. Jonathan Pugh, Oxford University Press (2020). © Jonathan Pugh.
DOI: 10.1093/oso/9780198858584.001.0001

> ... interference with self-determination can involve interference with people's deciding for themselves, *but also interference with their acting as they have decided they want to act.*[1]

This negative obligation suggests that there is a practical dimension to the concept of autonomy as we understand it in bioethical discussion, a dimension that pertains to the agent's ability to act in pursuit of their ends.

This understanding of the practical dimension of autonomy overlaps to some extent with well-known conceptions of freedom in political philosophy. Isaiah Berlin famously outlined a conception of negative liberty that we use in attempting to answer the question 'What is the area within which the subject—a person or group of persons—is or should be left to do or be what he is able to do or be, without interference by other persons?' For Berlin, negative liberty contrasts with a positive sense of liberty, a sense that pertains to the kind of freedom required for what I have called decisional autonomy, or what Berlin suggests is the sense of freedom involved in being 'the source of control or interference that can determine someone to do, or be, this rather than that'.

Whilst Berlin's conception of negative freedom has been highly influential, the conception of the practical dimension of autonomy that I shall outline departs from it in some important ways, as I shall explain below. Briefly here, rather than being concerned with what or who is preventing the agent from acting, I shall suggest that the practical dimension pertains to an individual's ability to act effectively in pursuit of their ends. Some initial clarifications of how we ought to understand this claim are immediately necessary. First, in claiming that autonomy requires that agents are able to act effectively in pursuit of their ends, I do not mean to claim that they must be *successful* in their endeavours; one can of course fail to achieve one's ends and yet still be autonomous. Rather, the point undergirding the practical dimension of autonomy is that being unable to act effectively in pursuit of one's ends is inimical to one's autonomy all things considered, if we understand 'being able to act effectively' to simply mean that an agent (or an authorized proxy for that agent)[2] is not precluded from achieving the goal that she autonomously wants to achieve by the absence of certain kinds of freedom. I shall say more about this below.

Second, the decisional dimension of autonomy is theoretically prior to the practical dimension with regards to our understanding of an agent's all things considered autonomy. If an agent lacks autonomy with respect to their decision about what to do, then they still lack autonomy all things considered, even if they have the freedom to act effectively on the basis of that non-autonomous decision. For instance, one would not be autonomous if one performed an act motivated by a manipulated desire, even if one was not hindered in successfully performing that act. Accordingly, although we might agree with the philosopher Thomas Hobbes that irrational beings may appropriately be described as free in the physical sense that he famously describes,[3] they may not appropriately be described as autonomous on the approach that I am defending, in so far as they lack decisional autonomy. For the purposes of

[1] Brock, *Life and Death*, 29. Emphasis added.

[2] In the interests of brevity I shall henceforth omit this qualification.

[3] Hobbes, *Leviathan*, 139.

this chapter, unless otherwise stated, I shall henceforth assume that the agents under discussion are autonomous with respect to their decisions.

Philosophers are sometimes sceptical of the claim that a theory of autonomy should incorporate conditions pertaining to what I am calling the practical dimension of autonomy. For instance, John Christman writes:

> The ability to act – successfully and as planned – cannot be (a necessary condition of autonomy). I am often prevented from acting or completing my plans .... Such circumstances make me less free (in a certain sense of freedom), but they do not make me less autonomous, at least if this latter term is to retain any of its conceptual distinctiveness.[4]

Christman is certainly correct to deny that autonomy cannot require that we are successful in achieving our goals. However, dismissing considerations pertaining to the agent's ability to act from one's theory of autonomy on this basis is to discount an important aspect of autonomy due to the inadequacies of an implausibly strong understanding of it. It is entirely plausible to deny that autonomy requires the ability to act successfully, whilst maintaining that it may yet require some lower threshold ability to act in pursuit of one's goals. This is the kind of condition that I shall defend in this chapter.

In fact, the failure to accommodate a practical dimension into one's theory of autonomy leads to an impoverished discussion of autonomy in bioethics. Three points speak in favour of this view. The first follows on from my above discussion of the principle of respect for autonomy; the way in which we use the concept of autonomy in bioethical contexts suggests that we implicitly understand it to incorporate a practical dimension. For example, we can coherently say that the fact that euthanasia is illegal severely undermines the autonomy of terminally ill individuals with decision-making capacity who wish to end their suffering. If we believe that a theory of autonomy for use in contemporary bioethics should be congruous with our widespread use of the concept in that context, then it seems that our theory of autonomy should accommodate a dimension of the concept that it is implicitly understood to incorporate in our bioethical discussions.

The second point in favour of this view is that acknowledging the practical dimension of autonomy seems to be necessary if we are to account for the high prudential value that we afford to autonomy. I shall consider the value of autonomy in greater detail in Chapter 9; at this point though we might observe that there would seem to be little prudential value in being autonomous with respect to one's decisions if one was perpetually frustrated in one's attempts to pursue one's autonomously chosen ends. If we believe that autonomy bears high prudential value because we

[4] Christman, *The Politics of Persons*, 154. Some philosophers are more explicit than others in this regard. For instance, Taylor rejects the claim that autonomy incorporates a practical dimension, and instead claims that being able to act effectively in pursuit of one's ends may increase the *value* of autonomy (Taylor, *Practical Autonomy and Bioethics*). Coggon and Miola explicitly draw a distinction between autonomy and what I call the practical dimension of autonomy in Coggon and Miola, 'Autonomy, Liberty, and Medical Decision-Making'. However, this tendency is also apparent in the more subtle way in which philosophical discussions of autonomy typically concern only what I have termed the reflective element of decisional autonomy. See Oshana, 'Personal Autonomy and Society', 83–6, for an analysis of this tendency in the philosophical literature.

have a fundamental interest in 'living a life that is our own' (as I shall claim in Chapter 9), then it seems that we should be able to *act* on the basis of our decisions, as well as making those decisions in an autonomous manner. John Harris puts the point in the following, typically forceful, way:

> Agents are quintessentially actors; to be an agent is to be capable of action. Without agency, in this sense, decision-making is... both morally and practically barren.[5]

The third and perhaps strongest point in favour of the view that autonomy incorporates a practical dimension is one that I shall develop over the course of this chapter. To put it simply here though, if we fail to acknowledge the practical dimension of autonomy in our overall theory of autonomy, it is not clear that we can adequately account for considerations that are important for cashing out elements of decisional autonomy. In the previous chapter, I noted that coercion serves to undermine decisional autonomy because the coercing agent subjugates her victim's will by controlling their practically available alternatives. In this chapter, I shall also argue that considerations pertaining to our practical freedoms should play an important role in understanding the boundaries of the cognitive element of decisional autonomy, and the way in which our beliefs about what we are free to do can have crucial effects on our choices. In this regard, whilst we should acknowledge Berlin's insight that considerations of decisional autonomy (or what he calls positive liberty) often conflict with considerations of practical autonomy (or what he calls negative liberty), we should not overlook the ways in which there can be other positive interactions between these two dimensions of autonomy.

The fundamental point that grounds this view is that, *we make our choices, and sustain our motivating desires in the light of our beliefs about what is practically realizable.* Indeed, the significant implications of these beliefs for motivation, agency, and choice have been empirically demonstrated in the literature of self-efficacy.[6] If one is to account for this crucial theoretical point, one cannot ignore considerations pertaining to the practical dimension of autonomy in one's overall theory. Moreover, a theory of autonomy that incorporates this feature will be better able to accommodate key insights of relational autonomy. Our ability and freedom to act, and our beliefs in our self-efficacy are not just a function of our own capabilities; they are also mediated by our social circumstances and relationships, as I shall explore below.[7]

This last feature suggests that in investigating the relationship between freedom and autonomy, we must distinguish the implications of one's freedom at the point of action from one's freedom at the point of decision. I return to this distinction below; first though, I shall explain two different senses of freedom that might be employed in this discussion.

[5] Harris, '"... How Narrow the Strait!"', 249.

[6] Bandura et al., 'Self-Efficacy Beliefs as Shapers of Children's Aspirations and Career Trajectories'; Axelrod and Lehman, 'Responding to Environmental Concerns'; Krueger and Dickson, 'How Believing in Ourselves Increases Risk Taking'; Bandura, 'Perceived Self-Efficacy in the Exercise of Personal Agency'. Further, for a discussion of how medical therapy can alter self-perceptions of authenticity and autonomy by enhancing agency, see Haan et al., 'Becoming More Oneself?'

[7] Oshana, 'Personal Autonomy and Society', 95.

2. Positive and Negative Freedom

If an agent is to be able to act effectively in pursuit of their ends, they will need to have certain sorts of freedoms. As such, a natural starting point for an investigation into the practical dimension of autonomy is to carry out a consideration of different understandings of liberty or freedom (like Berlin I shall use the terms interchangeably).[8]

As I outlined in the previous section, it is commonly claimed that there are two separate understandings of freedom. First, freedom understood as the absence of constraint represents a negative conception of freedom; negative freedom may broadly be construed as freedom from interfering debilitating forces that prevent the agent from acting. This description of negative freedom represents the first way in which my conception of practical autonomy departs from Berlin's conception of negative freedom; unlike Berlin, I do not claim that the freedom in question here can only be negated by *agential* forces. On the conception that I am developing here, forces of hazard, such as disease or disability,[9] can be understood to restrict an agent's practical autonomy in the sense that they can impede agents from being able to act effectively in pursuit of their ends. In this sense, the conception of practical autonomy that I am developing is apolitical; I have noted the relevance of agential intentional influences on decisional autonomy in previous chapters.

There is a second sense in which my conception of practical autonomy is broader than negative freedom as it is commonly construed. On some occasions, we may have the requisite negative freedoms to pursue our goals, but still be unable to do so because we lack certain abilities.

Such cases suggest that we also have a positive conception of *practical* freedom, in which freedom is constituted not by the absence of restraint, but rather by the presence of capacities or conditions that enable the agent to be effective in the pursuit of their ends.[10] Again, I shall depart from Berlin's terminology and follow others in using the term 'positive freedom' to refer to this element of practical autonomy, rather than to considerations pertaining to the control required for decisional autonomy.

Bernard Berofsky aims to capture the essence of this alternative conception of positive freedom by claiming that this sense of freedom is constituted by those personal traits that are '... essential or highly useful to the satisfaction of a wide range of activities and decisions'.[11] However, this conception of positive freedom is too broad. Whilst it is true that many abilities are generally useful for the pursuit of a wide range of goals, an agent's ability to pursue her ends may require very specific

[8] Berlin, 'Two Concepts of Liberty', 34. See Pitkin, 'Are Freedom and Liberty Twins?' for a discussion of ways in which one might distinguish between the two terms.

[9] For a discussion of how mental disorder can undermine practical (and also decisional) autonomy, see Bolton and Banner, 'Does Mental Disorder Involve Loss of Personal Autonomy?'

[10] Of course, Berlin famously understood positive freedom in a broader sense; however, as Miller points out, Berlin's concept of positive freedom incorporates 'a number of quite different doctrines' (Miller, 'Introduction', 10). In order to avoid a lengthy exegesis of Berlin's essay here, I shall instead consider Berofsky's narrower conception of positive freedom.

[11] Berofsky, *Liberation from Self*, 16.

freedoms that are not essential to widely pursued activities. For instance, although having 20/20 unaided vision is not useful for the pursuit of a *wide* range of goals (assuming that we have easy access to visual aids such as spectacles and contact lenses), a person with slightly impaired vision who wants to become a military fighter pilot nonetheless lacks a physical capability that is necessary for them to achieve their goal. Agents can thus lack positive freedoms that are important for the pursuit of *their* goals, but that are not essential for the pursuit of a wide range of activities.

Conversely, agents might lack freedoms that are important for the pursuit of a wide range of goals, and yet still have the positive freedom to act in pursuit of what it is that they want to do. To illustrate consider the case of the slave-philosopher Epictetus. In view of the fact that he was born a slave, Epictetus clearly lacked negative freedom of the sort that is necessary for the effective pursuit of the vast majority of life-plans. Yet, even supposing this, Epictetus was nonetheless free, in both the negative and positive sense, to pursue his goal of living a life of philosophical reflection. *Pace* Berofsky, positive freedom of the sort that is central to an agent's practical autonomy is constituted by those traits and capacities that she requires in order to pursue an end that she herself is motivated to achieve.

Although the distinction between positive and negative freedom is widely adopted, it is somewhat problematic. In some cases, it may be unclear whether some factor is an element of positive or negative freedom; for example, it may not be clear whether we should understand intelligence as a constituent of positive freedom, or a lack of intelligence as a barrier to negative freedom.[12] In questioning the utility of the distinction, Joel Feinberg argues that we can have a comprehensive understanding of freedom as being constituted by freedom from preventative causes, given a sufficiently nuanced analysis of such causes, and the constraints to which they give rise. He suggests that we should analyse preventative causes as giving rise to the following two sorts of constraint:

(1) A negative constraint = A preventative cause constituted by the absence of some enabling factor.
(2) A positive constraint = A preventative cause constituted by the presence of some debilitating factor.[13]

Once these distinctions are made, it seems that we might obviate the need for a distinction between positive and negative freedom; freedom is just constituted by freedoms from different sorts of constraints.[14]

I am sympathetic to this view. Nevertheless, since I lack the space to further defend this alternative conception, and given the prevalent use of the vocabulary of positive and negative freedom, I believe that the clarity of the following discussion will be best served by adhering to an understanding that employs this distinction. However, I shall use the language of positive and negative freedom in the attenuated sense that Feinberg suggests is harmless, whereby positive freedom is characterized as the

[12] Ibid., 42. See also MacCallum, 'Negative and Positive Freedom'.
[13] See Feinberg, *Freedom and Fulfillment*, 5–6.
[14] This sentiment is shared by MacCallum's account in MacCallum, 'Negative and Positive Freedom'.

absence of a negative constraint, and negative freedom is characterized as the absence of a positive constraint.[15]

The conception of the practical dimension of autonomy is thus broader than Berlin's conception of negative freedom. It can be impeded by non-agential forces, and it incorporates elements of a sense of 'positive freedom' which is quite distinct from Berlin's understanding of that term. To conclude this part of the discussion, we can observe that a better historical precedent for the element of autonomy that I am seeking to identify here is Hobbes' understanding of physical freedom rather than Berlin's conception of liberty, where 'physical freedom' is defined in the following way:

> a Free-man is he that, in those things which by his strength and wit he is able to do, is not hindered to do what he has a will to.[16]

3. Autonomy, Freedom at the Point of Action, and the Modal Test

The question of how much freedom autonomy requires is a complex one, not least because of the difference between the two conceptions of freedom identified in the previous section. A further difficulty arises due to the fact that the question can be raised at two salient points.[17] First, we might raise it at what we may term 'the point of action', when the agent has *already* decided to act in some way. Raised at this point, the question of freedom is primarily relevant to the practical dimension of autonomy. However, the question may be raised prior to the point of action, at what we might term the 'point of decision', that is, prior to when the agent has decided what it is she will do. Raised at this point, an agent's beliefs about what she is free to do may also impinge on the decisional dimension of their autonomy, as I shall go on to explain.

As such, in order to answer the question of how much freedom autonomy requires, we must carry out two separate investigations. In this section, I shall begin by considering how much freedom an agent requires at the point of action in order to be able to act effectively in pursuit of their ends. I shall consider how much freedom may be required at the point of decision in section 5.

We can begin by observing that practical autonomy cannot require absolute negative freedom (at the point of action), that is, the absence of all possible positive constraints on action, since we can be positively constrained from doing something without that constraint being inimical to our ability to achieve our ends. For instance, consider this example:

> Harry has been asked by Jane to look after her dog. Suppose that Harry would instead like to visit the nearby pub. However, Harry decides to stay and look after the dog because he wants to prove his dependability to Jane. Now, suppose that Jane locks Harry in the house with the dog,

[15] Feinberg, *Freedom and Fulfillment*, 7. [16] Hobbes, *Leviathan*, 139.

[17] This distinction maps onto Berofsky's distinction between freedom of action and freedom of decision. Berofsky, *Liberation from Self*, 26–7.

because she is aware that Harry will have spotted the pub on his way in. However, Harry does not realize he is locked in, having *already* resolved to stay in the room looking after the dog.[18]

In this example, Harry is positively constrained from leaving the room. However, although he seems to lack a significant negative freedom, Harry still has the negative freedom to *do what he is motivated to do*; he is not positively constrained from looking after the dog. Now, although it might be correct to claim that Harry would enjoy greater freedom if he were not locked into the room, it is not the case that having this freedom would render him more able to effectively pursue his end. Assuming, as is the case in the above example, that prior knowledge of a lack of negative freedom is not impinging on Harry's decision about what to do, his lacking the freedom to leave the room does not seem to reduce his autonomy in any significant way.

The contrast between freedom at the point of action and autonomy is also highlighted by cases in which agents sacrifice certain negative freedoms as an expression of their autonomy. To illustrate this, consider the case of Odysseus and the Sirens:

Not wanting to be lured onto the rocks by the sirens, (Odysseus) commands his men to tie him to the mast and refuse all later orders he will give to be set free. He wants to have his freedom limited so that he can survive.[19]

Here, if the crew removed the positive constraints preventing Odysseus from leaving the ship, this would hinder his ability to pursue his goal of hearing the sirens' song without being lured from his ship. We can interpret this case as one in which the agent autonomously decides to limit their own negative freedom to do certain things, on the basis that having such freedoms would hinder their effective pursuit of their chosen goal. Far from enhancing his practical autonomy, removing the positive constraint on Odysseus' action whilst the ship sailed past the sirens would have been inimical to his practical autonomy, and allowed him to act instead on a compelled desire to swim to his death, a desire with respect to which he would not be autonomous. Similarly, in order to participate in civilized society, we may also have to sacrifice a number of freedoms as part of our social lives. However, we may be understood to implicitly consent to the sacrifice of certain freedoms (such as the freedom to commit acts of violence), on the basis that our doing so is a condition of the social contract that affords us a number of strong and important protections that better enable us to pursue our own independent goals.

These cases suggest that what is important with regards to the negative freedom that practical autonomy requires at the point of action is not the number of options that one has the negative freedom to pursue, but rather whether one has the particular negative freedom to pursue the end that one has decided to pursue. In order to be able to act effectively in pursuit of their end, an agent cannot be positively constrained from doing so.

[18] This is a Lockean variant of a so-called Frankfurt example. See Frankfurt, 'Alternate Possibilities and Moral Responsibility' and Locke, *An Essay on Human Understanding*, Book II, Chapter XXI.

[19] Dworkin, *The Theory and Practice of Autonomy*, 14–15.

There are perhaps some limits to this; for instance, we might claim that we should not allow an agent the negative freedom to completely abandon their future negative freedom, by selling herself into slavery say. However, we should be clear about why this matters for autonomy. On the account that I am defending, the reason that selling oneself into slavery is problematic is that in doing so, the agent abdicates their negative freedom to act in accordance with a *future* desire that they might develop to not live as a slave.[20] Whilst respecting the agent's locally autonomous decision here requires that we do not positively constrain her from becoming a slave, we might still positively constrain her from doing this in the name of her *global* autonomy. This, I suggest, is a case in which respecting local and global autonomy might require different things of us; I shall consider other such cases in Chapter 9. However, the mere fact that the slave desires to subjugate herself to another's authority for the rest of her life is not *necessarily* incompatible with her global autonomy on the view I am defending in this book, as some theorists have maintained.[21]

As is the case with negative freedom, lacking certain positive freedoms need not always be inimical to our practical autonomy. After all, we all lack certain capabilities, but this does not necessarily preclude the possibility of our practical autonomy. Most obviously, some freedoms are just irrelevant to our ability to pursue our ends. For example, if I do not enjoy listening to or playing music, the fact that I lack perfect pitch does not seem to prevent me from being practically autonomous. My above discussion of positive freedom also suggests that different agents might require different positive freedoms to act in pursuit of their goals. Whilst there may be certain abilities that most agents require to do this, it seems that an agent with suitably esoteric goals could require very different sorts of positive freedoms from other agents.

With these reflections in mind, and being mindful of the fact that a plausible theory of autonomy cannot require that agents are always successful in achieving their ends, I am now in a position to explain what it means for an agent to be able to act effectively in pursuit of their ends in the sense that I invoked when introducing the practical dimension of autonomy. In some cases, positive constraints that take away an agent's negative freedom will preclude the agent from pursuing a certain goal in *any* sense; for example. The question of whether an agent has the requisite negative freedom for practical autonomy may thus seem to be a binary question; it is either the case that a debilitating factor that precludes the pursuit of a goal is present, or it is not.

An analogous claim could be made with regards to *some* positive freedoms; if an agent lacks certain enabling factors, they may be precluded from acting effectively in pursuit of their goals in *any* sense. For instance, I shall argue below that an agent may lack practical autonomy if they are informationally cut-off from achieving their goals by virtue of holding certain false beliefs. Call these sorts of freedoms *discrete*

[20] This is how Dworkin explains the wrongness of selling oneself into slavery. See Dworkin, 'Paternalism'.

[21] See Oshana, 'Personal Autonomy and Society', 86–9; Waller, 'Natural Autonomy and Alternative Possibilities'. For a similar reply to the one given above, see Sneddon, 'What's Wrong with Selling Yourself Into Slavery?'

freedoms. With regards to discrete freedoms, we may say that an agent is only able to act effectively in pursuit of a goal whose achievement requires certain discrete freedoms, if they actually have those freedoms.

However, many of our freedoms admit of degrees. For instance, it seems plausible to claim that the pursuit of different goals might require different degrees of intelligence. Scalar freedoms such as intelligence present something of a theoretical problem with regards to practical autonomy, since it cannot be the case that an agent must have the *maximum* degree of some particular scalar positive freedom in order for it to be appropriate to claim that they are able to act effectively in pursuit of their ends; this would make the standards of autonomy far too demanding. Therefore, in cases in which the pursuit of some goal requires a scalar freedom x, it seems that we must stipulate that there is some threshold level of x that the agent must reach in order to be practically autonomous. However, as I pre-empted above, in stipulating the relevant threshold here, we must also allow for the possibility that an autonomous agent could have the threshold level of this scalar positive freedom and yet fail to achieve their goal. If practical autonomy is not to be too demanding, it cannot require that the practically autonomous agent must always *succeed* in their endeavours.

One plausible way of cashing out the notion of 'having the necessary positive freedom to be able to act effectively in pursuit of some goal' in a way that meets these criteria is to apply a modal test. First, we may appropriately be said to have such freedom, if there is some nearby possible world in which we have the same degree of positive freedom, and in which we *do* successfully achieve our goal. However, if there is *no* nearby possible world in which the agent has the same degree of freedom under consideration, and in which they successfully achieve their goal, it is plausible to claim that their failure to achieve their goal in the real world may be attributable to their lacking this freedom.[22] We may say that lacking the degree of freedom in question is thus sufficient (although perhaps not necessary)[23] for establishing that the agent lacks practical autonomy; they are modally precluded from successfully achieving their goal by the lack of this particular freedom. This formulation gives substance to what it means to have the necessary scalar positive freedom to be able to act effectively in pursuit of some goal, without committing us to the view that being practically autonomous requires that the agent must *succeed* in the pursuit of her goals, or that she has the maximum degree of a particular scalar positive freedom.

Accordingly, at the point of action, the freedom (in both the positive and negative sense) that is required for practical autonomy is the freedom to act effectively in pursuit of one's own ends in the manner that I have delineated above.[24] This view

[22] For a seminal discussion of the role of possible worlds in the logic of counterfactual conditional statements, see Stalnaker, 'A Theory of Conditionals'.

[23] I am leaving open the possibility that agents who are not modally precluded from success could nonetheless lack practical autonomy for other reasons.

[24] One potential objection to this account is that it might be understood to entail that agents who have a preference to achieve an outcome that cannot possibly be achieved (say of flying unaided) can be said to lack practical autonomy. I am prepared to accept this point, but only because it has limited force. The reason for this is that on the account of autonomy that I developed in Chapter 2, agents will not be autonomous with respect to such preferences, in so far as preferences are understood to be action-guiding. Recall that on the theory that I developed in Chapter 2, preferences are understood to be rational desires for

resonates with relational and embodied approaches to understanding autonomy. We act in the world as embodied agents, and this unavoidably shapes the boundaries of our freedoms in quite obvious ways; consider the example of a patient suffering from locked-in syndrome.[25] Furthermore, many of the resources and freedoms that we require to live in accordance with our autonomous desires are socially mediated.[26] Whilst it is true that we all need social resources such as education to enable us to pursue our goals, as Anderson and Honneth point out, vulnerable individuals may be particularly reliant on social conditions for their practical autonomy, as this discussion makes clear:

Consider, for example, the autonomy of people with mobility-limiting disabilities. Unless physical accommodations are made for such persons—wheelchair ramps, accessible vehicles, and so on—their ability to exercise their basic capabilities will be restricted in a way that constitutes a loss of autonomy. In general, the argument here is that the commitment to fostering autonomy—especially of the vulnerable—leads to a commitment, as a matter of social justice, to guaranteeing what one might call the material and institutional circumstances of autonomy.

It is important to acknowledge the exact extent of the claim that practical autonomy requires the freedom to act effectively in pursuit of one's ends. First, this claim pertains only to the freedom required at the point of action, and only to ends that the agent decides to pursue in accordance with the conditions of decisional autonomy.

Second, in making the above claim, I am seeking only to give an account of the freedom required for practical autonomy, and not an account of the nature of freedom itself. This is important, since defining freedom *itself* as relative to an agent's desires or motives seems to involve a conceptual confusion. To see why, consider the example of Tom Pinch discussed by Joel Feinberg.[27] Tom Pinch is gifted with the freedom to do everything but act effectively in pursuit of the one end that truly matters to him. Feinberg points out that Tom Pinch does not lack freedom per se; after all, *ex hypothesi*, Tom Pinch enjoys almost every conceivable freedom. Rather, Feinberg claims that Tom Pinch lacks only contentment.[28] In view of my arguments above, whilst we should agree that Pinch is free, we should also note that Feinberg conflates contentment and the practical dimension of autonomy in claiming that Pinch lacks only contentment. In addition to my arguments regarding the practical dimension above, two further points speak against Feinberg's interpretation of the

a certain motivating desire to be *effective* in moving one to act. I also argued in Chapter 2 that an agent's preferences must cohere with their non-irrational acceptances. The problem then with the preferences that I am considering here is that they will fail to cohere with an important set of the agent's acceptances; namely, their beliefs concerning their freedom at the point of decision. I shall discuss this in section 5. Notice that this view is compatible both with the claim that agents may autonomously harbour 'pipe-dreams' in a non-action-guiding sense, and the claim that they can be autonomous in pursuing these goals if they (non-irrationally) believe that they can be achieved.

[25] For further discussion of the significance of embodiment to autonomy, see Christman, *The Politics of Persons*, 10.

[26] Oshana, 'Personal Autonomy and Society'; Anderson and Honneth, 'Autonomy, Vulnerability, Recognition, and Justice'; Young, *Personal Autonomy*.

[27] Feinberg, *Freedom and Fulfillment*, 38. [28] Ibid., 38–9.

example. First, one can fail to achieve one's goal despite having the freedoms necessary to its effective pursuit; thus, having the requisite freedom does not entail contentment in the way that Feinberg's interpretation seems to suggest. Second, one may be mistaken in thinking that achieving a certain goal will bring contentment; having the freedom to do what one most wants to do is thus not guaranteed to bring contentment.

The problem for Tom Pinch is that he lacks a freedom that is necessary, at the point of action, for his practical autonomy. This is not to say that the freedom that autonomy requires at the point of action exhausts the concept of freedom; the nature of freedom goes beyond the freedoms that are necessary for practical autonomy. Although we may say that Tom Pinch is generally free, he is not practically autonomous because he lacks the freedom to act effectively in pursuit of the one end that he actually wants to achieve. If this conclusion is correct, then we might observe one of its corollaries, namely the implication that our freedoms can be increased in ways that are inconsequential to our practical autonomy at the point of action. For example, recall the example of Harry above. Suppose that Jane returned to her room after half an hour and, again unbeknownst to Harry, unlocked the room that Harry was in. This would increase Harry's freedom, but it is far from clear that it would increase his autonomy in staying in the room.

This suggests something interesting about the relationship between practical autonomy and freedom. If, as the above discussion suggests, all that matters at the point of action is whether the agent has the freedom to act effectively in pursuit of the ends that they have decided to achieve, then the agent's freedom to do otherwise is inconsequential to their practical autonomy *at the point of action*. One might worry that this claim is in tension with another popular view, namely the view that autonomy requires freedom of choice. For example, Hurka assumes that 'autonomy involves choice from a wide range of options',[29] and Raz claims that an autonomous person must have 'adequate options available for him to choose from'.[30] Although I shall suggest that Raz and Hurka are not entirely correct here (for reasons that I shall explain in section 5), their claims above are not in tension with my conclusion that the agent's freedom to do otherwise is inconsequential to their autonomy *at the point of action*. Indeed, Raz and Hurka might agree with this conclusion; instead, they would claim that freedom of choice is crucial for autonomy at the *point of decision*.

Before considering the relationship between autonomy and choice at the point of decision, it is prudent to address the way in which holding certain true beliefs seems to be necessary for the effective pursuit of many of our ends. In doing so, I shall consider one way in which considerations pertaining to the practical dimension of autonomy have implications for our understanding of decisionally necessary beliefs that play a central role in the cognitive element of decisional autonomy.

[29] Hurka, 'Why Value Autonomy?', 362.

[30] Raz, *The Morality of Freedom*, 373. See also Oshana, 'Personal Autonomy and Society'.

4. True Beliefs, Autonomy, and Modality

An agent's beliefs play an important role in decisional autonomy. In order for an agent to regard an outcome *x* as good in a reason-implying sense in the manner that reflective autonomy requires, she must hold certain beliefs about the descriptive features of *x*, and about the good. In Chapter 2, I argued that an agent must meet a minimum threshold of theoretical rationality in holding these beliefs if she is to qualify as being autonomous with respect to the motivating desires that she sustains on their basis.

However, in the introductory chapter, I suggested that decisional autonomy also incorporates a cognitive element pertaining to the agent's understanding of their action or decision. This element reflects the Aristotelian claim that actions performed from reasons of ignorance are non-voluntary; the thought here is that decisional autonomy requires that agents hold certain *true*, and not merely theoretically *rational* beliefs.

In bioethical contexts, it is natural for theorists to suppose that there is some important relationship between autonomy and true beliefs, by virtue of the commonplace assumption that autonomy is closely related to the doctrine of *informed* consent, and the criterion of understanding incorporated into the standard account of autonomy in bioethics. However, the claim that there is an important relationship between autonomy and true beliefs is not universally endorsed in the recent philosophical literature.[31] Wilkinson captures a common sentiment when he writes:

> A person may have false beliefs about his or her options without his or her autonomy being affected; who has true beliefs about all their options?[32]

Wilkinson uses this observation to motivate his claim that an agent's lack of autonomy may only be attributable to their holding false beliefs if they have been intentionally deceived into holding them. What matters for Wilkinson is how the agent comes to hold these beliefs, and not the content of the beliefs themselves.[33] I argued against this view in Chapter 3. Here though, I wish to reiterate the point that the quoted observation provides insufficient support for Wilkinson's own position. The mere fact that autonomy is compatible with *some* false beliefs does not entail (and provides little support for) the claim that decisional autonomy is compatible with *all and any* false beliefs.

What is needed then is a nuanced account of the different sorts of beliefs that can affect our decisional autonomy. Aristotle also recognized this in his discussion of the sense of voluntariness that is undermined by ignorance. Aristotle does not make the mistake of over-generalizing this claim, taking care to note that not all forms of ignorance undermine voluntariness. First, he notes that ignorance does not undermine voluntariness if the agent herself is responsible for her state of ignorance; this

[31] For two examples of theorists who claim that false beliefs do not undermine autonomy, see McKenna, 'The Relationship between Autonomous and Morally Responsible Agency', 208–9; Arpaly, 'Responsibility, Applied Ethics, and Complex Autonomy Theories', 175; Wilkinson, 'Nudging and Manipulation'.

[32] Wilkinson, 'Nudging and Manipulation', 345.

[33] Ibid.

amounts to acting *in* ignorance, rather than acting *from* ignorance.[34] More pertinently for my purposes here though, on the Aristotelian conception, only ignorance of *particulars*, that is, of 'the circumstances of action and the objects with which it is concerned'[35] can undermine voluntariness. This is to be contrasted with ignorance of *proharesis*, which has been translated by some commentators as 'moral purpose', and ignorance of universal truths, neither of which undermine voluntariness for Aristotle.[36]

Instead, Aristotle lists a number of examples of particulars, an agent's ignorance of which would undermine the voluntariness of their action; these include ignorance of who one is, of what one is doing, of the sphere in which or to what one is doing it, what it is that one is doing it with, of what it is for, and of the way in which one is doing it.[37] However, he does not provide a principled basis for including these particulars but not others. Yet, it is clear that voluntary decisions can be made from ignorance concerning some particulars of one's decision; Wilkinson is absolutely correct on this point. For instance, we can clearly make voluntary decisions despite our ignorance of what future states will actually obtain. The fact that I do not know whether a coin will land heads or tails does not preclude the possibility that I may voluntarily make a bet that it will land heads.

We thus need to provide an account of the limitations to the scope of forms of ignorance that can undermine voluntariness. The claim I want to make in this section is that there is a principled way in which we can appropriately delimit this scope, grounded in considerations of practical autonomy. I shall claim that ignorance of particulars is sufficient to undermine voluntariness if the particulars in question are such that the agent *must* hold true beliefs about them if her action is to be appropriately connected to the pursuit of her intended end. Such a claim, if true, shows that there is an important relationship between the decisional and practical dimensions of autonomy, and thus that an adequate theory of autonomy *in toto* should incorporate at least some considerations pertaining to practical autonomy.

In order for an agent to be able to act effectively in pursuit of the end that she is motivated to achieve, it is clear that she must have certain true beliefs about how to go about achieving that end. Indeed, if an agent acts in a manner that she is incorrect in believing will serve as a means to achieving her chosen end, her action will be importantly disconnected from that motive, and the values underlying it. Thus, as Suzy Killmister observes in discussing the significance of false beliefs to autonomy:

> No matter how autonomous an agent's motivations are, the action itself cannot be autonomous unless it is appropriately connected to the motivation behind it.[38]

Since our decisions are made partly on the basis of our descriptive beliefs about the world, if these beliefs are false they can serve to sever the connection between our actions and our underlying motivations and values. Alfred Mele also captures this sort of thought when he suggests that being 'informationally cut-off' precludes one from autonomous agency. He writes:

[34] Aristotle, *Nicomachean Ethics*, 1110b 25–9. [35] Ibid., 1110b 34–1111a.
[36] Ibid., 1110b 30–1111a. [37] Ibid., 1111a 3–6.
[38] Killmister, 'Autonomy and False Beliefs', 521.

> [A] sufficient condition of S's being informationally cut-off from autonomous action in a domain in which S has intrinsic pro-attitudes is that S has no control over the success of his efforts to achieve his end, *owing to his informational condition*.[39]

To illustrate this thought, consider the following example, which I considered in an earlier chapter (but for a different purpose this time). Suppose that Sheila wants to quench her thirst, and pours a clear liquid from her kitchen tap into her glass. Accordingly, let us assume that Sheila has decisive apparent epistemic reason to believe that the glass contains water, and that the water will quench her thirst. However, suppose that she is mistaken in her belief; the liquid is, in fact, contaminated.

In view of my arguments in the previous chapter, Shelia meets the conditions of reflective autonomy with respect to her motivating desire here: She does what she believes she has strong self-interested reason to do. She is also theoretically rational with respect to the beliefs that ground this desire. However, her (theoretically rational) false belief undermines her ability to act effectively in pursuit of her intended end, by severing the connection between her chosen end, namely to alleviate her thirst, and how she actually attempts to achieve it.[40] She is not wholly self-governing in her conduct because we can plausibility attribute her failure to achieve her desired end to the fact that she held that particular false belief.

Some theorists are critical of informational conditions on autonomy because they take them to entail that one must be *successful* in one's actions in order to be autonomous with respect to them.[41] This of course would make the standards of autonomy far too demanding. However, the claim that I am advancing here is compatible with the claim that an agent can be autonomous when she fails to achieve her end. The point is that the agent's poor informational condition should not *thwart* the possibility of her being successful in achieving her end, by virtue of disconnecting her act from her intention. Successful action can be thwarted by false beliefs, and a failure to hold certain key true beliefs.

To illustrate why this is not problematic, consider Suzy Killmister's example of a woman, Jill, who attempts to intentionally kill a man, Jack, by hitting him over the head with a crowbar.[42] Although Jill fails, Killmister claims that she is nonetheless autonomous, because her failure to achieve her end is not *due* to her poor informational condition. Killmister herself does not elaborate further on how Jill differs from someone like Sheila in my earlier example with regards to her poor informational condition, and why Jill is autonomous when Sheila is not. On the approach that I am advocating here though, this is a crucial point; in order to ascertain when ignorance

[39] Mele, *Autonomous Agents*, 181, emphasis added.

[40] One can describe Shelia's actions in ways that make it appear that she is practically autonomous. If we describe the end that Shelia is hoping to achieve as 'getting the liquid in the glass to her mouth', then her act of picking up the glass and putting it to her mouth is clearly connected to her motive in an appropriate way. However, to the extent that we identify the end that 'getting the liquid in the glass to her mouth' itself serves as a means to (i.e. alleviating her thirst), we see that this act is not appropriately connected to her motive, given that the glass contains contaminated liquid. This illustrates the importance of precision in how we individuate the agent's acts when we are assessing her autonomy.

[41] See McKenna, 'The Relationship between Autonomous and Morally Responsible Agency'.

[42] Killmister, 'Autonomy and False Beliefs', 525.

undermines voluntariness, we need to have some way of establishing that the agent's failure to achieve her end is due to her poor informational condition, and when it is not.

Here, I suggest that we can militate the sort of modal test that I described above regarding positive freedom. We may say that Jill's failure is not attributable to her false beliefs if there is a nearby possible world in which Jill holds the same set of beliefs in the relevant circumstances, and in which she successfully achieves her end. Whilst this is true of Jill, it is not true of Sheila. The modal test thus allows us to identify the sorts of beliefs that can preclude autonomy by severing the vital connection between the actions we take to realize the ends that we value.

False beliefs about future states of affairs that we nonetheless previously had strong epistemic reasons to think would obtain, do not pass this modal test. To illustrate, suppose that I rationally believe that some bad future outcome of very low probability will not occur, say an extremely adverse side-effect of a medical treatment with a <1 per cent chance of occurring. On the basis of this belief, I consent to the treatment because I believe that it will be effective, and that it is necessary for safeguarding my health. Let us suppose that, unfortunately for me, the improbable negative side-effect does in fact occur; my belief that it would not occur turned out to be false. The point about the modal test is that this is not the sort of false belief that precludes my decisional autonomy in consenting to the procedure. The reason for this is that there are a large number of nearby possible worlds in which I held the same belief (that the side-effect would not occur), and in which I was successful in achieving the goal I had chosen to pursue by initiating this course of action.[43]

We can use the modal test to identify other particulars that the agent must hold true beliefs about if her action is to be appropriately connected to the pursuit of her intended end. If there is a nearby possible world in which the agent either holds false beliefs about some particular (or is simply ignorant of true information about that particular in the relevant circumstances), but is nonetheless successful in achieving her desired end, then her ignorance about this particular in reality does not provide sufficient grounds for her failure to achieve her end. If, however, there is *no* nearby possible world in which this is the case, then ignorance about that particular is sufficient to undermine voluntariness. The particular in question can then be said to be the object of a *decisionally necessary belief*.

Two further things are worth noting. First, autonomy may plausibly be undermined even when an agent is not completely ignorant of some decisionally relevant particular. An agent may be aware of some relevant piece of information, but fail to adequately grasp its implications for their decision. This is particularly salient in the medical context; the understanding that autonomy requires is not the mere awareness of material information about one's condition or proposed treatment, but also the *appreciation* that this information applies to oneself. Accordingly, we might

[43] There may be some cases in which a very rare side-effect is a guaranteed product of some extremely abnormal unknown feature of one's physiology (such that it would obtain in every world in which one's physiology remains the same). Would a failure to believe that the side-effect will occur in one's circumstances amount to being modally precluded in the sense I have outlined? I believe not, on the basis that there are very nearby possible worlds in which this abnormal physiological feature does not obtain.

further suggest the understanding that autonomous decision-making involves might require the 'vivid imagination' of what future states of affairs that may be brought about by our choices will be like *for us*.[44]

Second, we may also note that instances of theoretical irrationality can similarly modally preclude agents from achieving their ends. Theoretical irrationality can also rupture the connection between the agent's decision and the values that are operative in their particular choice context. I explored how such irrationality can undermine decisional autonomy in Chapter 2 in my discussion of Rebecca Walker's illuminating examples. Failures of theoretical rationality can undermine one's ability to accurately assess the extent to which a particular belief coheres with one's other beliefs about both descriptive and evaluative features of the world; this too can preclude one from acting effectively in the sense that I have been outlining here.

I noted at the beginning of this section that contemporary philosophers and bioethicists are divided over the question of whether holding false beliefs undermines autonomy. The framework that I have adopted in this book may help to explain why this is the case. I have explained that holding false beliefs can render an agent ineffectual in pursuing the ends that she is motivated to achieve. I have also claimed that this phenomenon can offer us insights into the forms of ignorance that may appropriately be described as undermining one sense of voluntariness, as identified in the Aristotelian distinction. However, whilst such false beliefs affect the cognitive element of decisional autonomy, they need not affect the *reflective* element of her decisional autonomy.

As such, it seems that the diverging intuitions concerning cases of false beliefs can be explained as follows. If one believes that the reflective element of decisional autonomy can tell the whole story of autonomous agency, then having epistemically rational false beliefs concerning the means that are necessary to achieving one's desired end need not undermine one's autonomy. On the other hand, if we claim that an adequate theory of autonomy also includes a cognitive element of decisional autonomy, whose boundaries should be informed by considerations pertaining to a practical dimension of autonomy (as I have argued here), then it is clear why even epistemically rational false beliefs can undermine autonomy; they will do so when they render the agent ineffectual in her pursuit of the ends that she is motivated to achieve, in the way that I have described in this section.

To conclude this discussion, it is important to be clear about the scope of the claims that I am making here. The modal test that I have outlined here is intended to identify a *sufficiency* condition for when ignorance about a particular undermines voluntariness. It does not identify a *necessary* condition. In other words, it leaves open the possibility that there may be forms of ignorance that would *not* entail an agent's failure to achieve her end in all nearby possible worlds, but which we may still find it plausible to claim undermine voluntariness.[45] For instance, ignorance of risks

[44] Recall that Savulescu stipulates vivid imagination as a condition of autonomous choice. See Savulescu, 'Rational Desires and the Limitation of Life Sustaining Treatment'.

[45] It might be further argued that there are some beliefs concerning which the following two statements can be true. First, an agent can be autonomous with respect to a decision without holding the belief in question (i.e. the belief is not decisionally necessary). However, it may also be the case that being

attending a medical procedure might plausibly fall into this category. I shall take up this question when I turn to the cognitive element of decisional autonomy and informed consent in Chapter 6. In the remainder of this chapter though, having established one relationship between decisional and practical autonomy, I shall return to the question of the freedom that autonomy requires at the point of decision, and describe another important relationship between these two dimensions of autonomy.

5. Freedom at the Point of Decision

At the end of section 3, I suggested that practical autonomy requires that the agent has, at the point of action, the positive and negatives freedoms that are necessary for them to act effectively in pursuit of their ends. In this section, I shall consider the freedom that autonomy requires *at the point of decision*. In considering the agent's freedom at the point of decision, we are considering the freedom that she believes herself to have prior to making a decision about what to do; as I shall explain, it is important to consider the agent's freedom at this point, because an agent's beliefs about their freedoms can impinge on their decisional autonomy.

Let me begin by again stressing the observation that we make our decisions about what to do in the light of what we believe to be practically realizable.[46] James Griffin puts this point as follows:

> We do not, as a matter of fact, form our plans of life as if they were, in effect, choices from a Good Fairy's List – 'whatever you want, just say the word'. Our desires are shaped by our expectations, which are shaped by our circumstances.[47]

When we are in the process of deciding what to do, our decision is informed by what we believe we are free and able to do. For example, when a person considers which career path they want to pursue, they will make their decision having assessed the capacities that constitute their positive freedom to pursue certain careers, and having considered any positive constraints on their negative freedom to pursue others. It may be the case that their beliefs about what they are and are not free to do are false; however, it is not the freedom that one *actually* has that one takes into

intentionally deceived to *not* hold the belief in question may nonetheless undermine autonomy. Some theorists seem to hold the view that this is true of all beliefs. See Wilkinson, 'Nudging and Manipulation', 345. For the reasons discussed here, I deny this claim, but the modal test suggests a reason for why this might be true of some set of beliefs. In some cases, when we fail to hold a particular true belief, there will be some nearby possible worlds in which we do come to hold it, by virtue of refining our beliefs in accordance with the requirements of theoretical rationality, or by discovering new evidence. However, intentional deception serves to narrow the scope of the possible worlds in which this will be the case; intentional deceivers will often make efforts to ensure that we do not come to hold the relevant beliefs. This is similar to the point that Yaffe makes with regards to intentional coercers and manipulators tracking compliance in their targets as discussed in the previous chapter. Yaffe, 'Indoctrination, Coercion and Freedom of Will'. The point here is that intentional deception may modally preclude agents from achieving their ends in a manner that mere ignorance does not.

[46] This is a point that Aristotle acknowledges in his assertion that prohairesis is a deliberate desire for things in our power. Aristotle, *Nicomachean Ethics*, 1113a 9–10.

[47] Griffin, *Well-Being*, 47.

consideration in one's practical deliberations. Rather, it is one's *beliefs* about the freedoms that one has.

This point is familiar from the empirical literature concerning self-efficacy beliefs. The phenomenon explained above has also been referred to as 'conscious character planning' in the philosophical literature.[48] Unless we are wholly sceptical of the possibility of autonomy, it seems that we must claim that conscious character planning does not undermine autonomy.[49] The fact that normal humans have limited freedoms and tailor their preferences in accordance with them cannot be inimical to their autonomy with respect to those preferences, if autonomy is to be possible. To claim otherwise would be to rule out the possibility of autonomy at the very outset, given the nature of the world we live in, in which environmental forces contribute to the shape and limits of our freedoms. The absence of certain freedoms at the point of decision merely shapes the contours of our choice domains.

In conscious character planning, an agent's awareness of the limitations of their freedoms *informs* their decisions about what to do, but it does not preclude their decisional autonomy. However, an agent's beliefs about their freedom can threaten their decisional autonomy if they believe themselves to have extremely limited freedoms. To see how, it is illustrative to contrast the case of Tom Pinch (considered above) with the example of Martin Chuzzlewit:

> Suppose that Martin Chuzzlewit finds himself on a trunk line with all of its switches closed and locked, and with other 'trains' moving in the same direction on the same track at his rear, so that he has no choice at all but to continue moving straight ahead to destination *D*... But now let us suppose that getting to *D* is Chuzzlewit's highest ambition in life and his most intensely felt desire. In that case, he is sure to get the thing in life he wants most.[50]

Whether or not Chuzzlewit is autonomous here depends on the extent to which his lack of freedom is the *reason* that he came to sustain his motive to go to *D*. For Chuzzlewit to be reflectively autonomous with respect to his motive to get to *D*, he must have come to adopt it on the basis of a (non-irrational) belief that his getting to *D* would be good in a reason-implying sense. However, our disposition to adopt motivating desires on the basis that their content is good in a reason-implying sense can be compromised in situations in which we believe that our freedoms (at the point of decision) are severely restricted. If we believe that *only* one course of action is available to us, our lack of alternative possibilities may dissuade us from engaging in any sort of reflection about the value of the available outcome; rather, we may adopt the motive to pursue that outcome on no other basis than the fact that it is the only option available to us.

In contrast to conscious character planning, this phenomenon is known as adaptive preference formation.[51] Adaptive preference formation may be defined as the 'unconscious altering of our preferences in light of the options that we have

[48] Elster, *Sour Grapes*, 117–19. [49] See ibid., and Friedman, *Autonomy, Gender, Politics*, 25.

[50] Feinberg, *Freedom and Fulfillment*, 38.

[51] Elster, *Sour Grapes*; see also Sen, *Development as Freedom*; Nussbaum, *Women and Human Development*.

available'.[52] To illustrate the phenomenon of adaptive preference formation, let us alter the case of Harry the dog-sitter above so that Harry forms an adaptive preference:

> Suppose that Harry forms the desire to leave the house and go to the pub upon Jane's departure. However, he then hears Jane lock him into the house. Upon hearing this, Harry resigns himself to staying in to look after the dog, but convinces himself that this was really his preference all along.

Unlike conscious character planning, adaptive preference formation *does* seem inimical to autonomy.[53] On the theory that I have developed over the course of the preceding chapters, the reason for this is that in cases of adaptive preference formation, the agent no longer endorses their motivating desire on the basis of a belief that the outcome of the desire is good in a reason-implying sense; rather they sustain this desire because the outcome it concerns is the *only* option available to them. However, the fact that an outcome is the only one available does not make that outcome good in a reason-implying sense. Moreover, the self-deceptive nature of the way in which this preference is formed may preclude later critical reflection on the value of the outcome.

Although lacking freedom at the point of decision is an obvious causal factor underlying adaptive preference formation, it is not clear that lacking such freedoms must *necessarily* lead to adaptive preference formation. After all, the fact that only one option is available to an agent does not make it impossible for them to endorse that option on the basis of its reason-giving content (rather than its mere availability). For example, it is (to all intents and purposes) practically impossible for a passenger to jump out of a commercial airplane in mid-flight. Yet, even if Smith believes that he has no alternative to staying in a plane for the duration of a flight, this does mean that he cannot regard the outcome of staying in the plane as good in a reason-giving sense. As long as Smith (non-irrationally) believes that the content of his motivating desire to stay in the plane is good in a reason-implying sense, then he can be reflectively autonomous with respect to that desire, even if he also believes that he lacks the freedom to do otherwise. However, Smith will lack autonomy in this situation if he adopts the motivating desire to do something, *just because* he believes he lacks the freedom to do anything else.

This has implications beyond this somewhat contrived thought experiment. Each of us has a number of attachments and commitments that it would be extremely costly for us to give up. We are in a meaningful sense not free to abandon them. However, as Christman highlights, it would be a mistake to deny that we can be autonomous with respect to these commitments on the basis that we are not free to

[52] Colburn, 'Autonomy and Adaptive Preferences', 52. Note that an agent's options can be restricted by virtue of social oppression. For this reason, adaptive preference formation has been of particular interest to theorists who are concerned with autonomy as a social ideal. See Mackenzie, 'Three Dimensions of Autonomy', 30.

[53] See also Elster, *Sour Grapes*, 20; and Colburn, 'Autonomy and Adaptive Preferences', 61–71.

give them up.[54] On the contrary, these commitments can represent our deepest values and strongest reasons. Similarly, in bioethical contexts, we are often considering whether people are making autonomous decisions in desperate circumstances, where they have severely restricted choice sets. Again, the fact that an individual is facing restricted choices, does not entail that they cannot decide rationally in that context. Nonetheless, when we believe we have *no* choices available to us (not even unattractive ones), we may find it difficult to summon the motivation to engage in somewhat otiose rational deliberation about what to do.

With this understanding of adaptive preference formation in mind, let us return to the question of Martin Chuzzlewit's autonomy. The way in which Feinberg phrases the example makes it ambiguous as to whether it is best to interpret Chuzzlewit's being motivated to get to *D* as an instance of adaptive preference formation. The fact that Chuzzlewit 'finds himself' on the particular trunk line does not tell us whether he regarded getting to *D* as being good in a reason-implying sense prior to finding himself on the track, or whether he forms the motive to get to *D* on the basis that he has found himself on the particular trunk line that leads to *D*. In the latter case, Chuzzlewit lacks autonomy because he does not adopt his motive on the basis of its reason-giving content, but rather on its mere availability; he has thus formed an autonomy undermining adaptive preference. However, if Chuzzlewit had formed a preference for *D* prior to finding himself in this curious position, and his lack of freedom had not otherwise impaired his reflective autonomy with respect to his motivating desire, Chuzzlewit could be reflectively and practically autonomous.

Of course, if we believe that we have more freedoms at the point of decision, then in many cases the extent to which we direct our choices through rational deliberative processes will be enhanced. Although it is possible for Chuzzlewit to view *D* as good in a reason-implying sense without having further freedoms, the absence of other freedoms may jeopardize the likelihood that he will rationally deliberate on the value of *D* in this way. In contrast, if other alternatives (*E*, *F*, and *G*) are eligible for choice, then the agents are more likely to be drawn to a justificatory evaluative stance. It is not just that the agent will choose *D* because there are reason-giving facts about *D*; rather she will choose *D* because she believes that it is *better* than the other available alternatives, and this is a choice for which she is responsible.[55]

There are of course limits to this, since having too many available choices can impede rational decision-making processes. I shall discuss this point further below. Whilst recognizing this limitation, it is nonetheless plausible to postulate that giving people choices can sometimes serve to increase the scope and power of their rational deliberation about what to do. In allowing individuals to choose from a greater number of alternatives, we can sometimes increase the extent to which their choice is a reflection of their values rather than their circumstances.

This represents a further important way in which autonomy is an inherently relational phenomenon, as the choices that are available to us at the point of decision

[54] Christman, *The Politics of Persons*, 160. As such, I believe that there are limitations to the extent to which Friedman is correct to claim that autonomy requires that we are able to envisage alternative possible courses of action, or to imagining oneself otherwise. Friedman, *Autonomy, Gender, Politics*, 9.

[55] Hurka, *Perfectionism*, 150.

will typically be socially mediated. Most obviously, the societies in which we live may provide us with more or less available options to choose from. For instance, women in Saudi Arabia have a far more restricted choice set regarding potential professions than their counterparts in the United Kingdom, due to the former's restrictive labour laws.

In the bioethical context, we may also note that physicians can exert a considerable degree of control over their patients' autonomy by virtue of the control they can exercise over the treatment options that are made available to a particular patient. Of course, considerations of justice and beneficence may considerably dictate these decisions; physicians will only offer treatment options that are in a patient's interests, and which can be provided in accordance with the constraints of a just allocation of scarce medical resources. Nonetheless, there are some cases in which medical professionals may limit autonomy with less convincing justifications. Consider, for instance, the fact there is evidence to suggest that young childless men with decision-making capacity are more likely to be accepted for sterilization surgery than young childless women with decision-making capacity.[56] Here it seems that broader social attitudes and expectations about women may be serving to influence medical professionals with regards to what sorts of medical treatments options are and are not appropriate for a particular demographic.

In this example, women's choice is restricted in a quite direct sense, in so far as certain women cannot access a medical procedure. However, social forces can shape an individual's available options in perhaps more insidious ways. They can serve to undermine an individual's self-esteem, and their capacity to view certain desired options as valuable in their social context. For example, Anderson and Honneth point out that in societies where being a 'stay at home dad' is regarded as a euphemism for 'unemployment', it is difficult for male members of that society to regard full time parenting as a valuable option that is eligible for choice.[57]

Another way in which a lack of freedom can negatively affect decisional autonomy is that restricting another's freedom can serve as a method for undermining forms of social recognition that play a key role in capacities that are plausibly necessary for autonomous decision-making.[58] For instance, in addition to self-esteem, Honneth and Anderson emphasize the importance of 'self-respect' and 'self-trust' for autonomy. The former concerns an agent's capacity to understand herself as an agent capable of rational deliberation and whose choices deserve moral consideration. The latter pertains to the agent's capacity to place trust in her own affectively mediated commitments, and to view these commitments as authentically her own.[59] Both self-trust and self-respect are acquired and maintained in the context of interpersonal relationships. Indeed, amongst the many ills of societal inequality, oppression, and discrimination, these features of society amount to failures to engage in forms of

[56] See McQueen, 'Autonomy, Age and Sterilisation Requests'. For further discussion of this phenomenon, see Mertes, 'The Role of Anticipated Decision Regret and the Patient's Best Interest in Sterilisation and Medically Assisted Reproduction'; Pugh, 'Legally Competent, But Too Young To Choose To Be Sterilized? Practical Ethics'.

[57] Anderson and Honneth, 'Autonomy, Vulnerability, Recognition, and Justice', 136.

[58] Ibid., 132–5. [59] Ibid.

social recognition that allow individuals to regard themselves as people whose choices matter, whose choices are their own, and whose choices deserve respect.[60]

The above interpersonal influences have been highlighted by those theorists who are particularly interested in how autonomy can be impeded in and by society in general. There are of course lessons for the role of autonomy in bioethics here;[61] as the example of voluntary female sterilization suggests, medicine can be susceptible to social forces that influence the opportunities for choice afforded to individuals. We may also note that the way in which we seek to safeguard autonomy in bioethics may already implicitly incorporate considerations of relational autonomy. For instance, when it functions correctly, the institution of informed consent may serve to facilitate the forms of social recognition stressed by Honneth and Anderson. It can serve as a formal recommendation that the patient is someone whose views about treatment matter, who is competent to make those decisions, and whose decisions warrant respect.

However, as I mentioned in the introduction, we need to take care not to simply assume that *all* of the conclusions regarding the nature and value of autonomy in broader social contexts transfer straightforwardly to the bioethical context. In particular, we might plausibly deny that a minimum threshold of autonomy for local decision-making in the bioethical context must require the same variety of choices stressed by social theorists of autonomy with regards to individuals' global autonomy in liberal societies.[62] We might agree with the latter that those in power have a duty to organize societies in a manner that enables their citizens to (equally) enjoy broad spheres of autonomy, with a variety of alternative options available to pursue different conceptions of the good. However, when we are talking about autonomy in the bioethical context, a plausible account must allow for the possibility that people can make locally autonomous decisions when they face very limited choice sets. For instance, recall the example or Alan from the previous chapter. More broadly, if we claim that agents can only make autonomous decisions if they have a variety of options available to them, then we may be committed to the view that a patient who will die unless they receive a life-saving medical intervention cannot autonomously consent to it; after all, even if the patient in such a case could choose to forgo treatment, if anybody lacks an adequate variety of options, surely this individual does.

6. The Enhancement and Development of Autonomy

In this chapter, I have argued that an adequate theory of autonomy in bioethics should incorporate a practical dimension pertaining to the agent's ability to act

[60] Mackenzie and Sherwin, 'Relational Autonomy, Self-Trust, and Health Care for Patients Who Are Oppressed'.

[61] For a broader discussion of extending the discussion of autonomy in bioethics to consider broader social and relational patterns, see Dodds, 'Choice and Control in Feminist Bioethics'; Jennings, 'Reconceptualizing Autonomy'; Sherwin and Stockdale, 'Whither Bioethics Now?'

[62] Raz, *The Morality of Freedom*; Hurka, 'Why Value Autonomy?'; Oshana, 'Personal Autonomy and Society'.

effectively in pursuit of their ends. In particular, I claimed that having certain sorts of true beliefs will often be necessary for practical autonomy. In turn, this illuminated an important relationship between practical autonomy and the cognitive element of decisional autonomy; the sorts of ignorance that undermine voluntariness are partly defined by considerations pertaining to the agent's ability to act effectively in pursuit of her ends.

I also claimed that there is an important relationship between decisional autonomy and the practical dimensions of autonomy, in so far as agents decide to sustain their motivating desires in the light of their beliefs about what is practically realizable for them. Taken together, these discussions suggest an important reason why an adequate theory of autonomy in bioethics should incorporate a practical dimension. A theory that does not incorporate a practical dimension may lack a principled basis for delimiting the forms of ignorance that undermine voluntariness, and such a theory cannot adequately explain the effect that our beliefs about what we are free to do can have on our decision-making. Below, I shall explain how this discussion also has important implications for considerations of how we can increase autonomy through increasing agents' freedoms.

This concludes my purely theoretical discussion of autonomy. I can now outline the following supplementary rationalist conditions on decisional autonomy and practical autonomy that I have developed over the course of the previous chapters. I have suggested that the two elements of the decisional dimension of autonomy should incorporate the following conditions:

> *Cognitive*: An agent must not be modally precluded from acting in pursuit of her ends by her informational condition, by virtue of theoretical irrationality or a failure to hold decisionally necessary beliefs.
> *Reflective*: The autonomous agent's motivating desires must be rational in the following sense:
> They must:
>
> (a) Be endorsed by preferences that are sustained on the basis of the agent's holding (non-irrational) beliefs that, if true, would give the agent reason to pursue the object of the desire.
> And
> (b) These preferences must cohere with other elements of the agent's character system.

I also suggested the following condition for the practical dimension of autonomy:

> *Practical Dimension*: An agent must have both the positive and negative freedom to act effectively in pursuit of the end that she is motivated to achieve.

To conclude, I shall offer some brief reflections on the extent to which we might seek to enhance autonomy beyond these thresholds by increasing freedom.

It may appear to be straightforwardly true that increasing an agent's freedoms will always serve to enhance their autonomy. In the bioethical context, this sort of assumption is often made by supporters of using biotechnologies for the purposes of human enhancement. For instance, Nick Bostrom claims that an individual who used enhancement technologies would '... enjoy more choice and autonomy in her life, if the modifications were such as to expand her basic capability set' since such blessings 'tend to open more life-plans than they block'.[63] However, there are reasons to doubt this apparently plausible claim.

(i) *Increasing Freedom and Enhancing Autonomy*

Prima facie, the question of how to enhance the practical dimension of autonomy seems quite straightforward; if we increase an agent's positive and negative freedoms so that they are able to act *more* effectively in pursuit of their ends, then this will serve to enhance their practical autonomy. Furthermore, since agents often come to change their preferences over time, they may come to require different sorts of freedoms in order to act effectively in pursuit of ends that they later decide they want to achieve. Accordingly, enjoying a diverse range of freedoms promotes practical autonomy, in so far as having such freedoms accommodates the possibility that agents may come to change their goals.

However, giving an agent additional freedoms or options can in some cases hinder their pursuit of their goals. Most obviously, providing an agent with additional extraneous freedoms may involve replacing their freedom to do what they want. For example, suppose that I have decided that I want to enjoy a particular brand of beer, but my local pub has stopped serving that brand in favour of serving fifty other beers that I do not like; here, increasing my overall positive freedom by increasing the number of beers that I can drink at this pub has failed to enhance my practical autonomy, since doing so has taken away my freedom to enjoy the beer that I actually want to have. Similarly, as I pointed out above, agents sometimes limit their own freedoms in order to enable them to effectively pursue certain goals. This was the point of the example of Odysseus and the Sirens; removing the positive constraints preventing Odysseus from leaving the ship would serve to hinder his ability to pursue his goal of hearing the sirens' song without being lured from his ship. Increasing a freedom that the agent herself has herself chosen to limit (in order to facilitate her pursuit of some goal) would then undermine, rather than enhance her practical autonomy.

Increasing an agent's general freedoms can also affect their freedom to pursue their preferred option without strictly making that option unavailable. The addition of new freedoms may bring with it the cost of a new responsibility, such that the failure to choose the newly available option may now count against the chooser when previously it did not.[64] In such cases, agents may feel unable to pursue their preferred option because of this burden of responsibility. Some have claimed that this sort of phenomenon might arise if voluntary active euthanasia were legalized; the thought here is that giving people the choice to undergo voluntary euthanasia would serve to undermine the practical autonomy of individuals whose preference is to stay alive *as a default option*.[65]

Increasing an agent's freedom to pursue one goal more effectively might also have a negative effect on their ability to pursue other goals. To illustrate, suppose that one

[63] Bostrom, 'In Defense of Posthuman Dignity', 212. See also Malmqvist, 'Reprogenetics and the "Parents Have Always Done It" Argument'.

[64] Dworkin, *The Theory and Practice of Autonomy*, 67.

[65] Velleman, 'Against the Right to Die'.

valued having a successful career in business, and that one would be able to pursue this goal more effectively if one were more ruthless. In this case, whilst becoming more ruthless might enable one to pursue a career goal more effectively, it might also be detrimental to one's pursuit of another valued goal, like being a good parent for example. Accordingly, if increasing an agent's freedom to pursue some goal x is to enhance their practical autonomy, this enhanced freedom must either not diminish their efficacy with respect to their pursuit of another of their goals, y, or, if it would diminish their pursuit of y, then the agent must believe that they have a sufficiently strong reason to pursue x more effectively, at the cost to their efficacy in pursuing y that this might entail.

Perhaps it might be claimed that increasing an agent's freedom will more plausibly serve to increase her decisional autonomy, by virtue of the fact that this will serve to increase the number of competing reasons that they consider in their practical deliberations. In many cases, the more alternatives we entertain when we make a choice, the more that our choice becomes a reflection of our own will, rather than of our restricted circumstances. Susan Wolf puts the point succinctly when she writes:

> The more options and the more reasons for them that one is capable of seeing and understanding, the more fully one can claim one's choices to be one's own.[66]

Of course, one way in which we could increase an agent's decisional autonomy in this sense is by enhancing their ability to compute a greater number of the possible courses of action open to them. Whilst bioethicists are typically interested in the use of biomedical cognitive enhancements to achieve this,[67] we might also do so in far more mundane and familiar ways through the use of traditional forms of education, interpersonal dialogue, and the use of external decision aids.[68] Indeed, in the next chapter, I shall note that one of the challenges we face in the context of informed consent is that human decision-makers are prone to error, irrational biases, and simply being overwhelmed by information. Naturally, if it were possible to reduce these obstacles, then it would be possible for individuals to attend to the reason-giving facts associated with a greater number of alternative options.

Another way in which we could plausibly increase the number of alternatives that an agent considers in their practical deliberations becomes clear when we attend to the relationship between the practical and reflective elements of autonomy. Since agents form their desires in the light of their beliefs about what is practically realizable, and since considering more competing reasons will often increase one's decisional autonomy, we might also seek to enhance an agent's autonomy simply by making more options practically realizable for them; this I take it is the main thrust of Bostrom's point, outlined above. Increasing an agent's freedoms might be understood to indirectly increase an agent's reflective autonomy in so far as it leads them to consider more competing reasons in their deliberations. This is a key mechanism via

[66] Wolf, *Freedom within Reason*, 144.

[67] Maslen, Faulmüller, and Savulescu, 'Pharmacological Cognitive Enhancement—How Neuroscientific Research Could Advance Ethical Debate'; Zohny, 'The Myth of Cognitive Enhancement Drugs'; Bostrom and Sandberg, 'Cognitive Enhancement'.

[68] O'Connor et al., 'Decision Aids for Patients Facing Health Treatment or Screening Decisions'.

which society can shape the limits and contours of individual autonomy, and it is one that is often overlooked in bioethical discussions of the potential impact of biomedical enhancements.[69]

However, it is implausible to claim that increasing an agent's freedoms will always serve to enhance an individual's decisional autonomy in this straightforward way. As I shall explore further in the next chapter, agents are often unable to process the large amount of information that is necessary to making rational choices amongst a vast number of options. Agents faced with a large number of options may simply be overwhelmed by their available choices, and thus become unable to make an autonomous decision;[70] this is the so-called paradox of choice.[71]

Furthermore, the additional choices that are made available will only serve to enhance an agent's autonomy if they are relevant to a choice domain of which the agent is part. For example, if a vegetarian is choosing between two different restaurants, the fact that one restaurant has a wider variety of meat dishes than the other has no direct bearing on which restaurant will offer the vegetarian more autonomy with regards to her decision about what to order. If greater freedom is to meaningfully enhance autonomy, it must make available choices that will enter into her deliberation as plausible alternatives. For that to be the case, they must thus concern outcomes that are good in a reason-implying sense for the agent in question.

Finally, having certain choices may undermine reflective autonomy in so far as they may invite social pressure to conform in a manner that threatens the voluntariness of one's choice.[72] To illustrate this, Gerald Dworkin provides the example of giving university students the option to live in mixed-sex dorms. Whilst it might be claimed that students who do not wish to live in mixed sex dorms could simply choose not to, this fails to acknowledge the point that this new option introduces a social pressure on those who do not want to live in mixed dorms to conform to the social expectation of their peers. Accordingly, having the freedom to choose some alternative may undermine the voluntariness of one's choice, if having that option leaves one open to social pressure that can serve to exert controlling influence over one's decisions. This is importantly related to the way in which changing an individual's option set can take away their preferred status quo default option, since social pressure can often be introduced as a result of that default position being altered (as in the dormitory case).[73]

(ii) *Freedom and the Development of Autonomy*

Freedom may be understood to play a particularly salient role in the development of autonomy in children. Many of the preferences and acceptances that come to constitute our character systems as adults were initially developed unreflectively in

[69] We might also note that increasing an agent's freedoms may serve as a guard against adaptive preference formation.

[70] Dworkin, *The Theory and Practice of Autonomy*, 66.

[71] Schwartz, *The Paradox of Choice*.

[72] Dworkin, *The Theory and Practice of Autonomy*, 68. For a discussion of this issue in the context of human enhancement, see Vincent, *Enhancing Responsibility*; Chandler, 'Autonomy and the Unintended Legal Consequences of Emerging Neurotherapies'; Goold and Maslen, 'Must the Surgeon Take the Pill?'; Juth, 'Enhancement, Autonomy, and Authenticity'.

[73] Velleman, 'Against the Right to Die'.

childhood. However, in accordance with my discussion in Chapter 2, we can nonetheless become autonomous with respect to these features of our characters if we later reflectively choose to sustain them as part of a coherent character system. Of course, it is highly unlikely that this decision will constitute a single, discrete epiphany. Rather, making these kinds of choices is best construed as a continuous (and integral) part of the developmental process. Joel Feinberg captures a similar idea when he writes:

> The child can contribute towards the making of his own self and circumstances in ever-increasing degree. Always the self that contributes to the making of the new self is itself the product of both outside influences and an earlier self that was not quite fully formed.[74]

Beyond aiding the development of the child's general cognitive abilities, parents may cultivate their child's autonomy in a number of other ways. For instance, advocates of the self-determination theory of motivation in psychology have suggested that key aspects of autonomy support include, *inter alia*, providing explanations and rationales for behavioural requests, demonstrating interest in the child's own feelings, and offering children structured choices that reflect their feelings.[75] Furthermore, whilst children clearly lack the capacity to make autonomous decisions in a number of important domains (for reasons I shall explore in Chapter 7) part of respecting the child's autonomy is to recognize that they may deserve some limited domain of autonomy, and to seek to facilitate the exercise of their autonomy when appropriate.

However, one of the most important influences that parents can exert over the development of their child's autonomy is by shaping their freedoms and options. Whilst we may have some autonomy-based reasons to respect some of a child's current choices, respect for a child's autonomy often requires that we do not prematurely foreclose their options. This is the insight underlying Feinberg's claim that children have a 'right to an open future'.[76] The right to an open future is a kind of 'right in trust'; it is a general right that safeguards sophisticated autonomy rights for the child that they cannot currently take advantage of due to a lack of sufficient capacity, but which are to be 'saved' for the child, until she is capable of exercising them later in life. Nonetheless, the right to an open future can be violated before this time if the child's future options are prematurely closed. For instance, although a young child cannot physically exercise the right to reproduce, he will be able to exercise that right in the future, so it would be possible to violate his right in trust to do so by sterilizing him.[77]

One sense in which observing a right to an open future safeguards an individual's autonomy is that it protects freedoms that they may require to pursue autonomously chosen goals at a later point. However, the right has a deeper role for the development of autonomy. One of the key themes of my discussion in this chapter has been that we form and sustain our preferences in the light of what is practically realizable;

[74] Feinberg, *Freedom and Fulfillment*, 96.

[75] Joussemet, Landry, and Koestner, 'A Self-Determination Theory Perspective on Parenting'; Mullin, 'Children, Paternalism and the Development of Autonomy'.

[76] Feinberg, *Freedom and Fulfillment*, ch. 3; see also Davis, 'Genetic Dilemmas and the Child's Right to an Open Future'.

[77] I take this example from Davis, 'Genetic Dilemmas and the Child's Right to an Open Future', 9.

accordingly, options that are foreclosed in childhood will not feature in the individual's later reflections on what sort of things to pursue in life. Furthermore, whilst I have suggested that autonomous choice is possible in the face of extremely limited option sets, I also noted that such limited option sets leave individuals vulnerable to adaptive preference formation, and make it less likely that they will come to reflect on the reasons they have to pursue what they are motivated to pursue. Accordingly, even if we agree that adult individuals can make locally autonomous decisions from a restricted range of option, this is quite compatible with claiming that having a wide range of options is crucial to the *development* of an individual's autonomy, in so far as it is necessary for prompting the development of the capacity to reflect on what one has reason to do, and to make a choice based on one's own reasons. If we are to later take ownership of the motivations and preferences that we develop uncritically in childhood, we must have the freedoms that prompt us to later consider 'why this, and not that'?

Despite its central role in the development of autonomy, the right to an open future should also be understood to be subject to the caveats that I have outlined above; *too* open a future may in fact be detrimental to the future adult's autonomy, for the reasons I have identified. Indeed, it is unrealistic to suppose that we can safeguard an *entirely* open future for any child.[78] The reason for this is that maintaining certain options will normally have the opportunity cost of foreclosing others; for instance, as a child progresses further through their education, they will usually drop certain school subjects (say in the arts) in order to specialize in others (say, in the sciences), thereby foreclosing certain future options. Maintaining some options requires a degree of time and commitment that necessitates ceding other options. Moreover, we might note that parents will quite naturally and perhaps even inadvertently restrict the availability of certain options by virtue of transmitting certain values to their child through their parenting style.

But how should parents make choices about how to shape the contours of a future that we might describe as 'reasonably' open? Above, I noted that individuals may decide to delimit their own future opportunities in this way as an expression of their autonomy. Yet, in the case of children, we must make such choices without knowing what the child will grow up to value. In light of this epistemic obstacle, one might be tempted to capture the spirit of an appeal to the individual's autonomy by invoking the notion of presumed consent. For instance, as part of a larger argument for the claim that prenatal genetic enhancements threaten the child's autonomy, Jürgen Habermas argues that there is a crucial moral difference between genetic therapies and genetic enhancements, on the basis that parents can presume consent for therapies that seek to avoid profound evils which are 'unquestionably extreme, and likely to be rejected by all',[79] but not genetic enhancements. We might similarly invoke the concept of presumed consent in order to determine the boundaries of how we may permissibly shape and delimit our children's future opportunities and capacities.

Notwithstanding other elements of Habermas' wide-ranging critique of prenatal genetic enhancements and their significance for autonomy,[80] let me conclude by

[78] Mills, 'The Child's Right to an Open Future?' [79] Habermas, *The Future of Human Nature*, 43.

[80] For a fuller discussion see Pugh, 'Autonomy, Natality and Freedom'.

explaining why this appeal to presumed consent fails to capture the spirit of autonomy in the manner that its adherents might think. When Habermas' considers whether we can presume consent for a genetic therapy, he asks us to consider whether 'all others' would be likely to consent to the intervention. However, if the concept of presumed consent is to capture the spirit of autonomy's value, then this is simply the wrong question to ask. If we are interested in facilitating the future child's autonomy, then we must consider not what 'all others' would think about the intervention, but rather whether the future child *herself* would consent. Yet, once we recognize this, it becomes clear that a presumed consent approach for interventions that delimit or expand the individual's sphere of freedom will almost inevitably prove both too much and too little. The reason for this is that the values that the child develops, and which would undergird her later retrospective endorsement of the intervention (for which we are now presuming consent), in some cases may depend on whether or not the intervention in question was carried out in the first place. That is, the performance and non-performance of the intervention in question may generate different future values, which in turn might respectively undergird a presumption of retrospective endorsement or repudiation.

The problem of invoking presumed consent to justify the manner in which we shape our children's freedoms is not merely the epistemic issue that we do not know what the child will come to value. Rather, the problem with using this theoretical apparatus to justify an intervention that will significantly affect the future child's freedom, is that whether or not the intervention is performed will likely have a significant influence on the values that the child will come to develop *and her view of the intervention itself.* Yet these are both things that we must ascertain if we are to be serious about 'presuming consent' on behalf of the future child. The theoretical apparatus of presumed consent is thus simply the wrong tool for the job. It can only serve as a useful guide for how to treat children once the child has developed some settled dispositions upon which we might base our presumption; the less developed the child, the less useful the apparatus of presumed consent. In the case of presuming consent on behalf of future children who are currently at an embryonic stage, I suggest that the apparatus of presumed consent can really tell us very little.

In light of this problem with the apparatus of presumed consent, I suggest that the most plausible strategy to adopt in shaping the child's freedoms is to prioritize a child's options to pursue goods that they will have impersonal reason to pursue when they have the capacity to exercise meaningful choice.[81] To safeguard an impersonal good x is not to presume that 'x is what the future adult will come to want, all things considered' or to presume consent per se, Instead, it is to presume that the future adult will have some defeasible reason to pursue x, and that we have reasons to retain that option in the individual's choice set over options associated with outcomes that the future adult may or may not understand to be reason-giving, depending on features of their future selves that are not yet evident to us.

[81] For defence of a broadly similar approach, see Maslen et al., 'Brain Stimulation for Treatment and Enhancement in Children'.

6

Informed Consent, Autonomy, and Beliefs

Over the course of the next three chapters, I shall explicate the implications that my rationalist account of autonomy has for informed consent. Informed consent requirements are ubiquitous in health care, and they are regarded as a cornerstone of ethical medical practice. It is also often treated as a truism that these requirements are to be justified by the principle of respect for autonomy. However, whilst this view is still widely accepted, it has recently been brought into question, with critics suggesting that informed consent requirements are neither necessary nor sufficient for safeguarding individual autonomy in the biomedical sphere.

In the first part of this chapter, I shall suggest that this objection is misplaced, though I shall claim that it suggests that we should revise our understanding of what informed consent requires. In doing so, I shall extend my previous discussion of the relationship between beliefs and autonomous decision-making. This will provide the foundation for the final part of the chapter in which I shall outline a rationalist test of materiality. I suggest that this ought to undergird an adequate standard of information disclosure for informed consent, drawing on the recent hybrid account evidenced in the 2015 Montgomery judgement in the UK.

1. The Structure, Definition, and Limits of Informed Consent

As Gerald Dworkin points out, the doctrine of informed consent is a 'creature of law';[1] it has been developed in various legal domains in which one party sanctions another to perform '... some course of action to which the consented to party would otherwise have no moral right'.[2] The fundamental idea that we aim to capture when we claim that '*A* morally ought to obtain *B*'s informed consent to *A*'s doing *x* to *B*', is that the moral permissibility of *A*'s doing *x* to *B*, is at least partly dependent on the following conditions being met:

(i) *B* must be sufficiently informed with regards to the relevant facts concerning *x* to understand what *x* is (and what consequences are likely to occur as a result of *x*).

[1] Dworkin, *The Theory and Practice of Autonomy*, 101.

[2] Kleinig, 'The Nature of Consent', 8. See also Miller and Wertheimer, *The Ethics of Consent*, for examples of the domains in which informed consent can be invoked.

Autonomy, Rationality, and Contemporary Bioethics. Jonathan Pugh, Oxford University Press (2020).
DOI: 10.1093/oso/9780198858584.001.0001

(ii) On the basis of this information, *B herself* makes the decision to allow *A* to do *x*.[3]

One reason that the moral permissibility of *A*'s doing *x* to *B* can be at least partly dependent on whether *B* has provided informed consent to *x*, is that *B* may bear a right against *A* performing an interference of the sort involved in *x*. For example, *B* could have a right to bodily integrity that affords her protection against *A* performing an injection on her. However, many rights that incorporate these sorts of claims of protection also incorporate a second-order power to waive the claim in question.[4] To authorize a medical treatment in accordance with the requirements of informed consent is to waive the rights of protection that might otherwise preclude the moral permissibility of the intervention. In providing informed consent to an injection, one waives one's claim right against the bodily interference that the injection involves. However, when *A* does *x* without *B*'s informed consent, *B*'s extant claim rights have not been waived, and are still 'in play'. In such cases, if *A* does *x*, *A* will have infringed (and perhaps violated) *B*'s right, and failed in her own duty to refrain from doing *x* to *B* (in the absence of *B*'s waiving that claim). We may also note that in some contexts, *A* may have a *positive* obligation to facilitate *B's* ability to make an autonomous decision about whether to consent to *x*.

For reasons I shall further explain in my discussion of the value of autonomy in Chapter 9, we should not understand the requirements of informed consent to generate or impose a positive obligation *to provide x* to *B*. Consent can involve the waiver of moral protections that would otherwise render a medical intervention impermissible, but there may yet be other moral reasons that can outweigh the autonomy-based reasons we might have to provide *x* to *B*. This is clearest in cases where doing *x* to *B* will have harmful implications for others, or when *x* cannot be provided within a just framework of resource allocation.

However, harm to others is arguably not necessary for the moral or legal impermissibility of doing certain things to *B* to which she has consented. Indeed, in the legal context, even when a person provides valid consent, anything that causes that person actual bodily harm constitutes a criminal offence '... unless it can be shown that the act falls into one of the exceptional circumstances in which consent can provide a defence'.[5] Naturally, 'proper medical treatment'[6] is one such kind of act; however, consent may not provide a legal defence (and perhaps not a moral defence) of certain kinds of harmful action, such as acts of violence within a sado-masochistic context,[7] killing, or medical procedures that fall outside the boundaries of 'proper medical treatment'.[8] In adopting this view, the law appears to accept that we either (i) hold certain claim rights that do not incorporate the corresponding power to waive

[3] There is a considerable debate about whether consent involves only a psychological state, or whether it also requires a behavioural expression. I lack the space to engage with this debate here, but note that medical law on informed consent and mental capacity implicitly reflects a behavioural understanding of consent. For discussion, see Hurd, 'The Moral Magic of Consent'; Kleinig, 'The Nature of Consent'.

[4] Wenar, 'The Nature of Rights'.

[5] Herring, *Medical Law and Ethics*, 150.

[6] For definition of this, see ibid.

[7] Athanassoulis, 'The Role of Consent in Sado-Masochistic Practices'.

[8] Herring, *Medical Law and Ethics*, 204–5.

the claim in question, or (ii) that we have overriding reasons in non-ideal contexts to avoid false positive assessments of decision-making capacity to waive claims against particularly significant harms.[9] However, as I shall suggest in Chapters 7 and 9, there are philosophical grounds for objecting to this understanding of the claim rights we enjoy.

Accordingly, *B* may not have a powerful positive right to medical intervention *x* in many cases, but she may hold a number of negative claim rights that generate a powerful duty for *A* to refrain from doing *x* to *B*, in the absence of *B*'s consent.[10] Since rights are typically understood to provide trumping[11] or exclusionary moral reasons,[12] it will typically take far stronger moral reasons (corresponding to competing rights) to justify overriding the negative obligation to refrain from performing non-consensual treatment on an individual, than it takes to justify overriding the moral reasons we have to provide treatment to which they have consented.[13] That said, even this negative obligation to refrain from non-consensual treatment can plausibly be overridden in certain contexts. For instance, in public health, there may be cases in which this negative obligation can be overridden by the competing rights of others.

I shall consider the strength of these obligations in greater detail in Chapter 9. Here though, I want to turn to a second aspect of informed consent. The moral and legal requirement to obtain *A*'s consent does not apply if *A* lacks the capacities that are necessary for providing valid consent.[14] To give a clear example, there cannot be any meaningful requirement to obtain informed consent to a medical intervention from a patient who is in a coma. Instead, the decision about whether to perform the intervention must instead be guided by alternative approaches, drawing on advance directives and proxy decision-makers (where applicable), and/or an assessment of what is in the patient's best interests.[15] Accordingly, our understanding of the conditions of decision-making capacity will have a considerable bearing on the scope of the requirement to obtain informed consent and to respect individual treatment decisions. I shall consider this aspect of informed consent in the next chapter.

With these limitations in mind, let us reconsider the constitutive conditions of informed consent. The conditions outlined at the beginning of this section can be understood to broadly map onto the two senses of voluntariness that are identified in the Aristotelian distinction outlined in the introductory chapter.

[9] Foster, *Choosing Life, Choosing Death*, 89.

[10] We may also note that an individual's positive rights are typically understood to be weaker than her negative rights. See Foot, *Virtues and Vices*.

[11] Dworkin, 'Rights as Trumps'. [12] Raz, *Practical Reason and Norms*, 35–48.

[13] This partly explains Foster's observation that '[a]utonomy in the medico-legal arena is (rightly) much more concerned with preventing unwanted violations than in guaranteeing a right to positive benefits'. Foster, *Choosing Life, Choosing Death*, 28.

[14] This is compatible with the claim that there is nonetheless a requirement to first take measures to enable the individual to attain decision-making capacity.

[15] In the legal context in England and Wales, these approaches are outlined in Mental Capacity Act 2005. For philosophical and legal discussions of these approaches, see Buchanan and Brock, *Deciding for Others*; Hope, Savulescu, and Hendrick, *Medical Ethics and Law*, 82; Herring, *Medical Law and Ethics*, 171–87.

Although my account of decisional autonomy departs from the standard account of autonomy in bioethics, the Aristotelian distinction can also be broadly understood to implicitly frame the latter. As I explained in the introductory chapter, on the standard view, an agent is autonomous with respect to a particular act if it is carried out:

(1) Intentionally,
(2) With understanding,
 And
(3) Without controlling influences that determine their action.[16]

Importantly for my purposes in this chapter, Faden and Beauchamp suggest that this account of autonomy can be used to undergird a theory of informed consent understood as a form of *autonomous authorization*.[17] On this view, to give informed consent is to perform a specific kind of autonomous action, one that '... authorises a professional to initiate a medical plan for the patient'.[18] A corollary of this is that in order to give informed consent, patients must have certain abilities (such as those required for understanding material information) that are *causally* necessary for meeting the above constitutive conditions of informed consent.[19] To have the abilities in question is to have decision-making capacity, or competence (I shall distinguish the two in the next chapter).

If a patient agrees to a medical procedure without sufficient understanding, unintentionally, or as a result of controlling influence, then their consent may be described as invalid. There is some debate as to whether the concept of invalid consent is morally meaningful. For instance, writing about coerced consent, John Kleinig claims:

> ... invalid consent no more counts as consent than an invalid vote counts as a vote. It has form but no substance. It is, I believe, more accurate to say that although *A* gave his assent, this did not amount to consent.[20]

I believe that Kleinig is correct to say this of coerced consent; the assent of the victim of coercion lacks moral substance because their assent reflects the coercer's authority over them, rather than their own autonomous authorization. However, it would be a mistake to assume that *all* kinds of invalid consent lack any moral substance. In some cases, mere assent can make some moral difference, even if it does not amount to the

[16] Faden and Beauchamp, *A History and Theory of Informed Consent*, 238.

[17] Beauchamp and Childress' *Principles of Biomedical Ethics* defends a similar view. I consider Faden and Beauchamp's *A History and Theory of Informed Consent* in this chapter rather than Beauchamp and Childress' view for two reasons. First, Faden and Beauchamp's work is solely on the nature of informed consent, and so represents a more focused discussion of the concept. Second, the views on informed consent that Beauchamp and Childress have espoused in *The Principles of Biomedical Ethics* have undergone significant revisions over the numerous editions of the book. However, as Walker acknowledges, Faden and Beauchamp's account is very similar to the view that is apparent in editions of *The Principles of Biomedical Ethics* that followed it. Walker, 'Respect for Rational Autonomy', fn. 3.

[18] Faden and Beauchamp, *A History and Theory of Informed Consent*, 278.

[19] Some accounts include competence itself as a condition of informed consent; however, I prefer to avoid this conflation of constitutive and causal conditions.

[20] Kleinig, 'The Nature of Consent', 15.

moral significance denoted by the full-blown authorization of valid consent. To illustrate, there is a stronger moral justification for treating a patient who lacks capacity if they assent to the treatment, than if they dissent to it.[21] One reason for this is that a treatment to which a patient has dissented is likely to be far more distressing for the patient. Furthermore, a process of assent can be important because it allows a patient who lacks capacity to have at least some sort of an input into a decision that affects them, an input that is commensurate with the capacities that they do have.[22]

Faden and Beauchamp distinguish informed consent as autonomous authorization from a second institutional sense of informed consent, which pertains to the rules and policies that actually govern informed consent in institutional contexts. What qualifies as an informed consent in this second sense, may or may not amount to the sort of act of autonomous authorization that the first sense means to identify.[23] For instance, there may be cases in which minors may have the capacity to autonomously authorize a medical procedure (and thus provide valid consent in accordance with the first sense), and yet this decision will not be legally recognized as a token of valid consent (in the second sense).[24]

The institutional sense can incorporate a wide range of conceptions of what 'informed consent' might require. For the purposes of my discussion in the second half of this chapter, it is important to be clear about two different institutional senses of 'informed' consent, which are required to provide sufficient protection against different kinds of torts in medical law, namely battery and negligence.[25] First, a physician can be liable to be charged with battery if she touches a patient *without* their valid consent. As I have discussed in the first part of this book, the voluntariness of a patient's decision can be undermined in a manner that may serve to invalidate their consent by controlling influences such as coercion, deception, and manipulation. This much is straightforward; the more complex question is what degree of understanding a patient must have in order to provide valid consent in this institutional sense. Following the case of *Chatterton v Gerson* (1981), the answer to this question in England and Wales is that the patient must be 'informed in broad terms of the nature of the procedure'.[26] As Maclean points out, it is relatively easy for physicians

[21] This is recognized in the law in various ways. In determining what is in the best interests of a patient who lacks capacity, physicians have to take into account the person's current views and feelings. Herring, *Medical Law and Ethics*, 177; Mental Capacity Act 2005, section 4. It is also particularly salient in the Scottish law regarding electro-convulsive therapy (ECT) for patients who lack capacity and who have been diagnosed with a mental disorder. Scottish Government, Mental Health (Care and Treatment) (Scotland) Act 2003 (2003), s. 237–9. https://www.legislation.gov.uk/asp/2003/13/contents.

[22] Sibley, Sheehan, and Pollard, 'Assent Is Not Consent'.

[23] Faden and Beauchamp, *A History and Theory of Informed Consent*, 276–7.

[24] This puts a somewhat simplistic gloss on the hugely complex question of when minors can provide valid consent to medical treatment. For further discussion, see Herring, *Medical Law and Ethics*, 187–94; Hope, Savulescu, and Hendrick, *Medical Ethics and Law*, ch. 10.

[25] It would be possible for a physician to be charged with the *criminal* offence of battery in extreme cases, where they have acted maliciously. However, most cases of battery in the medical context are civil rather than criminal cases. Hope, Savulescu, and Hendrick, *Medical Ethics and Law*, 71; Herring, *Medical Law and Ethics*, 150–2.

[26] *Chatterton v Gerson* at 265.

to satisfy this informational requirement in disclosure, and the law allows for considerable leeway in its interpretation of the 'broad nature' of medical interventions.[27]

However, whilst consent grounded by this minimal degree of understanding can be legally valid, and thus invoked to avoid liability to a charge of battery, it is not sufficient to avoid liability to medical negligence. A claim of medical negligence can be raised against a physician if (i) she has failed in her duty of care to the patient and (ii) this failure resulted in the patient suffering a harm. In most cases, actions of battery and negligence can often be distinguished quite easily, because considerations of whether a patient has provided valid consent are often quite distinct from whether the physician harmed a patient by failing to observe her duty of care. However, this distinction can be somewhat muddied by the fact that the physician's duty of care is understood to incorporate a duty to inform her patient of features of the treatment that go beyond its 'broad nature'. For instance, a claim of negligence may be grounded by the fact that the physician neglected to inform the patient of certain risks of a medical procedure, or alternative treatment options. Such information goes beyond that which is required for understanding the treatment in 'broad terms'.

There are interesting questions about these different requirements of information disclosure across these two institutional senses of informed consent, and how they might relate to our understanding of autonomous decision-making. I shall consider these questions in the second half of this chapter. At this point though, we may acknowledge that it is possible to draw a distinction between the 'valid consent' that is grounded by the minimal understanding of the broad nature of a proposed treatment and (ii) the 'substantially informed consent' that can be absent in this case, and which may provide partial grounds for a claim of medical negligence.[28]

This distinction is not always recognized in bioethical discussions of informed consent.[29] However, it is important to clarify it here, as it represents a source of potential confusion given the different ways in which scholars use the language of consent. Following the judge in *Chatterton v Gerson*, some scholars use the term 'real consent' to refer to what I have termed 'valid consent', and the term 'informed consent' to refer to the sort of consent that must be obtained in order to forestall claims of medical negligence.[30] This later terminology is somewhat unfortunate, as it may be thought to have the implication that valid or 'real' consent is not 'informed'. As I have explained above though this is a mistake; valid consent must be informed to *some* (albeit lesser) degree.

As such, when I need to refer specifically to the institutional sense of informed consent in my discussion below, I shall instead distinguish the two forms of consent that are operative in discussions of battery and negligence as 'valid consent' and 'substantially informed consent' respectively. Crucially though, in England and

[27] Maclean, 'The Doctrine of Informed Consent', 392–3. [28] Ibid.

[29] For one notable exception, see Walker, 'Informed Consent and the Requirement to Ensure Understanding'.

[30] Maclean, 'The Doctrine of Informed Consent'.

Wales, consent can be valid without being what I have called 'substantially informed'.[31]

2. Autonomy-Based Justifications of Informed Consent

The above discussion indicates that it is important to be clear about the sense of consent that one means to invoke, when seeking to justify a particular criterion of informed consent by appealing to the principle of respect for autonomy. In defining the provision of consent as a specific kind of autonomous action in the first sense, Faden and Beauchamp draw an inextricable link between consent and the principle of respect for autonomy. However, this sense is not co-extensive with the second institutional sense of informed consent, and we should not assume that they share the same justification.

Indeed, the development of the institutional sense of informed consent in the legal context raises significant challenges for any philosophical investigation into the topic. As Richard Ashcroft notes, we should not expect to find elusive, abstract philosophical concepts such as autonomy in the law, as the law requires more concrete concepts that can be tested and consistently applied in litigation.[32] We might also add to Ashcroft's claims that the philosophical bioethicist has something of an easy way out of complex debates in medical law; upon finding that the law fails to reflect a philosophical principle upon which it purports to be based, they can simply say 'so much the worse for the law'. However, this is not a particularly useful practical avenue for the medical lawyer who has to address these issues whilst working within this framework, which is shaped by a number of competing and conflicting justifications beyond philosophically pure abstract principles. In particular, the institutional sense of informed consent may need to serve a wide range of purposes whilst being constrained by the practical realities of the clinical encounter. In turn, this may legitimize employing lower thresholds for understanding, disclosure, and capacity than might be required for a decision to qualify as an autonomous authorization.[33] However, whilst acknowledging this, the concept of autonomy can still coherently play some, perhaps non-exhaustive role in its justification. It can serve as a guiding value that we may invoke to shape the contours of the institutional requirements of informed consent, so that they better serve the autonomy of patients, amongst the other purposes that they are intended to fulfil.

With that said, I shall begin by framing my discussion by considering the relationship between autonomy and the first sense of informed consent as a form of autonomous authorization. On this first sense, the relationship between informed consent and autonomy is straightforward; to provide informed consent is just to make a certain kind of autonomous decision, a decision to authorize a particular medical treatment. The positive obligation imposed by the requirement to obtain informed consent can be understood to amount to an obligation to help facilitate

[31] As such, this jurisdiction does not observe the so called 'doctrine of informed consent'. Herring, *Medical Law and Ethics*, 158.

[32] Ashcroft, 'Law and the Perils of Philosophical Grafts'.

[33] Beauchamp and Childress, *Principles of Biomedical Ethics*, 123.

autonomous decision-making, and the negative obligation to ensure that medical interventions do not involve the infringement of rights that have not been waived by their holders.

The rationalist account of autonomy that I have developed is meant to supplement the standard account of autonomy. Indeed, one of the strengths of the rationalist approach that I have developed over the course of the preceding chapters is that it can add further explanatory depth to the conditions laid out in the standard account. For instance, in the previous chapters, I have explained how my rationalist approach can provide a principled account of how the different forms of controlling influence captured by condition (3) above undermine voluntariness. Consider also condition (1). Faden and Beauchamp claim that an action must be intentional in order for it to be autonomous, and that '... an intentional action is action willed in accordance with a plan'.[34] Among the category of non-intentional acts, they include:

> ... things that persons do inadvertently, certain habitual behaviours, and instances of so called occurrent coercion in which a person is physically forced by another to do something.[35]

Intentional action understood in this way can also be interpreted as a necessary condition of autonomy on the account that I have defended. To will an action in accordance with a plan, can be understood as willing action in accordance with one's beliefs about what one has reason to pursue; moreover, the non-intentional actions delineated in the above quotation are also inimical to acting on the basis of this sort of rational deliberation.

The criterion of understanding is also congruous with the account that I developed in the first half of the book. To recap, I have argued that there can be decisionally necessary beliefs, in the sense that one must hold certain true beliefs about central features of one's choice in order to make an autonomous decision in that context. Furthermore, I have argued that failing to abide by norms of theoretical rationality can undermine the sort of understanding that autonomy requires, in the sense that it jeopardizes one's ability to assess the extent to which a particular belief coheres with one's other beliefs about both descriptive and evaluative features of the world.

One of my aims in this chapter is to provide more details about the implications of my theory for the scope of the criterion of understanding. Here though, we may simply acknowledge that Beauchamp and Childress claim that in order to autonomously authorize a medical procedure, the patient must have *substantial*, but not full understanding. They note that the patient's understanding of 'diagnoses, prognoses, the nature and purpose of the intervention, alternatives, risks and benefits, and recommendations' is 'typically essential' for such understanding.[36] Notice then that the criterion of understanding employed by Beauchamp and Childress for autonomous authorization goes beyond that required by 'valid consent' in the institutional sense. Instead, it bears a resemblance to that which is required by the doctrine of informed consent in the institutional sense, or what I have called 'substantially informed consent'. I shall return to this point below.

[34] Herring, *Medical Law and Ethics*, 187–94. [35] Ibid.

[36] Beauchamp and Childress, *Principles of Biomedical Ethics*, 132.

Despite this significant degree of congruence with the standard account, my rationalist theory of autonomy departs from this view by advocating that we should supplement the standard account with rationality conditions of the sort set out in Chapter 2. Thus, I suggest that the following ought to be understood as a necessary condition of the voluntariness element of informed consent:

> *Rationality Condition*: If an agent is to provide informed consent to some intervention, then they must also endorse their desire to undergo that intervention with a personally authorized preference.

The condition has significant implications for what we should want the informed consent process to achieve, if it is to facilitate autonomous decision-making. Merely ensuring the sufficient understanding of material information is not enough to facilitate autonomous decision-making, if that understanding remains unconnected to the patient's values. The condition thus speaks against viewing the patient as a passive recipient of disclosure who is 'to be informed'; instead, it speaks in favour of the patient actively contributing to the process, so that physicians can tailor disclosure to what matters to the patient, given her values. Of course, by adding this condition, I am implicitly widening the gap between what informed consent as an autonomous authorization should look like, and what informed consent in the institutional sense currently requires.

Informed consent in this first sense can thus facilitate autonomous decision-making, in so far as the process of informed consent helps to enable individuals to decide to authorize medical procedures in accordance with the above sorts of conditions. However, it also has an important role to play in respecting the agent's autonomous preferences. It has this role by virtue of the negative obligation the requirement to obtain consent imposes on others to refrain from certain kinds of action, in the absence of consent. In this chapter, I shall be interested primarily in the justification of informed consent in the context of medical practice, when that is understood to refer only to the provision of medical therapy but *not* the performance of non-therapeutic research.[37] However, by distinguishing the ways in which individuals can face both internal and external impediments to autonomy, and by stressing the importance of the rational endorsement of one's preferences to autonomy, the account that I have delineated serves to highlight an illuminating contrast between the justification of informed consent requirements in the context of non-therapeutic medical research, and the justification of informed consent requirements in medical practice.

It is commonly claimed that there is an important distinction between medical research and therapy due to the primary aims of each activity.[38] For instance, the

[37] The research context raises different questions about appropriate standards of understanding and disclosure. For analysis, see Sreenivasan, 'Does Informed Consent to Research Require Comprehension?'; Bromwich, 'Understanding, Interests and Informed Consent'; Bromwich and Millum, 'Disclosure and Consent to Medical Research Participation'.

[38] See Miller and Brody, 'Clinical Equipoise and the Incoherence of Research Ethics' for a discussion of the different ethical norms governing medical research and therapy. However, see Beauchamp, 'Viewpoint' for an argument against drawing a hard and fast distinction between research and therapy.

Belmont Report defines medical therapies (in part) as 'interventions . . . designed solely to enhance the well-being of an individual patient . . . ' whilst it defines medical research (in part) as 'an activity designed to test a hypothesis, permit conclusions to be drawn, and thereby to develop or contribute to generalizable knowledge'.[39]

The prioritization of generalizable knowledge in scientific research suggests that the intended primary beneficiaries of an individual's participation in a research study are the third parties who stand to benefit from this knowledge. The value of 'generalizable knowledge' in this context may be understood as a proxy for the interests of society at large, and future patients. Accordingly, it seems that one of the primary purposes of informed consent in the research context, is that it affords some protection to potential subjects from being put at risk of harm (broadly construed), or having their rights violated on the basis of broadly consequentialist justifications of research.

This is clearest in Phase I trials of a novel medical intervention, in which healthy volunteers are provided with sub-therapeutic doses of an intervention in order to establish its safety. Participants in such trials are put at risk of harm without any real possibility of benefiting from the intervention itself, although they may be benefited indirectly by payment for their participation.[40] In this way, informed consent requirements can be understood as safeguarding autonomy, in so far as they help to ensure that it is the individual herself who determines whether she wants to waive her claim rights against bodily interference (amongst others), and thereby put herself at risk of the harm that the research might entail for the benefit of others (or, if payment is offered, for indirect benefit). When the individual subject's autonomy conflicts with the interests of future patients, the former trumps the latter.[41]

Informed consent in the context of medical practice partly plays a similar role, in so far as it serves to protect patients from being forced into receiving treatments that might serve another party's interests rather than their own.[42] However, informed consent also plays a further role in medical practice that is not applicable in the context of non-therapeutic medical research, in so far as the interventions for which consent is being solicited in the former context are primarily intended to directly benefit the patient herself. Indeed, we may notice that the definition of medical practice quoted above stresses that the aim of a therapeutic intervention is to enhance the recipient's own *well-being*. Part of the reason that respecting autonomy is important in this context is that it gives the patient a say in the matter of what is really in their own interests, in the light of their own desires and values.

The importance of this is made clear once it is observed that patients can differ from their physicians in their conclusions about what they have strongest self-interested reason to do, even in view of the same relevant descriptive facts. To illustrate, consider this example:

[39] The Belmont Report.

[40] As I explored in Chapter 4, such payment can raise the spectre of coercion; see Emanuel and Miller, 'Money and Distorted Ethical Judgments about Research'.

[41] World Medical Association Declaration of Helsinki.

[42] For a relevant legal example of this, see *Appleton v Garrett* – Case Summary.

Suppose that Joe is undergoing an operation to remove a tumour from his diaphragm. An anaesthetist consults him regarding his post-operative analgesia. The efficiency of analgesia in Joe's case is crucial, since if the analgesia is not effective, it is likely that Joe's lung will collapse and lead to the development of a potentially fatal pneumonia. Joe is given the choice between an analgesic that poses a very small risk of spinal cord damage (such as a thoracic epidural), and one that is considerably less effective but which poses no such risk (such as an intravenous narcotic infusion).[43]

Here, the thoracic epidural is medically indicated; however, Joe might still rationally choose to receive an intravenous narcotic infusion instead, if he places sufficient weight on the value of pursuits that involve physical activity. For example, suppose that Joe is a professional athlete, and believes that his life would not be worth living if he became paralysed. In such a case, the possibility that the more effective analgesia could paralyse Joe might give him reason to believe that the less effective analgesia, which did not pose this risk of paralysis, was the preferable treatment option.

This case suggests that the role of informed consent requirements in medical practice is not merely to protect the patient from competing third-party interests, but also to ensure that the treatment that the patient receives is in accordance with what they want for themselves; and this may or may not coincide with what the physician believes is in the patient's best interests. Even if rational agents agree that they have some reason to purse an outcome, this does not entail that they will agree on the strength of that reason, relative to their reasons to pursue other outcomes.[44]

This observation goes some way towards explaining the intuitive pull of the claim that informed consent in medical practice can be justified in large part by an appeal to the principle of respect for autonomy, at least on the broadly Millian understanding that I have been developing in this book. Informed consent requirements can be understood as facilitating the patient's self-governance, not just because they protect the patient from controlling forces, or from their being exploited in the interests of others. They also give the patient the power to make their own treatment decisions, in accordance with their assessment of the strength of the reasons that they have to pursue different outcomes. At least part of the importance we attribute to informed consent can thus be construed as a reflection of the Millian thought that I highlighted in the introduction of this book, namely that we value laying out our own mode of our existence, even if our way of doing so is not prudentially optimific by third-party standards.

The view that the moral significance of informed consent is to be justified by an appeal to the value of patient autonomy has often been treated almost as a truism in bioethics. Indeed, as I illustrated above, Faden and Beauchamp simply define informed consent as a type of autonomous authorization, whilst autonomy has elsewhere been described as the 'ultimate moral foundation'[45] of informed consent. However, it is important to be clear about the extent of this claim, at least as I shall understand it in this chapter. As I suggested above, the moral significance of

[43] Savulescu, 'Rational Non-Interventional Paternalism', 327.

[44] For a discussion of how this point featured in the justification of the Montgomery judgement discussed below, see Herring et al., 'Elbow Room for Best Practice?', 8–9.

[45] Young, 'Informed Consent and Autonomy', 441.

informed consent in this sense can be grounded in large part by the broadly Millian conception of autonomy that I have been developing in this book. Yet, there are two important mistakes that we must avoid here.

First, it would be a mistake to assume that the Millian conception of autonomy provides the *only* justification for the first sense of informed consent that I have primarily been considering so far. There is a considerable literature that seeks to explore the ways in which Kantian conceptions of autonomy can also ground informed consent requirements. These approaches particularly focus on the role that such requirements play in ensuring that individuals are respected as ends in themselves, in a manner that is consummate with their human dignity.[46] The Kantian approach thus focuses on the role that informed consent plays in respecting the supreme moral status of rational agents; in contrast, the Millian approach places emphasis on the manner in which informed consent facilitates the agent's pursuit of their own conception of the good life. Nonetheless, these different forms of justification can both plausibly lend support to informed consent in its non-institutional sense.

Second, and perhaps more importantly, it would also be a mistake to claim that either (or indeed both) of these conceptions of autonomy can provide the sole justification of informed consent in its second *institutional* sense. Autonomy-based justifications of informed consent have sometimes been criticized on this score, with philosophers pointing to examples in which it appears that our reasons to abide by informed consent requirements are not best understood as being grounded by considerations of autonomy.[47] For example, one clear legal function of informed consent in the medical context is that it serves to provide physicians with a record of what has occurred in the course of providing treatment, a resource to which they can appeal to in cases of litigation.[48] It has also been suggested that informed consent procedures are integral to establishing a relationship of trust between doctors and patients,[49] or safeguarding a personal sphere of self-ownership that is not best understood in terms of autonomy.[50]

Although there is a great deal of truth in this general criticism, it is somewhat perplexing as an objection to autonomy-based justifications of informed consent. The fact that there may also be non-autonomy based justifications of informed consent in the institutional sense, speaks little against the claim that it may nonetheless derive an integral part of its justification from the fact that it *does* facilitate and enable us to abide by the principle of respect for individual autonomy, in a considerable number of cases.

To illustrate this point, consider David Archard's criticism of the relationship between autonomy and informed consent. Archard offers the example of 'inserting a

[46] Donagan, 'Informed Consent in Therapy and Experimentation'.

[47] See Taylor, *Practical Autonomy and Bioethics*, 133; Dworkin, *The Theory and Practice of Autonomy*, 103; Archard, 'Informed Consent'.

[48] Brock, *Life and Death*, 47–8.

[49] O'Neill, *Autonomy and Trust in Bioethics*, 145; see also Bok, *Lying*, 11, 26–7, and 63; Jackson, 'Telling the Truth', 491. For recent challenges to this view, see Eyal, 'Using Informed Consent to Save Trust'.

[50] Archard, 'Informed Consent'.

swab into someone's mouth without her agreement, yet harmlessly, painlessly, and without coercion or deception'.[51] He suggests that a Millian conception of autonomy cannot provide a sufficient explanation of the wrong involved in this failure to observe the requirements of informed consent because 'the value of autonomy is to be found in *the leading of lives*'.[52] As such, we only have autonomy-based reasons to respect decisions regarding 'critical life-choices'. Accordingly, we must thus appeal to a right against bodily trespass to cash out the wrong involved in the swab example.

I am somewhat sceptical of Archard's suggestion that a putative right to bodily trespass can be entirely divorced from such an autonomy-based justification. This might be true of some rights, particularly those that incorporate the Hohfeldian incident of a *claim* but not the *power* to waive that claim.[53] The thought underlying such putative unwaivable rights is that both autonomous and non-autonomous individuals have a very strong interest against certain kinds of interference that might justify affording them this unwaivable claim to protection. However, many rights (including the right against bodily trespass) incorporate both a claim to protection *and* the second-order power to waive that claim, at least in so far as the right is held by an autonomous individual.[54] Crucially though, it is difficult to see how the *powers* incorporated in these rights can be justified without some appeal to the value of autonomy (even if the claims themselves might be so justified). Indeed, it seems that the power to waive one's claim should only be granted authority if the right-bearer has decided to waive their claim in a locally autonomous fashion. In this way, considerations of local autonomy seem highly relevant to our understanding of aspects of these rights and their justification.[55]

Notwithstanding this point about the relationship between rights and autonomy, even if we agree with Archard that the wrong involved in cases of minor bodily trespass is entirely divorced from considerations of autonomy, it is clear that the requirement to obtain informed consent can be, and indeed *is* invoked in many critical life-choices that do generate strong autonomy-based reasons. The example of Joe above is just one case in point, in which the value of respecting Joe's choice is integral to the value of his leading his own life.

Accordingly, we should qualify the autonomy-based justification of informed consent with the caveat that autonomy is not the *only* justification of the informed consent in its institutional sense, even if it does provide a strong justification for it in many cases. Yet, even when the view is qualified with this caveat, some philosophers have further objected that informed consent in the institutional sense cannot be justified by an appeal to respect for autonomy, because it is not and cannot be sufficient for that purpose. For instance, Neil Manson and Onora O'Neill have argued that this is a decisive problem with justifying informed consent procedures by appealing to the principle of respect for autonomy. The problem is that such requirements fail to ensure that patients will choose autonomously; they only require that physicians respect the choices that the patient actually makes, whether or not

[51] Ibid., 19. [52] Ibid., 21. [53] Wenar, 'The Nature of Rights'. [54] Ibid.

[55] One explanation of this might be that the power incorporated into the right is grounded by considerations of agential authority, whilst the claim itself is justified by considerations of interest. For discussion of the basis of rights, see ibid.

this choice is autonomous or rational.[56] Not only that, but Manson and O'Neill also claim that if informed consent requirements were reformulated so that they would protect only rational, autonomous choices, then they would become too demanding for the vast majority of patients.[57]

Manson and O'Neill invoke a broad understanding of 'rational choice' here, claiming that theories of autonomy can understand rational choice as 'reflectively evaluated, or endorsed by second order desires';[58] we may note that this understanding is compatible with many of the theories that I surveyed (and rejected) in Chapter 2. However, it is clear that the standard view of autonomy, which is the primary target of their attack, does not incorporate conditions pertaining to the rationality of the patient's choice, even on this broad understanding. Indeed, advocates of the standard view of autonomy explicitly reject the suggestion that a theory of autonomy should incorporate a condition that requires that the patient's choice be consistent with their reflectively accepted values, because such a condition would, they claim, make autonomy too demanding.[59]

As the preceding chapters of this book should make clear, I believe that Manson and O'Neill are correct to claim that the standard view of autonomy and informed consent is inadequate. If we are to claim that a primary purpose of informed consent requirements is to safeguard patient autonomy, then we should incorporate conditions pertaining to the *rationality* of the patient's choice into our theory of informed consent. In view of the fact that Manson and O'Neill reject this solution (because it would, they claim, make the standards of informed consent too demanding), two strategies are possible. First, we could abandon the project of justifying informed consent requirements by an appeal to the principle of respect for autonomy. This is the strategy that Manson and O'Neill adopt; they argue that we ought to view an agent's provision of consent to a procedure as a waiver of an ethical and/or legal norm against performing the act in question, in limited ways in a particular context.[60] On the other hand, we might maintain that informed consent requirements are to be justified by an appeal to the principle of respect for autonomy, and supplement informed consent requirements with conditions that will facilitate rational choice, but which will not render informed consent requirements too demanding.

Over the course of the next two chapters, I shall adopt the latter strategy.[61] Again, it is important to be clear about the scope of what I shall attempt to claim. *Contra*

[56] Manson and O'Neill, *Rethinking Informed Consent in Bioethics*, 21. More recently, in a similar vein, Shlomo Cohen has claimed that 'conceptions of autonomy cannot provide practical ethical guidelines generally or specifically for informed consent'. Cohen, 'A Philosophical Misunderstanding at the Basis of Opposition to Nudging', 39.

[57] Manson and O'Neill, *Rethinking Informed Consent in Bioethics*, 21.

[58] Ibid.

[59] Faden and Beauchamp, *A History and Theory of Informed Consent*, 262–4; Beauchamp and Childress, *Principles of Biomedical Ethics*, 103.

[60] Manson and O'Neill, *Rethinking Informed Consent in Bioethics*, 72. See also 69–84.

[61] Though I cannot argue fully for why I reject Manson and O'Neill's strategy here, I shall sketch my main points of disagreement. First, it is not clear that their theory really divorces autonomy from informed consent in the way that they claim; after all, if consent transactions are meant to signify the patient's waiving a significant legal or ethical norm, it must surely be the case that the patient should still be autonomous with respect to their decision to waive that norm. Manson and O'Neill do warn against the possibility of bogus consent, in which consent is solicited in ways that violate ethical norms; they give the

Manson and O'Neill, requiring that an adequate conception of informed consent must *ensure* that patients make autonomous choices is an unreasonably high bar. Such a view overlooks the fact that the individual herself has an indispensable role to play in their own autonomy; disclosure, and the absence of controlling influences on choice means nothing for the patient's autonomy, if she herself is either unwilling or unable to contribute to the decision-making process. It is thus unfeasible to demand that informed consent in the institutional sense must alone *ensure* that patients make autonomous decisions; the best that we can hope for is that it will *facilitate* the patient's making an autonomous decision, and ensure that the autonomous decisions that she does make are respected.

As I suggested above, the main source of objection to the sort of rationality condition that I have proposed is that it would make the conditions of informed consent too demanding. This is a serious objection that the account must answer. However, it is an objection concerning the *causal* conditions of autonomy and the standards of capacity that they imply, rather than an objection to the rationality condition itself as a *constitutive* condition of autonomy and informed consent. As such, I shall postpone my consideration of it until I am in a position to discuss the issue of capacity in the following chapter. In the next section, I shall turn to further consider the role of autonomy in justifying informed consent in the institutional sense, by considering its relationship to 'valid consent' and 'substantially informed consent', as they are distinguished in the context of medical law governing claims of battery and negligence.

3. Battery, Negligence, Beliefs, and Decisional Autonomy

In the legal domain, questions pertaining to informed consent have been framed not so much in terms of what patients need to *understand* in order to be autonomous with respect to their treatment decision, but rather in terms of what physicians need to *disclose*.[62] Whilst it is easier to enforce a legal requirement to disclose information than it is to enforce a requirement to ensure understanding, the former receives only limited justification from considerations of autonomy. First, disclosing information to a patient may not be necessary for safeguarding autonomous decision-making in some cases. Most obviously, this can be so if the patient is *already* aware of that information. For example, it seems that I could provide valid consent to a physician's application of a bandage to my wound, without their having disclosed to me that I am bleeding profusely, and that applying a bandage to a wound will help to stop the bleeding.

examples of consent following coercion, force, and duress as examples of bogus consent. See ibid., 92. However, what, we might ask is the basis for *these* ethical norms? Whilst Manson and O'Neill appeal to a principled Kantian sense of autonomy to ground such norms, an alternative plausible explanation would be that coercion, force, and duress are wrong because they violate the patient's autonomy in the Millian sense that I have outlined (see also O'Neill, *Autonomy and Trust in Bioethics*, ch. 4, especially 83–6).

[62] See Beauchamp and Childress, *Principles of Biomedical Ethics*, 2nd edition, 67.

This example suggests that the sort of understanding that is required for patients to make autonomous decisions can sometimes be implicitly assumed with some justification, and patients can in some cases provide tacit consent that authorizes a procedure, without going through the rigmarole of institutional procedures of informed consent. Of course, given the expertise gap between physicians and their patients, and since physicians cannot be certain about their patients' prior knowledge, patients will often need to have information disclosed to them. However, it would also be a mistake to assume that disclosure of relevant information is *sufficient* to ensure the degree of understanding that is necessary for autonomous decision-making. Even competent patients may struggle to process the information presented to them if it is not adequately explained to them. Indeed, this speaks to a considerable tension in informed consent with which I shall be concerned in this chapter. The disclosure of information that may be material to a patient's decision may also serve to undermine the patient's ability to make an autonomous decision in that same context, for reasons I shall explain.

Disclosure, then, is neither a necessary nor sufficient condition of ensuring the degree of understanding that is required for autonomous decision-making. That said, it is perhaps the most powerful tool at our disposal when thinking about how best to facilitate autonomous decision-making in the institutional context. This is particularly so in the context of medicine, in which there is a significant expertise gap between the parties soliciting and providing consent.

As I explained above, informed consent in the institutional sense draws a distinction between the amount of information that must be disclosed (and understood) in order for a patient to provide 'valid consent', and that which must be disclosed (and understood) in order for the patient to provide 'substantially informed consent' to the intervention. Recall that a physician's receipt of the patient's 'valid consent' to an intervention can be invoked as a defence against battery, whilst a physician must have obtained 'substantially informed consent' in order to defend themselves from claims of negligence.

The torts of battery and negligence can cover quite separate kinds of action, and I do not have space to list the various differences between the two here.[63] However, these two legal categories somewhat overlap when it comes to the question of information disclosure in the medical context.[64] Indeed, the kind of information of which the patient is ignorant when they agree to undergo a procedure, can make all the difference between whether the patient has given valid consent or not. The question I want to consider in the remainder of this section is whether there are any autonomy-based reasons to support the way in which the law stipulates the lower threshold of understanding required for valid consent, in comparison to the standard deployed for claims of negligence.

Without discounting the possibility of other justifications, I want to suggest that considerations of autonomy do lend support to the distinction between what I have called 'valid consent' and 'substantially informed consent'. To recap some arguments

[63] For discussion, see Herring, *Medical Law and Ethics*, 152–3.

[64] For an argument that the Montgomery judgement represents a way in which the legal distinction between risk disclosure and consent is breaking down, see Herring et al., 'Elbow Room for Best Practice?'

I made in the preceding chapters, I have argued that there is a cognitive element of decisional autonomy; if an agent holds certain false beliefs, or fails to hold certain true beliefs, they may be precluded from making certain decisions voluntarily in that context. This will be so if the beliefs in question are decisionally necessary; I also suggested a modal test that may be employed to identify some of these beliefs.

The individual's failure to hold such beliefs undermines their decisional autonomy, regardless of how this came to be the case, be it through intentional third-party deception, or the non-intentional omission of true information. Accordingly, on the account that I have developed, if a physician performs a medical procedure on the basis of a token of consent that is grounded by a lack of understanding of this key information, it can be plausible to say that the physician has not only failed to act in accordance with their duty of care; they have also performed a medical procedure on the basis of a non-voluntary, and thus invalid token of consent.

Crucially though, I argued that the absence of many true beliefs is compatible with decisional autonomy. Our decisional autonomy is not undermined by our lack of true beliefs about future states of affairs, or the actual, rather than predicted, consequences of our choices. Of course, our practical autonomy may be enhanced by holding such beliefs; we will be more likely to achieve our goals if our beliefs about these matters are true. However, our ignorance of these matters does not render our decisions at the point of choice non-voluntary.

In light of the above recap, the key question for my purposes here is whether the legal distinction between valid consent and substantially informed consent maps onto the distinction between beliefs that are decisionally necessary, and those that are not. I believe that it does. To see why, recall that in order for a patient to provide valid consent to a medical procedure, the law states that they must be informed 'in broad terms of the nature of the procedure'. On my view, the reason that such ignorance can be said to be incompatible with valid consent, is that it modally precludes the patient from achieving their ends, by divorcing the decision they make from the values that are actually operative in their particular choice context. A patient who agrees to undergo a vasectomy without understanding that it will render him infertile does not provide valid consent to the procedure, because their understanding of the intervention is so poor that their informational condition precludes them from choosing what to do in accordance with their own values.[65]

In contrast, the sort of further information that is required for 'substantially informed consent' (but not merely 'valid consent') is not captured by this modal test. In previous chapters, I have argued that the concept of valid consent must be compatible with the fact that many patients must make treatment decisions in the light of severely restricted choices. As such, it seems that ignorance about alternative treatment options can be compatible with valid consent, even if not substantially informed consent. Furthermore, most information pertaining to risk will not be captured by the modal test that we can use to identify decisionally necessary beliefs, since there is typically a close relationship between modal possibility and probability.

[65] This also accounts for why the therapeutic misconception is such a problem for consent in medical research. See Henderson et al., 'Clinical Trials and Medical Care'.

This means that ignorance about risk cannot be understood to modally preclude an individual from acting effectively in pursuit of their ends, as I defined this in the previous chapter. Even though the risk-event that actually occurs in this world might have precluded the individual from achieving their ends in this world, there is another nearby possible world in which this risk-event does not eventuate. Indeed, Duncan Pritchard argues that very low-probability events can nonetheless be modally close.[66] Thus, one is not modally precluded from achieving one's ends by ignorance about the degree of risk attending different courses of action.

That said, in discussing how beliefs about risk can affect the voluntariness of our decisions, it is important to be clear that 'ignorance about risk' can cover two importantly different types of ignorance. First, it can relate to ignorance that one is assuming *any* risk by engaging in an activity; alternatively, it can relate to ignorance about the *particular degree* of risk that one is assuming. The first sense outlined above is incompatible with decisional autonomy. The reason for this is that in consenting to a medical procedure, a patient is not simply being asked to consent to the procedure itself; they are also being asked to consent to the assumption of risk. If we agree with the Aristotelian claim that ignorance of particulars can undermine voluntariness, then it seems that ignorance that there are risks associated with a medical procedure can undermine the voluntariness of a patient's consent to that procedure, simply by virtue of the fact that this form of ignorance means that they do not understand a significant part of what it is they are consenting to, namely, assuming a risk. However, this does not entail that ignorance about the degree of risk you are taking on, or indeed ignorance about future states of affairs, similarly precludes decisional autonomy.

Accordingly, I believe that the distinction between valid consent and substantially informed consent can be philosophically grounded by considerations of autonomy, by virtue of the fact that some beliefs are decisionally necessary, whilst others are not. Notice though that this is quite compatible with the claim that holding these further true beliefs may nonetheless serve to enhance an agent's autonomy. Indeed, it would be a mistake to conclude from the above discussion that questions pertaining to the disclosure required for 'substantially informed consent' are divorced from considerations of autonomy. Such a conclusion might seem tempting, since the law treats a failure to secure substantially informed consent as a breach in the doctor's duty of care, rather than an issue with the patient's autonomy per se. Yet, even if this is so, one must still account for *why* this amounts to such a breach in the doctor's duty of care. To my mind the most plausible answer is that the doctor has a positive duty to facilitate their patient's ability to make autonomous decisions. This includes facilitating autonomy beyond that which is required for the minimum threshold of understanding that is necessary for consent to be valid. In addition to enhancing the agent's decisional autonomy by increasing their understanding of their options, and indeed the number of options available to them, such disclosure can serve to facilitate the patient's autonomy by facilitating their own self-trust.

[66] Indeed, Pritchard argues that very low-probability events can nonetheless be modally close. See Pritchard, 'Risk'.

However, deciding on how one can best act in accordance with the positive obligation to increase decisional autonomy beyond that which is minimally required for valid consent is complex. Physicians cannot be expected to disclose *all* the available information about the risks attending a medical treatment, and patients cannot be expected to understand it. Medical conditions, procedures, and their attendant risks often admit of exceedingly complex descriptions, which, however accurate they might be, are unlikely to aid the patient in their decision-making.

This has important implications for disclosure. If physicians understood the obligation to facilitate autonomy to require that they aim for full understanding amongst their patients, they would be likely to overwhelm them with an excess of information that they could not reasonably be expected to compute, especially given that many patients will be less able to deal with complex information because of their illness. There is thus an important balance to be struck between (i) providing patients with the information that can enable them to identify the values at stake in their decision, and to form an impression of the strength of their apparent reasons, and (ii) refraining from providing so much information that the patient is unable to utilize it in a process of rational deliberation.

The theoretical apparatus we may appeal to in seeking to strike this balance is the concept of materiality; to adequately facilitate substantially informed consent, and to thus discharge their duty of care to their patient, we may say physicians must only disclose information that is *material* to the patient's decision. I shall conclude this chapter by considering how we should understand this concept of materiality, and the relationship between different standards of disclosure and autonomy.

4. Standards of Disclosure

According to a *physician*-oriented view of materiality, it should be solely up to the physician, in their professional capacity, to decide which information is material to their patient's decision. In turn, the physician's decision here is understood to be governed by a standard of disclosure endorsed by the professional community, according to which information ought to be disclosed if the majority of physicians within that community would customarily make such a disclosure. Until recently, this view was enshrined in the law in England and Wales in the form of the so-called 'Bolam test', named after the judge's assessment in *Bolam v Friern Hospital Management Committee* (1957) that 'a doctor is not guilty of negligence if he has acted in accordance with a practice accepted as proper by a responsible body of medical men skilled in that particular art'.[67] This test was then deemed to determine the boundaries of the physician's duty to disclose information to their patient in a later case.[68]

[67] *Bolam v Friern Hospital Management Committee* at 1 WLR 583.

[68] *Sidaway v Board of Governors of the Bethlem Royal Hospital* [1985]. For discussion, see Miola, 'On the Materiality of Risk'. In the US, see *Robinson v. Bleicher* (559 N.W.2d 473) 1997.

The Bolam test has been widely criticized as a paternalistic standard of information disclosure.[69] Part of the problem with the test is that a 'responsible body of medical men' might find it proper to omit information on the basis of considerations of beneficence alone, rather than patient autonomy. That is, the professional body could plausibly seek to justify the omission of certain information disclosure on the basis that such disclosure would lead patients to refuse treatments that are in their best interests. Indeed, on this justification, a physician could even refrain from disclosing information that the patient explicitly requested.

Extending the Bolam judgement to the context of risk disclosure was to leave the door open to this kind of paternalism. The natural rebuke to doing so was that this sort of paternalism runs contrary to the underlying autonomy-based justification of informed consent; part of the purpose of the informed consent requirements is to empower patients to make their own decisions about what happens to them, and to avoid paternalistic interference.[70] Partly on this basis, other patient-centric standards of materiality, which purport to emphasize patient autonomy over the paternalism of the physician-oriented approach, have been mooted.

In their philosophically grounded approach to substantially informed consent, Faden and Beauchamp explicitly advocate a purely subjective account of materiality. They claim that:

> ...a person must understand those propositions about (some medical intervention) *R* and about authorizing *R* that are germane to the person's evaluation of whether *R* is an intervention the person should authorize. This criterion is entirely subjective.[71]

Call this the subjective patient-oriented account of materiality.

The justification for adopting a subjective approach is that different patients are likely to regard different information to be pertinent to their treatment decision. Yet, one problem with the subjective account is that it fails to explain precisely *how* patients are to subjectively assess whether or not certain information is pertinent; Faden and Beauchamp simply point out that a person's long term goals and values can affect how individuals value various act descriptions.[72] However, it seems that in order for information to qualify as material to a patient's decision, even if only subjectively, there must be some plausible basis upon which the individual understands the information to be pertinent to her decision. Call this the subjective assessment problem.

One way in which the subjective assessment problem raises a difficulty for the subjective account arises when we recall that understanding some information is decisionally necessary. That is, certain information is so fundamental to the nature of a decision that one cannot make that decision voluntarily if one remains ignorant of it. Crucially, this is so regardless of whether an individual deems the information to be material or not. For instance, suppose Jerry feels ill and continually takes antibiotics because she believes that they are the only thing that will cure her; she does

[69] Brazier, 'Patient Autonomy and Consent to Treatment'; Jones, 'Informed Consent and Other Fairy Stories'; Miola, 'On the Materiality of Risk'; Brazier and Miola, 'Bye-Bye Bolam'.

[70] Indeed, this anti-paternalistic argument can be found in the judgement in *Chester v Afshar* at 18.

[71] Faden and Beauchamp, *A History and Theory of Informed Consent*, 302.

[72] Ibid.

not believe that the fact that she is suffering from a viral rather than a bacterial infection is material to her decision. Irrespective of her own views regarding the materiality of this information, Jerry's failure to appreciate the significance of this precludes her from receiving an effective treatment. Similarly, it is difficult to imagine how a patient could be autonomous with respect to their decision to undergo an anaesthetic if they failed to understand that undergoing an anaesthetic will render them unconscious.

One might defend the subjective standard on this score by saying that the standard is only meant to apply to information disclosure beyond that which is necessary to secure valid consent. However, the subjective assessment problem raises its head in other ways. In view of the fact that patients are normally not experts in medicine, and may be in a vulnerable state owing to the nature of their condition, they may make mistakes about what information is and is not material to their treatment decision. Indeed, as I shall explain below, empirical evidence suggests that patients are subject to a number of cognitive biases that can distort their understanding of their condition and treatment options. A second problem then with the subjective account, is that a particular patient may attach significance to information, but not in a manner that bespeaks an adequate understanding and processing of that information in rational deliberation.

Finally, it is not clear that a purely subjective account of materiality is practically realizable; first, it will often be difficult for practitioners to know what information a patient believes to be relevant to their decision, and it is the physician who has to decide what information to disclose to their patient. Crucially, since physicians are liable to negligence if they fail to disclose information deemed to be material by the standard invoked in medical law, a requirement that doctors must disclose any and all information that a patient could deem to be material would leave doctors highly vulnerable to litigation. Moreover, we might also be concerned that requiring physicians to disclose *any* risks a patient deems to be material, is to overlook the potentially detrimental effect that informational overload can have on the individual's ability to make autonomous decisions, and potentially overestimating patients' ability to process that kind of information.[73]

The failings of the subjective account in this regard might be claimed to lend support to a purely objective patient-centric account, which appeals not to what the particular patient deems material, but rather to what a hypothetical reasonable person would deem to be material. The way in which we ought to understand what constitutes such a hypothetical 'reasonable person' has been the subject of considerable debate. Briefly though, we may note two prominent interpretations outlined by

[73] It has also been claimed that the subjective element of the Montgomery ruling (discussed below) will encourage defensive medicine, by requiring doctors to disclose more information (to ensure their legal protection) than will actually facilitate their patient's decision-making. Chan et al., 'Montgomery and Informed Consent', are correct to point out that here the Montgomery ruling simply brings medical law into line with the GMC recommendations regarding the importance of communication. However, this simply means that a similar charge may be raised against these recommendations.

Dunn et al.[74] They note that one might interpret the reasonable person standard to mean that information ought to be disclosed simply if the *majority* of people think it ought to be disclosed in a specified set circumstances. However, as the authors note, there is little support for this interpretation in medical law. Not only do judges lack empirical support for what most people think about the significance of different kinds of risks, but a significant reason for invoking the concept of reasonableness in one's criterion of materiality is to avoid reliance on capricious, and potentially unreasonable opinions held by the population at large.[75] Accordingly, Dunn et al. favour an interpretation of the 'reasonable person' as invoking a concept of 'reasonableness as normatively justifiable'.[76] On this interpretation, information ought to be disclosed if it concerns information that warrants weighting in a rational agent's decision-making process, by virtue of its significance for individual well-being.

I agree with these authors that the 'normatively justifiable' interpretation of reasonableness in the 'reasonable person' standard is the most convincing; indeed it is congruous with the concept of impersonal reason-giving facts that I discussed in Chapters 1 and 2. But the reasonable person standard, so construed, cannot alone provide a standard of disclosure that is sufficient for adequately facilitating patient autonomy. The problem with such a proposed standard is that a particular patient's preferences may seldom be exhausted by what is normatively justifiable in this way. Even if we assume that there are certain impersonal goods that all rational agents have reasons to pursue, to presume that material information is wholly constituted by information that a reasonable patient (in this sense) would want to know presumes that our self-interested reasons are exhausted by a certain set of our impersonal reasons. As I explored in Chapter 2, this sort of claim seems to implicitly assume an overly objective conception of well-being. Rational individuals can and do disagree about the weight of the reasons that they have to pursue different goods, and individuals can have personal self-interested reasons to instrumentally value certain goods which may not be shared by a hypothetical rational patient.

There are thus significant gaps in both the subjective and objective patient-centric standards of disclosure that suggest that they are each insufficient for adequately facilitating patient autonomy. Of course, an obvious answer to this problem is to combine the two approaches in a hybrid approach. This is just the approach taken by

[74] Dunn et al., 'Between the Reasonable and the Particular'. For other detailed discussions, see Miller and Perry, 'The Reasonable Person'; Gardner, 'The Many Faces of the Reasonable Person'; Kennedy, 'The Patient on the Clapham Omnibus'.

[75] Dunn et al., 'Between the Reasonable and the Particular', 8. The authors also consider an interpretation of the reasonable person criterion according to which 'it is reasonable to inform a patient of risk when there is logical coherence between the patient's values concerning risk and the patient's beliefs about the significance of the risk in these circumstances'. Their reason for dismissing this interpretation is that on this interpretation, the reasonable person criterion would simply serve as a constraint on the exercise of the 'particular patient' limb; yet, since the reasonable person criterion represents a separate limb to the Montgomery test of materiality, the authors conclude that this interpretation is not what the judges had in mind. Nonetheless, this interpretation could potentially serve as an objective standard in its own right.

[76] Dunn et al., 'Between the Reasonable and the Particular'.

the UK Supreme Court judgement on *Montgomery v Lanarkshire*.[77] Paragraph 87 of the judgement states that physicians are:

> . . . under a duty to take reasonable care to ensure that the patient is aware of any material risks involved in any recommended treatment, and of any reasonable alternative or variant treatments. The test of materiality is whether, in the circumstances of the particular case, a reasonable person in the patient's position would be likely to attach significance to the risk, *or* the doctor is or should reasonably be aware that the particular patient would be likely to attach significance to it.[78]

The Montgomery judgement thus offers a two-pronged disjunctive test of materiality that incorporates both objective and subjective patient-centric elements. The benefit of this hybrid approach is that it allows the judgement to overcome the respective insufficiencies of the purely subjective and purely objective patient-centric approaches noted above. Furthermore, we may notice that by appealing to what 'the doctor is or should reasonably be aware that the particular patient would be likely to attach significance to', the subjective limb of this test avoids concerns about the practicalities of Faden and Beauchamp's subjective condition of materiality. On the Montgomery standard, physicians can only be charged with negligence if they are aware, or could reasonably be aware, that a patient would attach significance to the information in question.

The Montgomery judgement has been described as a triumph of autonomy over paternalism, in that it epitomizes a shift of the balance in medical law regarding disclosure away from the paternalism of the Bolam approach, towards the protection of patient values.[79] However, in the remainder of this chapter, I want to suggest, from a philosophical perspective, that the manner in which the Montgomery ruling frames both the subjective and objective elements of its test of materiality is somewhat problematic, at least if the goal of the ruling is to facilitate patient autonomy.[80] This is not intended to be a criticism of the judgement as a legal ruling. Such rulings have to strike a careful balance between ethics, jurisprudence, and practical realities; in particular, it has to set the boundaries of the physician's liability to negligence. However, I shall argue that it might be possible to better capture the spirit of Montgomery, of prioritizing patient values, by reconceptualizing its two-pronged test of materiality.

[77] In the following I shall be interested in the Montgomery judgement's implications for risk disclosure. For a more general overview see Herring et al., 'Elbow Room for Best Practice?'

[78] *Montgomery (Appellant) v Lanarkshire Health Board (Respondent) (Scotland)*, paragraph 87. Emphasis added.

[79] Bolton, 'The Montgomery Ruling Extends Patient Autonomy'; Heywood, 'R.I.P. Sidaway'; Edozien, 'UK Law on Consent Finally Embraces the Prudent Patient Standard'; Farrell and Brazier, 'Not so New Directions in the Law of Consent?'

[80] Interestingly, Dunn et al. point out ways in which elements of the Montgomery judgement cannot be adequately grounded by an autonomy-based justification, and argue that its justification is better understood in terms of the value of patient-centric care. Dunn et al., 'Between the Reasonable and the Particular'. Whilst I agree with these authors that parts of the Montgomery judgement do not optimally facilitate autonomy, I believe that standards of disclosure have greater significance for patient autonomy (as opposed to patient-centric care alone) than these authors envisage, for reasons that I have outlined over the course of the last two chapters.

As I suggested at the end of the previous section, any standard of disclosure has to strike a delicate balance between providing too little information to adequately facilitate patients' autonomous decision-making, and providing too much for that purpose. At the same time, the standard also has to establish practically realistic boundaries of the doctor's duty of care. This is a tall order, and I suggested that the purely objective and subjective patient-centric accounts erred in the first way; they risk providing patients with insufficient information for autonomous decision-making. In order to avoid this error, a hybrid approach incorporating both objective and subjective elements is necessary. In the final section, I shall suggest that the manner in which the Montgomery phrases the subjective element of its hybrid approach means that it is in danger of erring in the second sense, of providing patients with too much information.[81]

5. Rational Materiality

The problem with the subjective limb of the Montgomery test is that it does not avoid the subjective assessment problem. True, it does stipulate *some* basis upon which the subjective assessment must be made; the patient must 'attach significance' to the information. However, it is far from clear that this is a suitable basis for identifying information that is material to the kind of rational decision-making that autonomy requires.

I shall explain this point in the remainder of this chapter. At the outset of this discussion though, I want to suggest an alternative test of materiality grounded in the theory that I have developed over the course of the book, one that draws an explicit link between the materiality of information, and rationality.

> *Rational Materiality*:Information is material to a particular patient's treatment decision if the physician is, or should reasonably be aware that:
>
> (i) the patient's understanding of that information is necessary for adequately appreciating facts that are likely to give that patient considerable reasons to choose or reject a certain treatment option;
> and
> (ii) average human decision-makers would not be incapable of understanding and incorporating that information in a rational deliberative process.

Even before elaborating on this account of materiality in more detail, it should be clear that this account departs from the subjective account of materiality in two ways. First, by virtue of (i), certain information will be material to the patient's decision, *regardless* of the patient's own assessment of the materiality of that information. Furthermore, information that a patient mistakenly believes to be relevant to their treatment decision will not be material if it does not concern reason-implying facts.

Criterion (ii) acknowledges that some information disclosure may be detrimental to autonomous decision-making, even if the information in question meets other

[81] I shall follow Dunn et al. in interpreting 'reasonableness' to mean 'normatively justifiable' in the objective limb of the Montgomery judgement. Dunn et al., 'Between the Reasonable and the Particular'.

conditions of materiality. I shall explore this further below. Here though we may note that this criterion of materiality links my account to considerations of decision-making capacity, in so far as the latter requires the ability to understand, use, and weigh material information. My suggestion here, to be fleshed out below, is that an adequate test of materiality should acknowledge that the degree of capacity required to make a decision can be influenced by the nature and degree of the information that is deemed to be material to it.

First though, let us consider criterion (i). In so far as reason-giving facts can pertain to our impersonal reasons, the above test of materiality can also be understood to incorporate the objective limb of the Montgomery test, if reasonableness in that context is interpreted in terms of normative justifiability. However, by explicitly focusing on the rational content of the information to be disclosed, rather than the rationality of a hypothetical subject of that disclosure (as per Montgomery), the objective element of my account avoids some important ambiguities with the reasonable person criterion. For instance, even when we agree that the 'reasonableness' criterion in the objective limb of Montgomery should be interpreted in terms of normative justifiability, it remains ambiguous as to how we should understand the nature of the individual for whom the information must be normatively justifiable. Must it be normatively justifiable to a patient who is able to rationally process all and any relevant information relevant to well-being, or should we interpret it to mean a patient who is able to engage in rational deliberation, but who is nonetheless limited in their capacity to process such information? On the latter understanding, must the information be normatively justifiable to one who is *aware* of the limitation to their capacity to rationally process such information? My approach avoids these ambiguities by appealing to the reason-giving content of the information itself, whilst acknowledging (in the second criterion) ways in which disclosure can threaten an agent's rational decision-making.

I will begin by exploring how this aspect of my test of materiality would apply in medical contexts, before explaining the manner in which it departs from the Montgomery judgement in further detail. On my proposed test of materiality, information pertaining to two broad aspects of a patient's treatment decision will concern reason-implying facts. First, information pertaining to the *nature* of the proposed intervention will be material. For instance, the fact that an intervention will be painful or invasive provides patients with reasons not to choose that treatment (although these reasons will often not be decisive). This sort of information is also captured by the modal test that I outlined in previous chapters; patients must understand the nature of what they are consenting to if they are not to be modally precluded from acting effectively in pursuit of their ends when making treatment decisions. Second, facts pertaining to the probability of an intervention's bringing about some outcome will also be reason-implying. Such facts will include not only those pertaining to the risks attending the intervention and possible side effects, but also those pertaining to the probability of an intervention's ameliorating the patient's condition.[82]

[82] In their discussion, Herring et al. note that a positive aspect of the Montgomery judgement is that it emphasizes the disclosure of benefits as well as risks. Herring et al., 'Elbow Room for Best Practice?'

I have thus far identified different *types* of information that will be material to a patient's decision. Consider now the *extent* to which patients should be made aware of these different aspects of their treatment. Whilst some information about the nature of the treatment might concern reason-implying facts (for instance, the fact that the intervention is painful), a great deal of information about the treatment will not. For example, information concerning the exact biological mechanism that explains why an antibiotic helps to destroy a bacterial infection will normally not be material to a patient's decision to choose to take antibiotics; such information does not itself concern facts that provide agents with self-interested reasons. However, corollaries of that information may; for instance, in Jerry's case above, the fact that antibiotics are not an effective treatment for viral infections is material to her decision.

Although a great deal of specific information about the nature of a patient's condition or treatment options is unlikely to be material to their decision, it might be claimed that information concerning the foreseeable outcomes of their treatment options and their attendant possibilities is *always* likely to be material to a patient's decision. The Montgomery ruling comes close to making this sort of claim when it states that physicians need to make patients aware of *any* material risks of the proposed procedure, and that:

> ...the assessment of whether a risk is material cannot be reduced to percentages. The significance of a given risk is likely to reflect a variety of factors besides its magnitude: for example, the nature of the risk, the effect which its occurrence would have upon the life of the patient, the importance to the patient of the benefits sought to be achieved by the treatment, the alternatives available, and the risks involved in those alternatives. The assessment is therefore fact-sensitive, and sensitive also to the characteristics of the patient.

I argued above that in order to provide valid consent to *x*, the patient must understand that they are assuming *some* risk in agreeing to undergo *x*. That you are assuming a risk in performing some action can be a reason-giving fact. However, the strength of the reason it connotes depends on the gravity of the risk in question; very low risks generate very weak reasons.

The problem that this raises is that autonomous decision-making in a medical context can sometimes be threatened by the disclosure of such risks, even if they generate (weak) reasons. The disclosure of the nature and magnitude of very small risks can serve to hinder, rather than promote the patient's autonomy, because it feeds into well-known cognitive biases that serve to distort the agent's perception of the strength of the reason that they have. It is for this reason that I suggest that the rationalist account of materiality must incorporate criterion (ii) above, as I shall now explain.

If it were the case that patients were always able to understand the nature of small risks, and to incorporate them into a rational decision-making process that facilitated the pursuit of their own goals, then perhaps we should endorse the Montgomery ruling's implicit suggestion that physicians ought to disclose even minute risks, in order to increase the patient's autonomy with respect to their treatment decisions. However, research on cognitive biases suggests that patients are not able to compute information about risks in such an unbiased manner.[83] As Cass Sunstein points out,

[83] See Ingelfinger, 'Informed (but Uneducated) Consent'. See also Levy, 'Forced to Be Free?', and Sunstein, *Risk and Reason* for analyses of relevant empirical evidence.

when people have to make a decision in an emotionally charged context such as health care, they:

> ...tend to focus on the adverse outcome, not on its likelihood. That is, they are not closely attuned to the probability that harm will occur.[84]

This is particularly problematic when patients are being asked to choose two potential means of achieving the same valuable end. To illustrate, consider the following:

> Being fit or active has been associated with a greater than 50% reduction in risk of all-cause mortality.[85] However, vigorous exercise has also been associated with a very small acute risk of suffering a cardiac event during exercise; one study reported one such event per 2,897,057 person-hours of physical activity amongst healthy adults.[86]

This is the so-called paradox of exercise.

> Suppose a patient visits his doctor, and reports that he is petrified of suffering a heart attack after a friend recently died following one. The patient also has young children, and is terrified of not being able to see them grow up. The physician consults with the patient, and observes that he is at moderate risk of a heart attack. The patient is scared and says he will do anything to reduce his risk. The doctor could suggest that the patient modifies his diet; however, she notes that the patient's diet is not particularly bad, and modifying it is unlikely to lead to great improvement for this patient. The doctor could prescribe statins; however, she notes that these drugs may have some unpleasant side-effects.
>
> She believes that the best way in which the patient can reduce his risk is to engage in an exercise program. However, she is also aware of the 'paradox of exercise', and that engaging in vigorous exercise will transiently cause an extremely small increase in the patient's acute risk of a heart attack, even though the long-term benefits to the patient's cardiac health far outweigh this small increase in their transient risk. Nonetheless, she prescribes an exercise plan without mentioning this risk, and tells the patient to take things slowly.[87]

In this case, the doctor has grounds for believing that the patient would attach significance to the information about the small acute risk associated with bouts of vigorous exercise. The patient has stated that he will do anything to reduce his risk of a heart attack, and the information in question pertains to the transient risk of a cardiac event associated with the doctor's recommended course of action. The Montgomery standard thus seems to speak in favour of disclosure of this risk. The problem with this is that it is far from clear that the patient would take such information to be significant because of the strength of the reason it implies. Rather, the information is significant for the patient because of the particular emotional salience he attributes to the (highly unlikely) adverse outcome.

To exacerbate matters, the patient is likely to attribute even greater (yet unwarranted) salience to this risk simply by virtue of the fact that it has been disclosed to

[84] Sunstein, 'Probability Neglect', 62.

[85] Warburton, Nicol, and Bredin, 'Health Benefits of Physical Activity'.

[86] Malinow, McGarry, and Kuehl, 'Is Exercise Testing Indicated for Asymptomatic Active People?'; Thompson et al., 'Exercise and Acute Cardiovascular Events'.

[87] Maron, 'The Paradox of Exercise'; I discuss ethical implications of this paradox and exercise prescription in Pugh, Pugh, and Savulescu, 'Exercise Prescription and the Doctor's Duty of Non-Maleficence'.

them by an expert authority; 'if the doctor is telling me this, she must think it's important!' This may serve to radically distort the patient's perception of the strength of the reasons that the information is intended to convey, and instead lead the patient to make their decisions on an emotional response to that information that is not adequately grounded in the reality of their situation. The reality of the situation is that adhering to an exercise programme that slowly progresses towards more vigorous forms of exercise will significantly reduce their long-term risk of a heart attack, despite the small increase in the patient's acute risk that attends vigorous exercise for previously sedentary individuals.

Crucially, the doctor's reluctance to disclose in this case need not be born from a paternalistic motive of the sort that the Bolam approach enabled, and for which that standard was criticized. The doctor's concern about disclosure here may be grounded in doubts about whether the patient will use the information in a process of rational deliberation, and not simply in a concern that disclosure will lead the patient to choose contrary to what she believes to be medically indicated. Her concern may be that disclosing this information will not help the patient to make a decision that will help them best pursue their own goals and values. Instead, it might result in him forgoing exercise that will facilitate his pursuit of the goal he wants to achieve, in order to avoid a minute, but emotionally salient risk of the outcome that he wants to avoid.

The problem that this example raises is not simply that disclosing information about low levels of risk will harm patients by causing them psychological distress. If that were the case, the omission of this information could plausibly be justified by an appeal to the so-called therapeutic exception, an exception typically grounded by considerations of non-maleficence.[88] Rather the point that this example raises is that the provision of this information, and the unwarranted alarm it causes the patient, may actually be detrimental to their autonomy, their ability to make a rationally grounded decision, and to choose in accordance with what they actually value, regardless of whether or not the disclosure significantly harms the patient.

Accordingly, when thinking about disclosure and facilitating autonomous decision-making beyond the standard of voluntariness required for valid consent, we are faced with a significant tension. Extending the scope of disclosure requirements in accordance with the subjective limb of the Montgomery judgement will mean that patients are given more opportunities to make decisions about the risks they are and are not willing to take. However, increasing the opportunity for such decisions will only serve to increase patient autonomy if patients are able to make those decisions in an autonomous manner. This may sound almost trivially true, but it contains an important truth that the subjective limb of the Montgomery judgement overlooks: whilst our understanding of risks is sometimes crucial to making decisions about what we have most reason to do, the disclosure of precise details about risks can also play into the hands of our irrational biases. These biases can lead us to make

[88] The Montgomery judgement does include a clause allowing for the therapeutic exception, but notes that this is only justified if disclosure would be seriously detrimental to the patient's health. *Montgomery (Appellant) v Lanarkshire Health Board (Respondent) (Scotland)*, paragraph 88.

decisions that run contrary to what we believe we have reasons to pursue, and to acting in pursuit of our long-term plans.

How can we resolve this tension? It might be argued that we could seek to resolve it without adding further criteria of materiality to criterion (i) in the rational materiality test. For instance, perhaps we could take measures to partly mitigate some of the cognitive biases to which patients are subject. Perhaps if disclosure about a particular risk is to be worthwhile, patients should be helped to contextualize that risk to the kinds of risk they take in their day-to-day life.[89] Physicians should also be informed of the various cognitive biases that they and their patients are prone to exhibit, and should seek to mitigate their influence; this lends support to the dialogical approach that the Montgomery judgement endorses.[90] We might also advocate the introduction of 'informed consent specialists' who have received specialist training in human rationality, to act as 'middle-men' between the physician and their patient in complex cases.[91]

Each of these proposals has merit, but they are unlikely to act as a panacea solution for the types or irrationality that I have discussed here. Even where it is possible to try to mitigate the influence of these biases, it is not clear that such efforts will always be successful.[92] Accordingly, rather than appeal to what patients (actual or hypothetical) attach significance to, as the Montgomery ruling implies, or even appealing to the rational content of the information alone, the test of materiality I have suggested maintains that we should acknowledge this tension and seek to resolve it by appealing to the underlying purpose of information disclosure in our test of materiality. If the purpose of information disclosure is to facilitate an individual's ability to make decisions that are an accurate reflection of their evaluative judgements rather than their irrational biases, our decisions about what to disclose should be sensitive to the kinds of abilities that typical humans have.

Let me pre-empt to two potential objections to the objective phrasing of criterion (ii) above, which seeks to capture this thought. First, it might be argued that it is the individual patient's ability to understand, weigh and use, information that is relevant in this context, rather than what standard human decision-makers are able to do. However, phrasing the criterion in subjective terms would entail a problematic circularity between definitions of materiality and decision-making capacity. The reason for this is that assessments of decision-making capacity are typically partly grounded by the individual's ability to understand material information; accordingly, our definition of the latter cannot incorporate considerations of subjective capacity without circularity. An objective phrasing of criterion (ii) avoids this circularity; moreover, as I shall explain in response to the second objection, an objective phrasing captures a key element of the relationship between capacity and information disclosure.

A second objection to the objective phrasing is that it appears to contradict my earlier rejection of interpreting the reasonable person standard of disclosure as appealing to claims about what the majority of people think. However, there is no

[89] Sunstein, 'Probability Neglect', 92. [90] Herring et al., 'Elbow Room for Best Practice?'.
[91] Levy, 'Forced to Be Free?', 299. [92] Ibid., 297.

contradiction here; my criterion concerns what the majority of people are able to do, not what they *value*. The claim that I am making is that the information that we decide to disclose to patients should be information that most people are *able* to understand, weigh, and use; I am not claiming that our decision should be determined by what most people value.

In fact, the claim that I am making simply extends a point that is implicitly accepted by anyone who accepts the need for an account of materiality to limit the scope of disclosure requirements. There is a tight connection between the information that we deem to be material for making a decision, and the standard of decision-making capacity that will be relevant to that decision, since decision-making capacity requires the ability to understand, weigh, and use material information. It is for this reason that *full* understanding is not deemed to be necessary for decisional autonomy; to claim otherwise would be to preclude individuals from having decision-making capacity, since we humans are not capable of processing all of this information. This then, forms part of the motivation for a theory of materiality; we want to strike a balance between ensuring informed choice, and ensuring that most patients will be capable of understanding the information that we stipulate as being necessary for providing an autonomous authorization to treatment.

The point I am making here is that similar considerations arise with respect to information concerning very low risks; declaring this information material threatens to raise the standard of capacity required to make a decision beyond that which standard human decision-makers are capable.

Criterion (ii) broadly concurs with one professional standard of disclosure according to which decisions about disclosure should give consideration to features of the 'man on the Clapham omnibus'. However, it departs from this (flawed) standard by stressing that the relevant consideration here is what the man on the bus is capable of, and not what he values. Let me now turn to consider the implications of this criterion. How can we tell whether average human decision-makers are capable of understanding, weighing, and using a particular piece of information? This is ultimately an empirical question; however, a rough plausible heuristic here may be that we should tailor our disclosure about risk to the strength of the reason it connotes, on the basis of the assumption that cognitive biases may plausibly have less of a hold on us when we are weighing considerations that we take to have considerable reason-giving force. Explicitly attending to strong reasons is one way in which we can reduce the influence of these biases.

The strength of a reason associated with information pertaining to a particular outcome of a medical procedure is a function of the (dis)value of the outcome it concerns, and its likelihood. The higher the (dis)value, and the more likely it is to occur, the stronger the reason. However, since risk is a comparative concept,[93] when we are thinking about the strength of an all things considered reason to assume a certain risk in undergoing a medical procedure, we must weigh both the disvalue and probability of the risked outcome, against the probability and value of the hoped-for

[93] Herring et al., 'Elbow Room for Best Practice?', 10.

outcome of the procedure which provides the rational justification for the assumption of risk.

Indeed, the Montgomery judgement implicitly reflects this in stressing that the material benefits of alternative procedures must be disclosed in addition to the material risks.[94] To illustrate, the strength of your reason provided by a 2 per cent mortality risk of a medical intervention depends on what you stand to benefit by assuming that risk in undergoing the intervention. This risk might give Patient *A* a comparatively weak reason not to undergo surgery, if the risk is posed by a surgery that is necessary for saving her life. In contrast, the same degree of risk might give patient *B* a much stronger comparative reason to not undergo the surgery, if the surgery is an elective procedure that is less valuable for that patient, such as the alleviation of considerable, but tolerable pain. Finally, Patient *C* might have very strong comparative reasons not to expose themselves to even small risks of catastrophic outcomes in order to undergo cosmetic surgery.

For this reason, my proposal does not entail that physicians should never disclose information about low risks, or that patients cannot incorporate such information into a rational decision-making process. The point is that risks of the same probability can imply reasons of different comparative strength in different contexts, and decisions about information disclosure should be sensitive to this point. We may also notice that although the likelihood with which an outcome will occur is an objective matter, the strength of some of the reasons represented by facts about aspects of particular treatments will depend significantly on the patient's *values*. More specifically, it will depend on the weight that the patient assigns to the reasons they have to pursue different goods. In order to determine whether information about a low degree of risk represents a reason that is sufficiently strong to be deemed material to the patient's decision, physicians must thus be aware of the patient's own values, and their own general attitudes towards risk. This does not imply that the responsibility for facilitating the patient's autonomous decision-making lies solely with the physician. On the contrary, the patient is in a far better epistemic position with regards to her own values; she has an important role to play in facilitating her own ability to make autonomous decisions by engaging with the physician about the values that are central to how she wants to live her life over the course of the clinical encounter, enabling the physician to tailor the information they disclose. Patients thus share in the responsibility to facilitate their own autonomy; as I argued in the previous chapter, this includes a degree of doxastic responsibility.[95]

The disclosure of material information pertaining to impersonal reasons should thus serve as a *starting point* of the physician's disclosure; patients should be made aware of the salient aspects about the nature of their procedure, and also reminded that medical procedures, like many other activities in life, unavoidably involve the assumption of some low risks. However, disclosure concerning the precise nature and degree of risks that connote very weak reasons can serve to hinder rather than facilitate the patient's autonomy.

[94] *Montgomery (Appellant) v Lanarkshire Health Board (Respondent) (Scotland)*; Herring et al., 'Elbow Room for Best Practice?', 5.

[95] Foster, *Choosing Life, Choosing Death*, 104; Kukla, 'How Do Patients Know?'

As such, an adequate informed consent procedure requires that the physician and patient engage with each other to establish the patient's values and their attitudes towards risk, and in doing so conjointly establish the threshold level of strength of reason that a risk would have to connote, in order to warrant full disclosure. Further disclosure of risk should be justified by the decision reached following such a dialogue. For this reason, it makes little sense to stipulate that risks of a certain percentage probability must always (or never) be disclosed; decisions about disclosure of risk have to be sensitive not just to the nature of the outcome to which they pertain, but also to how and in what way that outcome matters for the particular patient in question.

In the exercise case above, because the doctor is aware that the overall goal that the patient places value on is avoiding a heart attack in order to be there for his young family, it is clear that the transient minuscule increase in acute risk of a cardiac event associated with exercise connotes an extremely weak reason for that patient. It is a risk that is clearly outweighed by the fact that the exercise programme will significantly decrease their long-term risk of such an event. Of course, as the degree of risk associated with a procedure under consideration increases, so too will the strength of the corresponding reason; in such cases, physicians may be required to engage further with their patient about the kinds of risk that they are willing to accept to achieve certain outcomes. Rational agents can come to different conclusions with regards to the appropriate attitude to take towards risk. Notwithstanding this point, discussions about attitudes towards risk need to be placed in the context of the kinds of risk to which the patient is already exposed, by virtue of her medical condition, and also those that she encounters simply by carrying out everyday activities.

The Montgomery ruling also advocates the importance of dialogue, in claiming that the doctor should act in an advisory role, and that this involves engaging in a dialogue with the patient that aims to:

> ... ensure that the patient understands the seriousness of her condition, and the anticipated benefits and risks of the proposed treatment and any reasonable alternatives, so that she is then in a position to make an informed decision.[96]

However, the account of autonomy that I have defended supports a stronger approach to this dialogue before the disclosure of risk. In order for informed consent to become a truly two-way informational transaction, the physician should not be limited to merely facilitating understanding. Rather, facilitating the individual's autonomy requires the elicitation and defence of the patient's values, and the physician advocating their own view, drawing on their own professional experience, about the kinds of risk disclosure that will facilitate the patient's autonomous decision-making.[97]

In abandoning the Bolam test, the Montgomery ruling denied the significance of the medical professional body's expertise in delimiting the scope of material

[96] *Montgomery (Appellant) v Lanarkshire Health Board (Respondent) (Scotland)*, at paragraph 90.

[97] Savulescu, 'Liberal Rationalism and Medical Decision-Making'. Decision aids can be a valuable tool in this model of the doctor–patient relationship. See O'Connor et al., 'Decision Aids for Patients Facing Health Treatment or Screening Decisions'.

information.[98] However, obviating *any* reference to medical opinion in thinking about disclosure fails to acknowledge that the medical profession does have something significant to offer to the facilitation of autonomous decision-making. Medical professionals have a great deal of experience in helping patients in medical contexts, and are aware of the effects that information disclosure can have on patient decision-making. The rationalist approach to materiality that I have developed here allows for this experience to be brought to bear on disclosure decisions by establishing a threshold strength of reason that is appropriate for a particular patient, without the professional body determining the boundaries of materiality in the overly objective manner of the Bolam test.

It might be objected that the approach I have advocated here is impractical, given the lack of resources available to health services. As I acknowledged at the outset of this discussion, my intention here has not been to criticize the Montgomery judgement as a legal instrument that has to balance a plethora of ethical, jurisprudential, and practical considerations. Rather, my aim here has been to use the Montgomery judgement as a legal model of disclosure that serves as the best starting point to think about the effects of disclosure for autonomous decision-making. The approach that I have outlined is naturally somewhat divorced from practical realities in a way that the Montgomery judgement cannot afford to be. The model outlined in the Montgomery judgement requires more time and resources than simply giving the patient a consent form to read and sign, and my proposed model arguably goes further still.

If resources do not permit this approach, this gives us strong reason to refrain from treating my approach as necessary to informed consent in the institutional sense outlined at the beginning of this chapter. Moreover, doctors should clearly not face sanction for failing to meet this standard if the resources do not allow them to spend the sort of time with their patient that this approach requires. However, this concern does not speak against my approach as the standard to be met in order for consent to play an operative role in facilitating autonomous authorization of treatment. Existing mechanisms are notoriously poor at ensuring adequate levels of understanding amongst patients,[99] and facilitating rational decision-making. We have reasons to try to improve upon this, and one step on the path to doing so is to think about how we could meet the challenges of facilitating autonomous decision-making *without* considerations of restrained resources. This is not to say that there are not other morally relevant considerations in play when we think about whether it would be justifiable to spend more scarce resources in order to better facilitate autonomous decision-making in the patient population, over other worthy goods.[100] These are important and difficult questions. However, these are questions about the weight we should attribute to different values in health care, and not simply a discussion about the nature of autonomy per se.

[98] Herring et al., 'Elbow Room for Best Practice?', 4.

[99] Flory and Emanuel, 'Interventions to Improve Research Participants' Understanding in Informed Consent for Research'.

[100] Chan et al., 'Montgomery and Informed Consent'.

Conclusion

In this chapter, I have begun to situate my rationalist account of autonomy in our understanding of the structure and justification of informed consent requirements. Having considered the cognitive element of decisional autonomy and its implications for understanding, and standards of materiality and disclosure, I shall in the following chapter continue my investigation of rationalist informed consent by considering the question of decision-making capacity. In doing so, I shall seek to respond to the demandingness objection that I highlighted in section 2 of this chapter.

7

Rational Autonomy and Decision-Making Capacity

In his judgement on a famous case concerning an adult refusal of treatment, Lord Donaldson of Lymington made the following observation:

> An adult patient who . . . suffers from no mental incapacity has an absolute right to choose whether to consent to medical treatment . . . This right of choice is not limited to decisions which others might regard as sensible. *It exists notwithstanding that the reasons for making the choice are rational, irrational, unknown or even non-existent.*[1]

This oft-cited judgement champions patient autonomy over medical paternalism; patients with decision-making capacity are afforded the right to make 'unwise' decisions with regards to their own health.

There are two notable features of this judgement. First, it implicitly acknowledges that the 'right of choice' is only afforded to those who do not suffer from mental incapacity. If mental capacity is closely related to considerations of autonomy (a claim I shall further defend below), then this suggests that the extent to which an individual is *able* to make an autonomous treatment decision has a considerable bearing on whether that decision should be respected. Second, this judgement also seems contrary to one of the central claims that I have advanced in this book, namely, that autonomous decision-making requires deciding on the basis of what one believes one has reason to do. The Donaldson judgement implicitly objects to this sort of account on the basis of an anti-paternalist concern: the worry that rationalist conceptions of autonomy will allow physicians to ignore a patient's wishes if they run contrary to medical opinion, on the basis that the decision is not rational and therefore not autonomous. According to this objection, rationalist autonomy pays mere lip service to the idea of individual self-government, and in fact simply amounts to indirect paternalism.

Part of my aim in this chapter is to respond to this anti-paternalist objection. I shall argue that we should reject the claim that a rationalist conception of autonomy (and *a fortiori* decision-making capacity) must have this sort of substantive connotation. In the next section, I shall begin by providing a brief general overview of capacity and competence, and outlining two prominent accounts. I shall then

[1] Re T (adult: refusal of medical treatment), my emphasis. For a philosophical approach to capacity that endorses this sentiment, see Draper, 'Anorexia Nervosa and Respecting a Refusal of Life-Prolonging Therapy', 125–6.

Autonomy, Rationality, and Contemporary Bioethics. Jonathan Pugh, Oxford University Press (2020).
DOI: 10.1093/oso/9780198858584.001.0001

introduce and critique a prominent view of the relationship between decision-making capacity and risk. In the second half of the chapter, I shall delineate and respond to two different versions of the anti-paternalist objection to a rationalist conception of decision-making capacity.

1. Competence, Capacity, and Competing Values in Their Assessment

The terms 'competence' and 'capacity' are sometimes used interchangeably in the bioethical literature. This is perhaps understandable, since in common usage, both concepts are used to broadly denote the ability to perform a certain task. For instance, outside of the bioethical context, we might describe someone as a competent driver if they are able to drive a car well; similarly, we might say that an Olympic sprinter has the capacity to run 100 m in under ten seconds.

However, it is important to acknowledge that the two terms can be used to mean somewhat different things in bioethics. For instance, in England and Wales, the concept of capacity is typically treated as a *legal* concept that is defined by the specific criteria set out in the Mental Capacity Act 2005. In contrast, 'competence' is understood to refer to a *clinical* concept, which may take into account a broader set of considerations than the legal conception of capacity.[2] Somewhat confusingly though, in the US context, the meanings of these terms are reversed. For instance, Beauchamp and Childress observe:

> Several commentators distinguish judgments of capacity from judgments of competence on the grounds that health professionals assess capacity and incapacity, whereas courts determine incompetence.[3]

This disagreement on the use of terminology is unfortunate. In the absence of any other convincing justification for adopting one use over the other, I shall follow the use employed in the English and Welsh context, which treats decision-making capacity rather than competence as the operative concept in the legal domain (of which I shall say more below).

Whilst the distinction between competence and decision-making capacity thus has some importance, it is important not to overstate this difference. First, as I shall explain, there is often a considerable degree of overlap between the two. Second, whilst only the courts have the authority to determine whether patients have decision-making capacity, they will typically defer to professional judgements. As such, the practical implications of the clinician's assessment of competence will typically be similar to a legal determination of decision-making capacity.[4] That said, the two are separate, and judges do not always follow the professional assessment.[5] Whilst acknowledging this distinction between competence and decision-making capacity, I shall phrase the remainder of my discussion in terms of the latter

[2] Tan and Elphick, 'Competency and Use of the Mental Health Act—a Matrix to Aid Decision-Making'.
[3] Beauchamp and Childress, *Principles of Biomedical Ethics*, 114.
[4] Grisso and Appelbaum, *Assessing Competence to Consent to Treatment*, 11.
[5] Re SB; for discussion, see Herring, *Medical Law and Ethics*, 164.

(which I shall abbreviate to 'DMC') alone. However, my claims should also be understood to extend to competence unless explicitly stated otherwise.

DMC can be understood as a range property in that it is a binary property that does not itself admit of degrees, even though we assign it on the basis of an individual's possession of certain abilities that do admit of degree.[6] As such, in considering whether a patient has DMC we are asking whether they have the requisite degree of the relevant abilities that are necessary to perform a certain task. The task in question in most discussions of DMC in the medical context is that of providing valid informed consent to (or refusal of) medical treatment.[7]

In understanding the relevant task for DMC in this manner, I am adopting a straightforward understanding of the relationship between DMC and local autonomy.[8] The reason that we limit the right to consent to or refuse medical treatment to those who have DMC, is that these individuals alone have the capacity to make an autonomous decision about this matter. This is important in cases of treatment refusal because only if a patient has DMC to refuse treatment will there be an autonomy-based justification for omitting to provide a treatment that could serve to outweigh considerations of beneficence that speak in favour of providing it. In the case of consent to treatment, DMC is significant in so far as we should only recognize the normative authority of waivers of rights that would otherwise preclude the permissibility of treatment, if the decision to waive the right (by so consenting) was autonomous. We may note that a significant virtue of this approach to understanding the relationship between autonomy and DMC is that it allows for a straightforward explanation of what the conditions of DMC are, and why DMC matters morally.

Of course, in light of the differences between the institutional and non-institutional senses of informed consent, we should also acknowledge that what it means to have DMC to give informed consent in the institutional sense may differ from what it means to have DMC to give informed consent in the sense of an autonomous authorization. In any case, though, one of the primary aims of an account of DMC is to outline the causally necessary conditions for an individual to make a decision to consent in accordance with the constitutive conditions of valid consent. If one holds that the conditions of autonomous decision-making map on to the requirements of informed consent, then there will be a close connection between the concepts of DMC, informed consent, and autonomy.

[6] McMahan, *The Ethics of Killing*, 250. For an exploration of why the possession of rationality conceived as a range property of agents is a sufficient basis of moral equality, see Carter, 'Respect and the Basis of Equality'.

[7] Buchanan, 'Mental Capacity, Legal Competence and Consent to Treatment'. It is also possible to talk about capacity in the more generalized sense of what capacities an individual requires in order to be a globally autonomous agent, as opposed to an individual who has the capacity to make an autonomous local decision. See Dworkin, 'Autonomy and the Demented Self', 10. Dworkin notes that global autonomy might require further diachronic evaluative capacities, and that it might also be understood to ground the general right to autonomy.

[8] I briefly consider and reject two alternative approaches to understanding the relationship between autonomy and DMC in the next chapter.

The fact that DMC is treated as a range property implies that in order to assess whether a patient has it, we must set a threshold level for the abilities associated with providing valid consent, such that an individual qualifies as having DMC to make a particular decision once they have passed that threshold for all the necessary abilities. Naturally, this raises the question of *where* we should set these thresholds. It is possible to ask this question in an abstract idealized sense, where the only relevant consideration is whether a particular ability is necessary for providing either an autonomous authorization or institutionally valid consent, depending on the sense of consent that we mean to invoke. However, this question is most typically asked in non-ideal contexts. An important implication of this is that non-ideal theories of DMC have a further aim of resolving a conflict between competing moral values that arise in light of the epistemic obstacles that arise in non-ideal contexts. To understand why this so, it is important to be clear about the moral values in question.

One of the most significant reasons underlying the claim that patients should be allowed to make their own treatment decision is that we attribute significant value to personal autonomy: following a long liberal tradition, it is widely held that individuals with DMC should be free to decide to act in ways that are not conducive to their well-being.[9] Indeed, we typically afford such individuals what has been termed 'legal capacity' in the medical context, in that we afford these individuals certain rights (and responsibilities), including the right to refuse beneficial medical treatment.[10] However, this right is often understood to be conditional on DMC. As I wrote above, one justification for limiting this right to patients with DMC is that only in such cases will there be an autonomy-based justification of omitting to provide a treatment that could serve to outweigh considerations of beneficence. Moreover, we might claim that the power to waive certain claims is also conditional on DMC, in so far as we should only recognize the normative authority of *autonomous* decisions to waive one's rights.

Although this link between DMC and legal capacity is widely endorsed, it is by no means universal; it has recently been challenged by the Convention on the Rights of Persons with Disabilities (CRPD).[11] Whether we should accept the link between legal capacity and DMC, or agree with the CRPD that legal capacity should be afforded on other bases is beyond the scope of my discussion here. I shall confine myself to the narrower question of the relationship between autonomy and DMC. However, my discussion concerning the role of autonomy and well-being in this chapter lends some indirect support to maintaining a relationship between DMC and legal capacity.

Returning to the role of the values of autonomy and well-being in the context of DMC, we may note that an ideal system of assessing DMC would be one that identified all and *only* those people who are able to provide valid consent as having DMC. However, there are a number of obstacles to employing such an ideal system of

[9] Kleinig, 'The Nature of Consent'.

[10] Re C (Adult: Refusal of Treatment); Craigie and Davies, 'Problems of Control'; Blumenthal, 'The Default Legal Person'.

[11] Convention on the Rights of Persons with Disabilities (CRPD); for discussion, see Bartlett, 'The United Nations Convention on the Rights of Persons with Disabilities and Mental Health Law'.

assessing DMC. One reason for this is that there is considerable disagreement about the nature of autonomy; this much should be clear from the first half of the book. As such, there is bound to be controversy in determining the abilities that our assessment of DMC should be aiming to identify. The second and perhaps more significant barrier though is that many of the abilities that we might plausibly agree are necessary for providing valid consent are mental abilities that do not admit of straightforward external assessment. We are thus likely to make mistakes in our assessments of these abilities with the relatively crude tools at our disposal.

In the light of these epistemic barriers and the errors that they make likely, our decision about where to set the relevant threshold for DMC in the non-ideal context must unavoidably make a moral judgement about how to balance the value of patient autonomy, against the moral reasons grounded in the duties of beneficence and non-maleficence. The benefit of setting a low threshold for DMC is that our assessment is likely to be more sensitive, in the sense that it will more reliably identify true positive cases; that is, on a low threshold approach, individuals who *are* able to make autonomous decisions will typically qualify as having DMC.

However, the cost of employing a low threshold is that our assessment is thereby unlikely to be particularly specific. Employing a low threshold increases the chance that our test of DMC will lead to false positive assessments; there is a higher chance that individuals will qualify as having the DMC to make a treatment decision, when they are *not* in fact capable of making the decision autonomously. The cost of such false positive assessments is that allowing such patients to make decisions that put them at risk of harm cannot be justified by an appeal to the value of their autonomy; we may be understood as harming them by allowing them to make their own decisions. Low threshold approaches to the assessment of DMC thus place greater emphasis on defending patients' decision-making authority, at the expense of protecting non-autonomous patients from harm.

In contrast, the benefit of setting a high threshold for DMC is that our assessments will be much more specific, in the sense that they will more reliably pick out true negative cases; that is, on a high threshold approach, individuals who are not able to make autonomous decisions will typically not qualify as having DMC. The cost of employing a high threshold is that our assessment is thereby unlikely to be particularly sensitive, in the sense that employing a high threshold increases the chance that our test of DMC will lead to false negative assessments; on such an approach, there is a greater chance that individuals will qualify as lacking DMC, when they are in fact capable of making a decision in an autonomous fashion. The moral cost of such false negatives is that prohibiting a person from making an autonomous decision about their treatment when they are capable of doing so runs contrary to the liberal tradition that affords greater weight to the duty to respect autonomy than to the duty of beneficence.[12] High threshold approaches to the assessment of DMC thus place greater emphasis on protecting non-autonomous patients from harm, at the expense of jeopardizing the decision-making authority of some patients.

[12] For a discussion of how this philosophical view is reflected in the Common Law regarding adult refusals of treatment, see Gavaghan, 'In Word, or Sigh, or Tear', 35. See also Clarke, 'The Neuroscience of Decision Making and Our Standards for Assessing Competence to Consent'.

With this discussion in mind, we may observe that in outlining criteria of DMC in non-idealized contexts, we have to answer three questions. First, is the criterion plausibly a necessary condition of autonomous decision-making or providing consent in its institutional sense? Of course, this question is also relevant when we are thinking about DMC in ideal contexts. Second, do we have the methods to reliably assess the abilities in question? Third, what are the implications of our criteria for the balance that we are aiming to strike between the competing moral reasons we face in making assessments of DMC in non-ideal contexts? Over the course of this chapter, I shall outline different permutations of the anti-paternalist objection to rationalist theories that place different emphases on these questions.

2. Two Cognitivist Accounts of DMC

Grisso and Appelbaum developed a particularly influential account of DMC which is largely echoed in the Mental Capacity Act in England and Wales. According to Grisso and Appelbaum, DMC requires the ability to:

1. Communicate a choice
2. Understand relevant information
3. Appreciate the situation and its consequences
   and
4. Manipulate information rationally[13]

These conditions bear a striking resemblance to those that are adopted in the Mental Capacity Act 2005 (henceforth MCA). A necessary (but not sufficient condition) for an individual's lacking DMC on the MCA is that she lacks *any* of the following abilities, as outlined in section 3(1) of the Act:

(a) The ability to understand the information relevant to the decision.
(b) The ability to retain the information for long enough to be able to make a decision.
(c) The ability to use or weigh that information as part of the process of making the decision.
(d) The ability to communicate their decision.[14]

Grisso and Appelbaum's theory and the approach evidenced in the MCA are similar in that they both emphasize cognitive capacities. However, it is worth highlighting three striking differences. First, the MCA does not adopt a criterion relating to the ability to appreciate information; appreciation goes beyond mere understanding of material information in requiring that individuals are cognizant of the fact that material information applies to them and their situation.[15] Second, although the MCA adverts to the need to weigh and use information, it makes no reference to the need to do so rationally, unlike the counterpart criterion in Grisso and Appelbaum's

[13] Appelbaum and Grisso, 'Assessing Patients' Capacities to Consent to Treatment'; Grisso and Appelbaum, *Assessing Competence to Consent to Treatment.*

[14] Mental Capacity Act 2005, 2(1), 3(1).

[15] Appelbaum and Grisso, 'Assessing Patients' Capacities to Consent to Treatment'.

approach. Third, the MCA supplements Grisso and Appelbaum's functional approach with a further diagnostic criterion. According to the MCA, the fact that a patient lacks one of the above abilities is not sufficient for establishing that she lacks DMC. For that to be the case, the patient's lacking the ability in question must also be attributable to 'an impairment of, or a disturbance in the functioning of, the mind or brain'.[16] The MCA thus incorporates both a functional and diagnostic test of DMC.[17]

I shall discuss whether these differences are philosophically warranted over the course of this chapter. Here though, we may note that the cognitive approach endorsed by both accounts is broadly compatible with the procedural analysis of autonomy that I have offered so far in this book. Indeed, section 1(4) of the MCA explicitly states that: 'A person is not to be treated as unable to make a decision merely because he makes an unwise decision'. In this regard, it echoes both Lord Donaldson's remarks quoted at the beginning of this chapter, as well as Buchanan and Brock's claim that standards of DMC should focus '... not on the content of the patient's decision but on the *process* of the reasoning that leads up to that decision'.[18]

The abilities outlined above are also all plausible candidates for abilities that are causally necessary for autonomous decision-making on my account. As I argued in the previous chapter, patients must be able to understand certain information about their decision in order to be autonomous with respect to it. Furthermore, being able to retain information is central to one's ability to make a decision on the basis of that information, and a criterion referring to the practical element of communication is also congruous with the practical orientation of my account of autonomy. Finally, my account also lends theoretical support to the criteria of appreciation and weighing and using information *rationally*; I shall make the case for this claim in section 3 where I shall also critically engage more broadly with these cognitivist approaches. Here though, I shall conclude my discussion of these two prominent approaches by highlighting two further general and widely accepted features of DMC.

The first is that DMC is typically understood to be contextually dependent.[19] Different local decisions will require different degrees of aptitude in the particular abilities relevant to DMC. Accordingly, although a patient may lack DMC to make certain sorts of decisions, this does not entail that they lack DMC to make *any* decisions for themselves. For example, whilst an agent may be able to understand material information pertaining to a decision about relatively simple treatments, such as whether she ought to have surgery on a broken bone, she may not be able to understand material information pertaining to more complex treatment options which could lead to various possible outcomes, such as in the treatment of cancer. Similarly, the fact that an individual is globally autonomous does not entail that they will make a locally autonomous decision.

The threshold level of DMC required to make a certain decision will depend upon the complexity of the information that is material to the patient. This is particularly relevant when we consider DMC in children. The majority of the provisions in the

[16] Mental Capacity Act 2005, 2(1). [17] Herring, *Medical Law and Ethics*, 157.
[18] Buchanan and Brock, *Deciding for Others*, 50.
[19] See also Brock, *Life and Death*; Herring, *Medical Law and Ethics*, 157.

MCA apply to children who are 16 and over;[20] once a person has reached this age, they are thus presumed to have DMC unless proven otherwise.

It would be a mistake to make the overly general claim that children simply lack the capacity for decisional autonomy, even though the law denies children the authority to make certain decisions for themselves. It is clearly the case that some children below 16 can hold and exercise the sorts of abilities discussed above with respect to at least *some* decisions. Indeed this is recognized in the legal concept of Gillick competence, according to which a child '... has a right to make their own decisions when he reaches a sufficient understanding and intelligence to be capable of making up his own mind on the matter requiring decision'.[21] Accordingly, in England and Wales, children who are under 16 but who are 'Gillick competent' can provide valid consent to some medical procedures; however, their refusal to consent to treatment that is deemed to be in their best interests may be overridden by someone with parental responsibility, by virtue of the Family Law Reform Act.[22] Notably, the latter is also true of children under 18.

This coheres neatly with a rationalist approach, since it seems plausible to claim that children are perfectly capable of recognizing and appreciating certain kinds of reasons. To give a simple example, consider the reasons grounded by an individual's hedonic likings and dislikings. Even very young children can recognize that they have stronger reasons to choose, for example, an ice-cream flavour that they have enjoyed previously (say chocolate) over one that they have disliked previously (say coffee). *Ceteris paribus*, it seems plausible to say that we ought to allow even a young child to make a choice between alternative ice-cream flavours, because doing so simply requires weighing two of the same kind of reasons (concerning the child's hedonic liking of a certain taste), reasons to which the child is well-equipped to respond. The child can thus make an autonomous choice in this circumscribed choice domain.

However, there are some reasons that children are not well-equipped to recognize and appreciate—even if it seems plausible to allow a five-year-old a degree of autonomy about which flavour ice-cream to have, we would be reluctant to allow her to make her own decisions about how often ice-cream should feature in her diet. The reason for this is that whilst a child of this age is able to recognize her reasons to eat ice-cream (namely, that she enjoys the taste), she is less able to appreciate and weigh facts that give her reasons to refrain from eating ice-cream, namely, that frequent consumption of ice-cream would be bad for her health. However, as a child's general cognitive capacities develop, so too will their ability to recognize and weigh more complex kinds of reason-giving facts.

A second notable general feature of capacity is that it has often been the case that the gravity of a decision has been understood to influence the relevant threshold of

[20] However, some provisions, such as those pertaining to advance directives, making a lasting power of attorney, and deprivation of liberty safeguards (amongst others), only apply to those who have reached the age of 18.

[21] *Gillick v. West Norfolk and Wisbech Area Health Authority and Department of Health and Social Security*, HL 17 Oct. 1985.

[22] Family Law Reform Act. For a useful overview of the law in this area, see Hope, Savulescu, and Hendrick, *Medical Ethics and Law*, ch. 10.

DMC that is necessary for making *that* decision: The more serious the consequences of a decision, the higher the threshold for DMC.[23] For instance, in the case of Re T, the Court of Appeal stated:

> What matters is that the doctors should consider whether at that time he had a capacity which was commensurate with the gravity of the decision. The more serious the decision, the greater the capacity required.[24]

Call this the 'sliding-scale view' of DMC.[25]

It should be noted that the sliding-scale view is often understood to operate only within certain thresholds. If an individual exhibits the abilities that contribute to DMC to a particularly high degree, then she should be understood to have the DMC to make her own medical decisions, no matter how detrimental the consequences of her decision are for her individual well-being. This reflects the liberal view that considerations of autonomy should trump those of beneficence.

More generally though, the sliding-scale view has somewhat puzzling implications. For instance, Culver and Gert note that in some situations, a choice to refuse treatment may have very serious consequences, whilst consenting to treatment may not. They note that the sliding-scale view thus has the somewhat puzzling implication that a patient might have sufficient DMC to choose option *B* (because it concerns a low-risk medical intervention and thus implies a relatively lower threshold for DMC), but lack capacity to choose option *A* (because the gravity of refusing consent implies a higher standard of DMC on the sliding-scale view). However, in making this choice between *A* and *B*, she has to understand and weigh the same information about her alternative options.[26]

Partly on the basis of this implication, Culver and Gert claim that the sliding-scale view conflates the distinct concepts of DMC and rationality, conceived in a substantive sense; patients only qualify as having DMC if they make decisions that are rational in the view of the medical profession.[27] One reason that this is problematic is that it unhelpfully conflates two separate concepts. Whilst this is Culver and Gert's particular worry,[28] it might be argued that this conflation is particularly concerning for those who endorse the anti-paternalist objection, because of the paternalistic connotations of conflating DMC with rationality (in this substantive sense). In the next section, I shall outline some ways in which the sliding-scale view might be defended, and consider whether these defences might be used to deflect this charge of indirect paternalism. I shall argue that the prominent justifications offered for standard interpretations of the view fail in this regard, but that we should not wholly disregard a revised version of the sliding-scale view. In section 4, I shall argue that,

[23] Buchanan, 'Mental Capacity, Legal Competence and Consent to Treatment'.

[24] Re T (Adult: Refusal of Medical Treatment).

[25] For support of the sliding-scale view, see Buchanan and Brock, *Deciding for Others*; Buchanan, 'Mental Capacity, Legal Competence and Consent to Treatment'; Eastman and Hope, 'The Ethics of Enforced Medical Treatment'; Drane, 'The Many Faces of Competency'.

[26] Culver and Gert, 'The Inadequacy of Incompetence', 636. [27] Ibid., 632.

[28] Culver and Gert do not themselves subscribe to this view, as they believe that it is permissible to overrule irrational decisions. Their complaint though is that the concepts of capacity and rationality should not be conflated.

contrary to Culver and Gert, the concepts of DMC and rationality do in fact overlap in some sense, but not in the manner that undergirds this particular criticism of the sliding-scale view.

3. Sliding-Scale, Risk, and Value

It might be argued that the sliding-scale view can be justified in both ideal and non-ideal contexts by considerations of autonomy alone. One such justification might claim that there is a positive linear relationship between the degree of risk that a decision concerns, and the degree of the requisite abilities it takes to make that decision autonomously.[29] Call this 'the linear justification' of the sliding-scale view.

The linear justification may seem appealing, because we can think of some examples that fit this picture of the relationship between risk and autonomous decision-making. The reason for this is that in some cases, decisions with more serious consequences can involve more complex information, and the weighing of a greater number of considerations and options. To illustrate, trivial decisions, such as deciding what to eat for lunch, typically do not require understanding the sort of complex information that might be involved in decision-making regarding a range of different cancer treatments.

Yet, this justification of the sliding-scale view is overly simplistic. There is not always a straightforward linear relationship of the sort it appeals to between appropriate requirements of DMC and the risks the decision concerns. In some cases, decisions can plausibly have grave consequences without necessarily requiring the individual to understand highly complex information, or to compute a large number of options. Choosing to refuse a blood transfusion when one is bleeding profusely has grave consequences, but it is not particularly difficult to understand why that might be the case. In stark contrast, one can also think of extremely low-risk decisions that might require understanding much more complex information and weighing of options; for example, those involved in playing a strategic board game.

As such, it is incorrect to assume that DMC to provide an autonomous authorization in an idealized sense will always vary in accordance with the risks associated with the outcome of a decision.[30] Although it might be plausible to endorse an attenuated version of the sliding-scale view on this basis (which calls for increased DMC for risky decisions when they concern more complex information and weighing of alternatives),[31] a full-blown version of the sliding-scale that forgoes this caveat cannot be defended by appeal to considerations of autonomy in this way.

An alternative plausible justification of the sliding-scale view appeals to claims about the *value* of the decisions in question, rather than claims about the nature of DMC they require. On what we may call the 'balancing justification of sliding-

[29] Buchanan and Brock, *Deciding for Others*, 52–5.

[30] Beauchamp and Childress also object to what I call the linear justification view. See Beauchamp and Childress, *Principles of Biomedical Ethics*, 76.

[31] As Craigie points out, although this full-blown sliding-scale view was previously endorsed in the Common Law in England and Wales, since the enactment of the MCA, it has only been adopted in this attenuated sense. Craigie and Davies, 'Problems of Control', 13.

scale',[32] our decision about setting relevant thresholds of DMC should seek to balance the values of autonomy and well-being.[33] On this approach, the degree to which an individual exhibits the abilities associated with DMC is understood as a proxy not only for their degree of autonomy, but also for the *value* that should be attached to respecting that autonomy. Accordingly, in order to justify respecting the individual's decision to expose herself to a significant risk of harm, that individual must exhibit the abilities associated with DMC to a high degree, since only then will the value of her autonomy be sufficient to outweigh the disvalue of the potential harm at stake.

This justification is problematic for different reasons. As Buchanan notes, the balancing approach runs contrary to the liberal principle that a person's autonomy is paramount, and cannot and should not be traded off against considerations of well-being; indeed, this view lies at the heart of the anti-paternalistic concern raised by Culver and Gert, which I consider below.[34] However, notwithstanding the problematic assumption that the value of autonomy can be measured against considerations of well-being in the straightforward manner that the balancing approach implies, the degree to which an individual manifests the abilities required for DMC is not a plausible proxy for the value of respecting their autonomy. It is far from clear that an increase in DMC can serve to increase the *value* of respecting the decision in question.

To see why, consider a decision that is not central to most individuals' conception of the good, such as one's decision about what to eat for lunch on a particular day. It is absurd to claim that increasing an individual's capacity to make that decision beyond the low threshold of DMC that it requires would increase the value of respecting that decision. The value of autonomy is more plausibly grounded by the importance of the decision to the individual's conception of the good, and living a life of their own. This is a quite separate question from the question of the extent to which the individual is capable of making that decision autonomously.

I suggest that both the 'linear justification' and the 'balancing justification' fail to provide a plausible justification for the sliding-scale view, let alone one that can help to explain how it can avoid the conflation raised by Culver and Gert. I shall conclude by considering an epistemic justification of the view that appeals to the greater need for certainty about DMC for making risky decisions in non-ideal contexts. Although I shall argue that typical understandings of this justification fail to adequately counter Culver and Gert's criticism, I conclude that epistemic considerations might yet lend support to either a repurposed sliding-scale view, or a version of the view with wider scope.

As I explained above, in non-ideal contexts, we face a number of epistemic barriers to assessing DMC. A corollary of this is that the lower the threshold of DMC we employ, the more likely it is that our test of DMC will be prone to false positive assessments. Moreover, we may note that as the risks associated with making a decision increase, so too does the harm of a false positive assessment. On the basis

[32] Buchanan, 'Mental Capacity, Legal Competence and Consent to Treatment'.

[33] Eastman and Hope, 'The Ethics of Enforced Medical Treatment'.

[34] For detailed discussion of issues facing the balancing account, see Wicclair, 'Patient Decision-Making Capacity and Risk'.

of these considerations, the epistemic justification of the sliding-scale view proceeds by pointing out that we should increase the threshold of DMC for risky decisions because we have stronger moral reasons to reduce false positive assessments in these cases, given the greater harms associated with them.[35]

Prima facie, it seems that the epistemic justification can allow the sliding-scale view to avoid conflating DMC with considerations of substantive rationality. The reason that we allow a patient to consent to but not to refuse a treatment that it would be very risky to refuse, is not because only the former decision is rational; rather, the justification is that we have moral reasons to require greater *certainty* in our assessments as the stakes of the decision rise.

Unfortunately for supporters of the sliding-scale view, whilst this epistemic justification avoids a direct conflation of DMC and substantive rationality, this conflation and its paternalistic connotations are nonetheless implicitly incorporated into the justification. The justification correctly acknowledges that epistemic barriers render our tests of DMC prone to false positive assessments, and that we can reduce these findings by raising the threshold for DMC. However, it overlooks the fact that these epistemic barriers also make our assessments of DMC prone to false *negative* findings.[36] This oversight is crucial, as it means the epistemic defence of the sliding-scale view does not sufficiently acknowledge that raising the threshold for DMC for risky decisions will serve to *increase*, rather than decrease, the likelihood of false negative findings.

Once we attend to this overlooked feature, it becomes clear that even if increases in the disvalue of false positive assessments of DMC plausibly track the increasing degree of risk involved in different decisions, this is not a sufficient basis for an epistemic justification of the sliding-scale view. The view can only be justified on epistemic grounds if there is *not* a similarly close relationship between the increasing degree of risk and the disvalue of the false negative assessments that are more likely when we raise the threshold of DMC for riskier decisions. However, if there is a close relationship between these degrees of risk and the disvalue of false negative assessments, then increasing the likelihood of the latter might plausibly offset the gain to be had by reducing false positive rates. If that is the case, simply increasing the threshold of DMC for riskier decisions would not unequivocally serve to increase our certainty about all of the morally relevant factors in this context.

One natural response to this worry is to appeal to the implications of each of these kinds of assessment for the individual's well-being. It might be claimed that individuals who are incorrectly denied the authority to make their own risky treatment decision (i.e. false negatives) may be benefited by this (in so far as they are protected from the risk of harm to which they would otherwise expose themselves), whilst those who are incorrectly given the authority to make such a decision (i.e.

[35] Buchanan, 'Mental Capacity, Legal Competence and Consent to Treatment', 417.

[36] Buchanan recognizes the implication that raising the threshold of capacity 'also increases the number of instances in which people are incorrectly assessed as not legally competent'. Ibid., 417. He suggests that advocates of the epistemic justification must simply assume that the severity of the harm of false positives does not increase with the severity of the harm at stake. My argument below is that this assumption is unjustified.

false positives) are quite likely to be harmed by their decision. On this approach, it might be argued that the increasing disvalue of false positives for riskier decisions is likely to outstrip the increase in the corresponding disvalue of false negative assessments for the same types of decisions.

However, such an argument moves far too quickly. Like the balancing justification, it implicitly assumes that considerations of well-being can be traded off against considerations of autonomy. Yet even if such trade-offs can be coherent, this defence of the epistemic justification of the sliding-scale view neglects the fact that in many cases, the value of an individual's exercising their autonomy plausibly *increases* in accordance with increasing degrees of risk that the decision may concern. That is, it may matter more for our autonomy that we make our own decisions concerning higher degrees of risk, because such decisions may have a far greater bearing on the extent to which our lives proceed in accordance with our own values. Risk is a function both of the probability of a certain event, but also the degree of its disvalue. Accordingly, a low-risk decision about what to have for lunch may concern outcomes with little disvalue (e.g. not enjoying a sandwich), or more dis-valuable outcomes with low probability (e.g. food poisoning). Such outcomes have little bearing on whether our lives proceed in accordance with our values. However, my decision to choose a very risky treatment for a non-life-threatening ailment may.

Accordingly, the sliding-scale view cannot be justified in epistemic terms merely by the fact that (i) we face epistemic barriers in assessing DMC, and (ii) the disvalue of false positive assessments increases as the risks associated with the decision increase. The simple reply to this is that the disvalue of false negative assessments of DMC may similarly increase as the risks associated with the decision increase. In neglecting this point, the epistemic justification of the sliding-scale view implicitly prioritizes the avoidance of false positive assessments of DMC over false negatives. It presume that it is more important to avoid harms that are not justified by appeal to the individual's autonomy, than it is to avoid preventing individuals from being wrongfully being denied the opportunity to exercise their ability to make autonomous decisions.

In this regard, the sliding-scale view somewhat bucks the anti-paternalistic tide, since we typically place greater emphasis on protecting patients' decision-making authority than considerations of beneficence and non-maleficence. Of course, one may raise a host of moral arguments about why we should emphasize one set of values over the over in seeking to resolve uncertainty in making decisions about setting the threshold of DMC. The point here though is that we lack justification for why our weighting of these moral values should be shifted *by considerations of risk alone*. In the absence of such a justification, we should reject the epistemic justification for the sliding-scale view as it stands.

However, this does not entail that we should wholly dispense with the epistemic justification of the sliding-scale view. It could be rendered more convincing by broadening the scope of what contributes to our understanding of proportionality in this context. The risk of harm associated with the consequence of a decision is only one relevant consideration; the importance to the particular patient of having the authority to make that risky decision is another. Taking into account both of these elements, and establishing that they do not offset each other is a necessary (although perhaps not sufficient) condition of having an epistemic justification for altering the threshold of DMC on the basis of the consequence of the decision concerned. Only then will our decision to resolve uncertainty about DMC by altering the threshold of DMC on the basis of risk be sensitive to both of the salient values in this context, rather than considerations of non-maleficence alone.

Whilst one might resurrect the epistemic justification of the sliding-scale view in this way, I suggest that the above considerations instead provide support for an alternative approach to our understanding of proportionality in this context, and the role the sliding-scale view should play. Recall that the epistemic justification of the view is grounded in the desire for greater certainty in our assessments of DMC for riskier decisions. This is an admirable sentiment; however, our desire for greater certainty can only be satisfied in a dangerously attenuated sense by raising the threshold degree of DMC required for risky decisions, for the reasons outlined above. It is misleading to say that raising the threshold of DMC leads to 'greater certainty'; rather, it leads to greater certainty about one morally relevant feature by raising doubt in another.

However, we have a strong moral justification for increasing our degree of certainty in assessments of DMC for risky decisions, when that is understood to refer to certainty *tout court*. The problem is that altering the threshold of DMC for making a risky decision is a poor mechanism for acquiring greater certainty in this sense. Increases in certainty about true positives evinced by raising the threshold alone will correspond to decreases in certainty about true negatives; vice versa when we lower the standards of DMC. However, it might be possible to acquire greater *tout court* certainty in this context by increasing the level of *evidence* required in making our judgement of DMC, rather than increasing the threshold of DMC per se.[37] Such an understanding would avoid the problems outlined above, on the assumption that we can rely on forms of evidence for DMC that would allow us to decrease the rate of false positive assessments, without correspondingly increasing the rates of false negative rates. Whether or not it is feasible to gather such evidence, it is clear that simply raising the threshold of DMC cannot serve this sort of purpose. I turn to the epistemic challenges of assessing DMC in section 5.

4. Rationalist DMC in the Ideal Context, and the Anti-Paternalist Objection

In the previous section, I considered the extent to which the widely accepted sliding-scale view of DMC has paternalistic connotations. I now want to consider whether similar charges could be raised against the implications that my rationalist conception of autonomy has for our understanding of DMC. In this section, I consider the implications that the theory has in the idealized context, where the only question we have to consider is whether the rationality criterion sets out a plausible necessary condition of DMC. I shall consider its implications in the non-ideal context in the following section. To begin this discussion, I shall explain the implications that my

[37] Beauchamp and Childress, *Principles of Biomedical Ethics*, 76–7.

theory has for the discrepancies between the two accounts of DMC that I outlined above.

The first discrepancy was that Grisso and Appelbaum's approach incorporates a criterion of 'appreciation' that is absent in the MCA test. Such a criterion is a highly plausible addition to an adequate set of criteria for DMC by the lights of the theory that I have outlined in this book.[38] Appreciation can clearly be a necessary ability for autonomous decision-making, since the failure to appreciate information in this way can clearly be inimical to an individual's holding decisionally necessary beliefs. For instance, if a patient fails to believe that they are seriously ill and will die without medical intervention when that is in fact the case, then they lack a belief that is crucial for making an autonomous decision in that context; in such an epistemic situation, they will be unable to perceive an important set of reasons, namely those in favour of undergoing medical treatment.[39]

In accordance with my earlier discussions in this book, we may also note that in addition to the ability to appreciate information in this sense, the ability to meet minimal standards of theoretical rationality will also be necessary for individuals to avoid some of the false beliefs that are inimical to their decision-making, and to use and weigh information in the manner that connotes autonomous decision-making.

The criterion of appreciation also represents a way in which the patient's evaluations feature in DMC criteria, since appreciation involves 'assigning values to information'.[40] This feature is also relevant to the second discrepancy between the two accounts, namely that Grisso and Appelbaum make explicit reference to the need to manipulate information *rationally* in one's deliberative process, whilst the MCA does not. Naturally, my view lends support to the former approach, and provides a theoretical basis for adding further content to this requirement.

Grisso and Appelbaum are predominantly concerned with the theoretical rationality that decision-making capacity requires, suggesting that this criterion requires that patients are able to '... reach conclusions that are consistent with their starting premises'.[41] Whilst I agree that this is an important part of DMC, I claim that we ought to understand this ability (and the ability to 'use and weigh' information to which the MCA refers) in a manner that reflects the rationality condition defended in the previous chapter. To have the ability to 'weigh and use' information in one's decision-making process is to have the ability to make a decision in accordance with what one values, that is, with one's personally authorized preferences. To weigh information in the manner that autonomy requires is to consider the bearing that material information has on ends that agents value (and their pursuit thereof), and to consider the strength of the relevant competing reasons. To do this, a patient must be

[38] Beauchamp and Childress take their criterion of understanding to incorporate appreciation. Ibid., 88–93 and fn. 32.

[39] Note that a patient can perceive these reasons, even if she only rejects the negative connotations of her illness. For instance, a patient who accepts the descriptive claim that she is not 'healthy' in a biostatistical sense, but who also denies that she has strong reasons to be healthy in this sense, may still be able to understand that she has very weak reasons to undergo medical treatment. For a detailed discussion of insight into mental disorder and implications for capacity, see Holroyd, 'Clarifying Capacity'.

[40] Appelbaum and Grisso, 'Assessing Patients' Capacities to Consent to Treatment'.

[41] Appelbaum and Grisso, 1636.

able to recognize that they have self-interested reasons to want certain things, and they must be able to use the information provided to them to decide what course of action to pursue, in the light of both descriptive facts and their own values. In short, DMC should incorporate considerations of practical, as well as theoretical rationality.

To further clarify the importance of values to DMC criteria, consider the following case:

Apathetic Andrea: Andrea suffers from clinical depression. Her physician explains to her that there are a number of treatment options available (including various anti-depressants, and forms of psychiatric counselling), and provides her with extensive information about each option and their possible outcomes. Andrea understands this information, retains it, and can compare how medically effective each option is against the other. However, Andrea is pathologically apathetic, and does not care at all what happens to her; she is convinced that everyone despises her, despite clear evidence to the contrary. Nothing can persuade her that her life is in any way worthwhile. Although she considers the information about each of her treatment options, she believes that this information is simply irrelevant. She simply does not care.[42]

In evidencing the ability to compare the relative effectiveness of each intervention, Andrea can plausibly be described as having the ability to 'weigh information'. However, if Andrea were to make a treatment choice in this scenario, it seems problematic to claim that her decision was autonomous, despite the fact that she meets the MCA criteria. The reason for this, I suggest, is that Andrea is unable to engage in rational deliberation about what to do, because she is unable to regard herself as having self-interested reasons to pursue her own well-being.[43] We might say that she is, in some sense, 'value-impaired'.[44]

Furthermore, Andrea's apathy is grounded by a theoretically irrational belief in her own lack of worth; she has what we might describe as an evaluative delusion.[45] To repeat claims I made in Chapter 2, this is not a claim about the truth or falsity of the content of the belief. Rather, there are grounds for claiming that Andrea holds this evaluative belief in a theoretically irrational sense, in so far as she holds it unshakeably in a manner that is immune to evidence. It is a form of an evaluative delusion, which, as I argued in previous chapters, can serve to undermine decisional autonomy.[46]

[42] I base this case on Appelbaum et al.'s observation that depressed patients may have decreased motivation to protect their interests, perhaps associated with feelings of hopelessness that may alter the nature of patients' treatment decisions. Appelbaum et al., 'Competence of Depressed Patients for Consent to Research', 1380. See also Rudnick, 'Depression and Competence to Refuse Psychiatric Treatment'.

[43] For discussion of similar cases and the MCA see Rudnick, 'Depression and Competence to Refuse Psychiatric Treatment'.

[44] Brock, 'Patient Competence and Surrogate Decision-Making', 130. In describing the depressed person as value-impaired, he notes that '[t]here may be no failure in their understanding or reasoning about this outcome'; he argues that 'mental illness that distorts what they value from what it would otherwise be can result in incompetence to decide about treatment'.

[45] Fulford, 'Evaluative Delusions'.

[46] It may also be understood as a particularly damaging form of evaluative delusion, in so far as it encapsulates a paradoxical identification with what one loathes rather than what one values. See Radoilska, 'Depression, Decisional Capacity, and Personal Autonomy'.

Grisso and Appelbaum's approach might partly capture Andrea's lack of DMC by adverting to the necessity of appreciation to DMC, and the importance of being able to assign value to information in the process of appreciation. However, as I have explored previously in the book, agents who are not value-impaired in this way can still fail to make autonomous decisions, because of the role their values are playing in their decision-making process. In some cases, an individual's decisions may reflect the force of a motivating desire that the individual does not rationally endorse. In others, we may be concerned that the values that ground the agent's decision are not authentic to her, and are thus not a suitable ground for her autonomy.[47] The problem in such cases is not that agents fail to assign value to information; it is that the values they assign do not really reflect what they want.

Such cases represent arguably the most challenging cases for any procedural theory of autonomy, as well as raising questions about how we should delimit the scope of the clinical category of evaluative delusions. This deserves its own discussion, which I shall postpone until the following chapter. Here though, I want to begin considering the anti-paternalist objection to incorporating considerations of theoretical and practical rationality into criteria of DMC even in *ideal* contexts.

The general thrust of this objection is that incorporating such considerations would render standards of DMC too demanding, and would lead to physicians being able to overrule patient choice. The anti-paternalist objection is arguably the most pressing objection facing the rationalist account to autonomy I have defended in this book. I have noted that it is implicitly incorporated within Lord Donaldson's judgement quoted at the beginning of the chapter. However, the objection as I have just phrased it captures two distinct but related concerns. Here, I shall consider the objection in its purest form, as an objection to rationalist criteria as elitist even in ideal contexts. In the next section, I shall consider an epistemic version of the objection that can be raised against rationalist criteria in non-ideal contexts, according to which such criteria make it more likely that physicians will be able to overrule patient choice because of limits to our ability to accurately identify rational decision-making.

The elitist version of the anti-paternalist objection has been raised explicitly by a number of philosophers. For instance, in defending the standard account, Faden and Beauchamp write:

> If conscious, reflective identification with one's motivation were made a necessary condition of autonomous action, a great many intentional, understood, uncontrolled actions that are autonomous in our theory would be rendered non-autonomous.[48]

Nelson et al. go further, arguing that to claim that authenticity of any stripe is a condition of voluntariness is '...both conceptually unsatisfactory and morally dangerous'.[49]

[47] This issue with cognitivist tests of capacity has sometimes been parsed as a failure to incorporate considerations of volitional control. Craigie and Davies, 'Problems of Control', 2. I shall consider this framing in my discussion of anorexia nervosa in the next chapter.

[48] Faden and Beauchamp, *A History and Theory of Informed Consent*, 264.

[49] Nelson et al., 'The Concept of Voluntary Consent'.

The first thing to acknowledge about this objection is that it is understood to pertain to all of the procedural theories of reflective autonomy that I surveyed in the first two chapters. This observation alone might seem to render the objection implausible. To see why, reconsider Frankfurt's view of autonomy; on Frankfurt's view, autonomy requires that one identify with one's first-order motivating desire with a second-order volition. Crucially for Frankfurt, human beings can be distinguished from other creatures by virtue of the fact that they alone are able to form second-order desires.[50] Accordingly, far from being elitist, Frankfurt might claim that the standards set in his theory of reflective autonomy are simply the standards for how we assess personhood.

However, it might be claimed that rationalist theories of autonomy of the sort that I have defended are particularly vulnerable to this objection.[51] For instance, John Christman writes that:

> . . . the property of autonomy must not collapse into the property of 'reasonable person', where the idea of being self-governing is indistinguishable from the idea of being, simply, smart.[52]

There are several things to say in response to this objection.[53] First, phrased in this way, the objection appears to assimilate rationality and 'smartness'; yet, one need not be 'smart' in order to be rational. On the theory that I have developed here, agents need only be able to pursue the outcome of their desire on the basis of their belief that the outcome is something that they have reason to pursue. It is not at all clear why this should be *intellectually* demanding; to suppose otherwise is to conflate the separate concepts of rationality and intelligence.[54]

One might instead interpret Christman's concern here to be that a rationalist approach to autonomy entails that it will be reserved only for those who think through their choices. I struggle to see why we should find it problematic to claim that an individual will only be able to make a locally autonomous choice if they think through it in basic ways. Indeed, this is just why we reserve the right to make one's own medical decisions for those who qualify as having decision-making capacity. In my view, the most plausible way of cashing out this concern is that we have reasons to be sceptical of a theory of autonomy that entails that individuals will only qualify as being globally

[50] Frankfurt, 'Freedom of the Will and the Concept of a Person'.

[51] Christman, 'Autonomy and Personal History', 14; Hyun, 'Authentic Values and Individual Autonomy'; Hill, *Autonomy and Self-Respect*, 49. Notably, Ploug and Holm, 'Doctors, Patients, and Nudging in the Clinical Context—Four Views on Nudging and Informed Consent' suggest that Christman's criticism can also be weighed against the form of rationality implied by the standard account.

[52] Christman, 'Autonomy and Personal History', 14.

[53] A closely related objection in this context is that rationalist conditions rule out the autonomy of individuals who prefer a life of non-reflection or spontaneity. Hyun, 'Authentic Values and Individual Autonomy', 199; Double, 'Two Types of Autonomy Accounts', 73; Blumenthal-Barby and Naik, 'In Defense of Nudge–Autonomy Compatibility'. However, this objection misconstrues the nature of procedurally rationalist theories by raising what is essentially a substantive complaint. The rationalist theory can quite easily accommodate the thought that an individual can autonomously live a life of non-reflection or spontaneity, as long as they do so because they believe that way of life is valuable—this is a procedural rather than substantive matter. For a similar reply to this objection, see Ploug and Holm, 'Informed Consent, Libertarian Paternalism, and Nudging'.

[54] See Baron, *Rationality and Intelligence* for an account of how the two differ.

autonomous if they think through every single one of their choices and make them in a maximally autonomous way. Yet a rationalist account does not require this—as long as one does not understand global autonomy as the aggregative accumulation of various locally autonomous choices (a suggestion I rejected in the introduction to the book), then it is quite compatible with an individual's making a considerable number of choices over their lives that are not locally autonomous.

That said, as I explored in Chapters 1 and 2, on a rationalist account, autonomy does require rational reflection in a way that other accounts do not, even if such reflection can be unconscious or dispositionally produced. I have suggested in previous chapters that accounts that do not appeal to actual reflection of this sort fail to accommodate paradigm cases of individuals who lack autonomy (i.e. the standard account), and that accounts appealing to hypothetical reflection (such as Christman's account) also face other challenges concerning their operationalization in bioethical contexts. Ultimately though, even if the rationalist has to bite the bullet and accept that autonomy is more challenging on his account than it is on others, this does not entail that it is beyond the capacity of most human beings. On the contrary, like Frankfurt, advocates of rationalist theories can suggest that having the abilities associated with rational decision-making is just part of what it is to be a person. Indeed, in the very first sentence of *On What Matters*, Parfit claims that humans are '... the type of animal that can both understand and respond to reasons'.[55] Similarly, in his defence against a similar objection, Joseph Raz points out that '[t]o want to be rational is to want to be a person'.[56]

Rationality conditions of decisional autonomy do not entail that autonomy-based protections will only be afforded to those who think through their choice with intellectual precision and accuracy, nor does it unduly preclude individuals from having decision-making authority. However, it might be argued that the rationalist account is elitist in a different sense, in that it places too much emphasis on cognitive elements of decision-making capacity and fails to acknowledge the importance of affective attitudes and emotional experience to DMC.[57] However, the rationalist account can be understood to incorporate affective elements of DMC in so far as many of our affective attitudes and emotional experiences can give rise to values, and ground certain sorts of reasons. Consider for example the experience of love; although the experience of love is not itself typically the output of rational deliberation (we 'fall in' love, rather than rationally deliberate ourselves into it), it can clearly give rise to other evaluative judgements that we come to reflectively endorse, and reasons to act in certain ways towards others. Moreover, as Nomy Arpaly has persuasively argued, emotions might plausibly be a source of reasons which may not be accessible at the time of deliberation, but which may nonetheless ground rational behaviour on a broadly coherentist approach.[58]

55 Parfit, *On What Matters*, 31.

56 Raz, *Engaging Reason*, 18.

57 Charland, 'Anorexia and the MacCAT-T Test for Mental Competence'; Vollmann, '"But I Don't Feel It"'; Christman, *The Politics of Persons*, 144; Mackenzie, 'Three Dimensions of Autonomy', 31; Kong, 'Beyond the Balancing Scales', 234–5.

58 Arpaly, 'On Acting Rationally against One's Best Judgment'. Marilyn Friedman also recognizes that features of emotion and character can constitute reasons. See Friedman, *Autonomy, Gender, Politics*, 9.

The rationalist account does speak against unreflective emotional states grounding autonomous decision-making and action, but this seems quite plausible; a person who acts in a fit of rage and later decides that this did not reflect their evaluative judgements is not appropriately described as having acted autonomously. This suggests that we need to have a nuanced understanding of the role of emotions in autonomous agency; it is neither the case that they alone can ground autonomous decision-making, nor that their mere influence impedes it. The issue turns on whether our emotional states are connected in the right way to our evaluative judgements.[59]

Similar remarks apply to relational influences on decisional autonomy. Cognitive tests of DMC have been criticized on the basis that they overlook relational (as well as emotional) influences on autonomous decision-making.[60] However, the approach to DMC that I am outlining here is quite compatible with relational influences. First, as I discussed in Chapter 5, many of the abilities that are necessary for decisional autonomy are socially mediated; accordingly, in claiming that decisional autonomy requires practical and theoretical rationality, I am implicitly accepting that the relational and social conditions that are necessary for individual rationality will also be necessary for DMC. We may also observe that relationships can be central to the content of our values. Nonetheless, whilst acknowledging these important points, it is best to maintain some conceptual distance between relational influences and DMC. The reason for this is that there are many interpersonal effects on the voluntariness of decision-making that do not adversely affect DMC, even if they undermine decisional autonomy in other ways. For example, I suggested that deceived agents and coerced agents may lack autonomy with respect to their decisions, but it can still make sense to describe them as retaining the abilities that are causally necessary for (counterfactually) making that decision autonomously. Indeed, as I explained in Chapter 5, it is only by virtue of the fact that the victim of coercion retains their rational capacities that coercion is able to dominate the victim's will.

Perhaps part of the explanation for why rationalist theories of autonomy are deemed elitist is that critics assume that these theories are *substantively* rational rather than *procedurally* rational.[61] This is one plausible way of reading Lord Donaldson's judgement; he seems to understand rational decisions as being co-extensive with decisions that *others* regard as rational, or with those that accord with impersonal reasons, ranked in a certain objective way.[62] However, on the theory that I have defended, agents may act on the basis of their beliefs about facts that

[59] For a nuanced discussion of how emotions can help us perceive practical reasons, see Tappolet, 'Emotions, Reasons, and Autonomy'. In cases in which an agent does not reflectively endorse their emotional states, then altering these emotional states may serve to enhance their autonomy. For example, see Douglas et al., 'Coercion, Incarceration, and Chemical Castration'.

[60] See Camillia Kong's recent defence of a relational approach to mental capacity in Kong, *Mental Capacity in Relationship*.

[61] Culver and Gert seem to understand rationality in this sense in disputing the role of DMC. Culver and Gert, 'The Inadequacy of Incompetence'.

[62] Similarly, when Draper calls for a distinction between incompetence and irrationality, she provides examples of decisions that appear irrational, but does not offer an account of irrationality per se. Yet, she endorses an account of competence that requires the ability to 'weigh information in a balance to arrive at a choice'. Draper, 'Anorexia Nervosa and Respecting a Refusal of Life-Prolonging Therapy', 126. As

provide them with either personal or impersonal self-interested reasons. This is crucial, since there is scope for considerable intersubjective variability in what agents have *personal* self-interested reason to do; moreover, rational agents may differ with regards to the weight that they place on different impersonal reasons. The upshot of this is that whilst we may agree with Lord Donaldson that patients should be free to make decisions that are irrational from the impersonal perspective, we should reject his claim that patients should be free to act in accordance with decisions that have *no* rational basis.

In a slightly different vein, Nelson et al. partly ground their criticism of authenticity-based accounts of voluntariness on the basis that we often make voluntary choices that are inauthentic. They write:

> Anomalous actions sometimes arise from choices that are out of character as a result of surrounding events that are unprecedented in the actor's experience, such as serious disease.[63]

To illustrate further, they appeal to the following example:

> A patient might request a highly invasive treatment at the end of life against his previous judgment about his best interests because he has come to a conclusion that surprises him.[64]

Whether or not this is a compelling objection to the accounts of authenticity that the authors have in mind, this example is not particularly problematic for the account that I have developed here. The reason for this is that the objection assumes that authenticity must require a far greater degree of stability than is necessary. It is true that autonomy requires a degree of stability in our overall evaluative nexus; we will be unable to adequately pursue the long-term plans that undergird our global autonomy if we frequently abandon the values that provide their basis. However, this is quite compatible with the claim that our local autonomous choices can run contrary to some of the evaluative judgements that we have long held dear. Such departures from a pre-existing value can be authentic if the change is *intelligible* to the agent, by virtue of its coherence in the overall nexus of her other acceptances and preferences; in short, her character. However, such choices may undermine autonomy if they are not a response to the agent's own judgements about what is good for her, but produced by other irrational drives (such as fear) that can disconnect the agent's motivation from her evaluative judgements. The crucial question is thus not whether or not the agent can autonomously choose contrary to a previously held evaluative judgement, but rather *why* the agent in question has chosen contrary to that judgement.

In contrast to the terms in which the objection above has been stated, we have little reason to believe that the patient in the above case, who changes her judgement about what is in her best interests, is acting contrary to her values generally, even if she is now deciding contrary to a particularly long-standing evaluative judgement. In fact,

such, it appears that she accepts the claim that competence is incompatible with some sorts of practical irrationality.

63 Nelson et al., 'The Concept of Voluntary Consent'. See also Beauchamp and Childress, *Principles in Biomedical Ethics*, 103.

64 Nelson et al., 'The Concept of Voluntary Consent'. The authors draw this example from Jaworska, 'Caring, Minimal Autonomy, and the Limits of Liberalism', 82.

we have good reasons to suppose that facing a serious medical condition will tend to prompt individuals to reconsider the values that undergird the reasons for their practical choices. Not only that, such agents will be carrying out this reflection at the same time as acquiring epistemic access to vital reason-giving facts about the precise nature of the situation that they now find themselves in. For instance, they may now be acutely aware of the fact that illness can drain a person of their reserves of determination.[65]

In contrast, the evaluative judgements that they had previously made about such situations were made without such awareness. In Nelson et al.'s case, the patient's understanding of the comparative strength of their reasons to avoid severe pain on the one hand, and to avoid death on the other, will naturally be sharpened and altered by being placed in a situation in which they are confronted with the reality of having to choose to act on the basis of one of these reasons. As such, the fact that the patient in question is now making a request that is in conflict with her previous evaluative judgement does not entail that it qualifies as non-autonomous on the rationalist view I have defended; it can instead be a rationally intelligible adaption to one's radically different circumstances.[66]

So, in phrasing their spin on the anti-paternalist objection, Faden and Beauchamp are quite right to claim that 'many intentional, understood, uncontrolled actions that are autonomous in our theory would be rendered non-autonomous' on a rationalist theory. But the reason for this is that many intentional, understood, and uncontrolled actions are not autonomous. The main remaining worry undergirding the elitist objection in the context of biomedical ethics is that incorporating the rationality condition I have suggested into a conception of DMC will serve to increase the number of patients who will lack DMC. I have in mind here patients such as those who suffer from conditions that render them unable to make treatment decisions in accordance with what they believe they have reason to do in light of their own evaluative judgements. Whilst such patients would lack DMC on the approach that I advocate, I do not take this to be a flaw of the theory. On the contrary, it is a flaw of the standard view that it finds such patients competent to make their treatment decisions, and regards their choices as autonomous. Whilst these patients are able to express a 'choice', it is one that is unconnected to what they themselves believe they have reason to do in light of their own values.

In fact, the standard theory itself comes very close to advocating a similar viewpoint in its stipulation that psychiatric disorders can represent internal forms of controlling influence that undermine autonomy. However, as I argued in previous chapters, in the absence of something like an account of authenticity, the standard account lacks a unified explanation of what it is that makes these disorders controlling in the sense that undermines decisional autonomy. As I shall discuss in the next chapter, my account allows for a far more nuanced understanding of the ways in which certain psychiatric disorders can, but need not, undermine autonomous decision-making.

[65] Gavaghan, 'In Word, or Sigh, or Tear', 249.

[66] See also Meynen, 'Depression, Possibilities, and Competence'; Gavaghan, 'In Word, or Sigh, or Tear', 246–9.

Strikingly, despite these philosophical objections to rationalist criteria of DMC, there is evidence to suggest that prominent accounts of DMC (including those invoked by the courts) seem to incorporate either a rationality constraint, or something similar in order to acknowledge ways in which volitional deficiencies can undermine DMC.[67] However, as I shall begin to explain in considering a different permutation of the anti-paternalist objection grounded by epistemic considerations, some versions of this view appear to place undue emphasis on unreliable proxies for procedurally rational decision-making.

5. Rationalist DMC in Non-Ideal Contexts and the Epistemic Anti-Paternalist Objection

Dispensing with the elitist conception of the anti-paternalist objection may suffice for justifying the adoption of a rationalist approach to DMC in ideal contexts. However, in accordance with my analysis above, in the non-ideal context we must consider two further questions about the application of a rationalist conception of DMC. First, do we have reliable methods to assess the supplementary abilities that I have considered so far? With regards to appreciation and theoretical rationality, it seems that the answer to this question is 'yes'. It is true that assessing these abilities requires going beyond the mere assessment of the individual's ability to understand information. However, these abilities plausibly admit of empirical assessment using similar methods to those that we use to assess understanding. Indeed, clinical tests for competence such as the Macarthur Competence Assessment Tool already use semi-structured interviews to assess appreciation.[68]

Whilst clinical assessment tools might plausibly assess appreciation and theoretical rationality, it is less clear that they will be able help physicians ascertain whether their patient is making their treatment decision in accordance with the requirements of practical rationality that I have outlined. It is one thing to establish that a patient can meet requirements of theoretical rationality in their deliberations in the manner that the MCA test and Grisso and Appelbaum's approach seems to imply. It is quite another to claim that they are weighing information rationally in accordance with their evaluative judgements, and making their decision in accordance with that weighting. In turn, this raises a further question about incorporating a rationality condition into our understanding of DMC in non-idealized contexts. Given that we are likely to make errors in our assessment of this ability, what implications might this criterion have for the balance that we are aiming to strike between the competing moral reasons at stake in setting thresholds of DMC? Is it justifiable to heighten the

[67] Craigie, 'Competence, Practical Rationality and What a Patient Values'; Craigie and Davies, 'Problems of Control'; Brock, 'Patient Competence and Surrogate Decision-Making'; Buchanan and Brock, *Deciding for Others*.

[68] Grisso, Appelbaum, and Hill-Fotouhi, 'The MacCAT-T'. For criticisms, see Baergen, 'Assessing the Competence Assessment Tool'; Kim, 'When Does Decisional Impairment Become Decisional Incompetence?'; Banner and Szmukler, '"Radical Interpretation" and the Assessment of Decision-Making Capacity'.

epistemic obstacles we face in making assessments of DMC by adding requirements of practical rationality?

One particular concern we might have in this regard is that medical professionals might exploit our epistemic limitations about the practical rationality of others to unjustifiably revoke patients' decision-making authority, in order to prioritize considerations of beneficence. The thought here is that in view of our epistemic limitations in this regard, adopting a rationalist criterion of DMC would most likely lead physicians to make judgements about the rationality of a patient's decision based on the *content* of the patient's decision, or their disease status.[69] Even if we agree that DMC should not be defined by appeal to such substantive considerations, perhaps the epistemic barriers we face in assessing rational DMC may leave us with little choice but to adopt a substantive approach to assessing capacity, inevitably increasing false negative assessments. This is in tension with both the proceduralist spirit of the MCA and the account of autonomy that I have defended, and it is precisely what Lord Donaldson was seeking to defend against in his judgement outlined at the outset of this chapter.

Indeed, there is some evidence to suggest that this sort of problem is already arising with respect to the manner in which the MCA is interpreted. Although the MCA does not make explicit reference to requirements of rationality or authenticity in its 'use and weigh' criterion, the manner in which the law has been interpreted in the context of refusals of treatment from patients suffering from anorexia nervosa suggests that the criterion has been understood to preclude individuals from qualifying as having DMC if their decisions are grounded by apparently 'compulsive motivations'. For instance, the MCA code of practice suggests that patients suffering from anorexia nervosa may lack DMC, not because of any deficiency in their ability to understand material information, but rather because 'their compulsion not to eat may be too strong for them to ignore'.[70] Furthermore, Jillian Craigie and Alisa Davies have highlighted a number of legal judgements that suggest that courts in England and Wales tend to view the desires that are symptomatic of anorexia nervosa as amounting to compulsions that are incompatible with DMC.[71]

The claim that compulsions undermine decisional autonomy is broadly compatible with my procedural account of autonomy, although I shall say more about this in the next chapter. In practice though, assessments of what constitutes a 'compulsion' in these contexts may be grounded by non-procedural considerations. As Camillia Kong has argued, the assessment of a compulsion can treat 'compulsion' as a thick concept;[72] it may incorporate substantive considerations either directly or indirectly through an appeal to the patient's diagnostic status. The concern here is that this interpretation of the MCA test coupled with our epistemic limitations threatens to unjustifiably collapse the ostensibly procedural test of capacity into a diagnostic status-based test, whereby anorexic patients are simply assumed to lack capacity because they are assumed to be subjects of compulsion in their decision-making.[73]

[69] Banner and Szmukler, '"Radical Interpretation" and the Assessment of Decision-Making Capacity'.
[70] *Mental Capacity Act Code of Practice*, 4.22. [71] Craigie and Davies, 'Problems of Control'.
[72] Kong, 'Beyond the Balancing Scales'. [73] Ibid.

I am sympathetic to Kong's concern about this in the specific context of anorexia nervosa, and I shall consider the issue in more detail in a case discussion in the next chapter. To conclude this chapter though, I want to consider this epistemic form of the anti-paternalist objection in a more abstract sense outside of this specific context. Do our epistemic limitations give us decisive reasons not to incorporate considerations of rationality into non-ideal assessments of DMC?

If Kong's critical analysis of the current interpretation of DMC is correct, then the flaw in this interpretation seems to lie in the fact that the courts are relying on individuals' disease-status, and perhaps even the content of the patients' decision, as an exhaustive and reliable proxy for procedurally rational decision-making. Before considering whether this mistake must be inevitable, it is important to note that the use of proxies to enable one to overcome epistemic barriers to accurate assessments of DMC is not problematic per se. It is quite coherent to claim that the content of an individual's decision can provide evidential support for an assessment of DMC, whilst denying that it can provide a sufficient ground for a judgement that an individual lacks DMC. To use Colin Gavagahn's memorable phrase the content of a decision can serve as a 'warning flag rather than a stop sign' in assessments of DMC.[74] Indeed, although the above discussion suggests that the MCA is not always interpreted correctly on the following point, the Act nonetheless implicitly endorses the view that substantive considerations can play a non-exhaustive role in assessments of DMC. Recall that the MCA stipulates that 'A person is not to be treated as unable to make a decision merely because he makes an unwise decision'. As Herring notes, the use of the word 'merely' here suggests that the fact that a decision is unwise can factor in one's assessment of DMC; it just cannot be the *only* factor.[75]

The account of autonomy that I have defended can help to elucidate why this approach to evidential proxies can be justified. When a patient has made their treatment decision autonomously, they should be able to justify that decision by appeal to what they understand to be the reason-implying facts about their treatment options, and its coherence with their other evaluative judgements. In many cases, the reasoning behind a decision will be quite transparent to third parties. In some cases though, the rationale for the content of a patient's decision may be opaque to others. If, in such cases, the content of a particular decision is contrary to what the patient has impersonal reason to do, or if it appears incongruous with other elements of the patient's character system, that gives us reason to investigate the patient's deliberative process in a deeper fashion. Crucially though, in such cases, the content of the decision should not serve as the end-point of an assessment of the patient's DMC. Rather, the fact that the rationale for the decision is opaque should act as a springboard for investigating the individual's reasons for making that decision, and also how it relates to her core preferences and acceptance.[76]

Proxies, however, *are* problematic if they are understood to be wholly sufficient for assessments of procedural DMC, or if they are in fact unreliable 'warning flags' for that which we are seeking to identify, in this case, procedurally rational decision-

[74] Gavaghan, 'In Word, or Sigh, or Tear', 252. [75] Herring, *Medical Law and Ethics*, 165.

[76] Gavaghan also defends further probing into the internal consistency of the patient's reasoning process in such contexts. See Gavaghan, 'In Word, or Sigh, or Tear', 247.

making. However, incorporating a rationalist condition into one's account of DMC does not entail that we must rely on unreliable proxies or indeed proxies alone.

This point has an important bearing on the broader epistemic concern that grounds this permutation of the anti-paternalist objection, namely the concern that incorporating judgements of rationality into assessments of DMC will unavoidably lead to more false negative assessments. This concern is only warranted if we accept that we lack evidential methods for accurately assessing the ability that we are attempting to capture here. Whilst one may plausibly object that we do not currently employ such methods, there is some scope for optimism about the possibility that we might accurately assess rational decision-making. First, there is currently a great deal of interest in using neuroscientific approaches to assessing the neural underpinnings of clear deficits in rational decision-making, and there have been calls to use such evidence in assessments of DMC.[77] However, this research is at an early stage, and may not be appropriate for many patients.

Yet there are other alternative methods we might adopt in tackling this epistemic barrier to assessments of practical rationality that have far greater clinical feasibility. For instance, Natalie Banner and George Szmukler's 'Radical Interpretation'[78] approach advocates that in assessing DMC, clinicians should focus not on the content of a belief or decision, but rather upon the relationships between that belief and decision to other elements of their 'mental economy':

> The epistemic standards of 'coherence' and 'correspondence' thus provide a framework within which decisions and behaviour, whether unusual or not, can be interpreted and understood. It is only in virtue of the implicit background structure of interconnected beliefs, actions, and so forth, that individual beliefs (or values) can be picked out as normatively inappropriate, and therefore potentially indicative of an impairment that could undermine capacity: a note of discord in an otherwise fairly coherent and harmonious symphony of intentional behaviour.[79]

As such, on the radical interpretation approach, and more generally on the view of autonomy that I have defended, a clinician's substantive assessment of a particular belief or decision should be understood to motivate a broader kind of enquiry into the agent's character system, rather than wholly constituting an assessment of DMC; substantive assessment here does not lend support to a substantive approach to autonomy or unwarranted paternalism.[80] The above discussion also suggests that, in situations in which there is disagreement between the physician and their patient about the best treatment option, it is not only appropriate for the physician to ask their patient to explain the reasons underlying their decision, but in fact necessary for establishing that the decision was made in the right way.

The concern that the manner in which the MCA is interpreted may currently lead to substantive assessments of capacity must be taken seriously. However, my suggestion is that this interpretation is a result of over-generalizations and misconceptions about both the nature of particular disorders and plausible demands of

[77] Clarke, 'The Neuroscience of Decision Making and Our Standards for Assessing Competence to Consent'; Peterson, 'Should Neuroscience Inform Judgements of Decision-Making Capacity?'

[78] Banner and Szmukler, '"Radical Interpretation" and the Assessment of Decision-Making Capacity'.

[79] Ibid., 385.

[80] Ibid., 389–92.

rationality, rather than a problem with incorporating considerations of rationality into assessments of DMC per se. It is possible to assess the extent to which a patient is making their decision in accordance with the kind of rationality condition I have outlined, without relying on the patient's disease status or substantive considerations alone as crude proxies.

Yet, it might finally be objected that engaging in radical interpretation is highly burdensome for health care teams, who simply do not have the time to engage in this sort of detailed discussion with every patient. However, my claim that radical interpretation is the best way to accurately assess 'rational DMC' and to thus facilitate our ability to afford decision-making authority to patients appropriately, is quite compatible with there being stronger moral reasons that outweigh those in favour of its use. Such reasons might include considerations pertaining to the just allocation of scarce resources in health care, including the medical team's time and energy. However, we cannot have our cake and eat it too. If we believe these other moral reasons are stronger, and therefore advocate an approach to patient decision-making that does not incorporate deep consideration of the patient's reasons and values, this only means that we must acknowledge that we are trading off the value of giving decision-making authority to the people who actually deserve it (and protecting those who deserve protection from harm) against other moral values. It does not mean that the radical interpretation approach does not facilitate our ability to make true positive and true negative assessments of DMC.

Of course, that is not to say that radical interpretation is a flawless evidential mechanism in this regard. Even if it is highly accurate, there is still the possibility that some individuals might unjustifiably be denied decision-making authority on the basis that they have incorrectly been assessed as lacking practical rationality in their decision-making. But, this cost has to be weighed against the costs of two features of the status quo. The first is that the low threshold approach to the DMC in the MCA means that it is likely that a number of individuals currently qualify as having DMC when they are *not* able to make autonomous decisions about treatment. Second, due to the vague wording of the 'use and weigh' criterion, there is scope for widely varying interpretations for the general applications of this criterion.[81] In addition to the concerns about how this may open the door to substantive considerations determining assessments of capacity, considerations of justice speak against leaving the interpretation of the 'weigh and use' criterion to the discretion and intuitions of different courts. The values of the individual either should or should not matter for *all* patients whose DMC is under consideration.

Ultimately, the question must boil down to how important we think rationality is to autonomy, and whether it is sufficiently important to include it amongst our criteria of DMC, given the costs of raising the threshold of DMC in a non-ideal context. My own view is that practical rationality warrants inclusion because of its centrality to autonomous decision-making. Practical rationality as I outlined it in the first chapters of this book is not just one ability among several that are relevant to DMC; it is central to the value of autonomous decision-making in so far as it allows

[81] Bartlett, *Blackstone's Guide to the Mental Capacity Act 2005*, 51.

us to direct our lives in accordance with our own values. It thus grounds the moral significance of all the other abilities that we typically accept are necessary to autonomous decision-making. Understanding information, retaining it, and 'weighing' it only matters for autonomy if we assume that agents have the ability to link that information (and how much weight it is given) to their own values; similarly we should only be concerned about the decision a patient communicates if it is a communication of a decision grounded by their values.

In the next chapter, I shall bring this theoretical discussion of DMC to bear on some practical cases that will serve to further elucidate features of my account. In doing so, I shall consider further the concern that assessments of DMC in the context of anorexia nervosa are in danger of collapsing the proceduralist test of the MCA into a status-based test that indirectly incorporates a substantive conception of autonomy.

8

Rational Decision-Making Capacity in End of Life Decision-Making

In this chapter I shall consider three cases of end of life decision-making that illuminate implications that my rationalist approach has for decision-making capacity (DMC). Although end of life decision-making is not the only medical context in which judgements of DMC can be contentious, the gravity of the consequences of refusing consent to medical treatment here makes the stakes of this debate particularly high.

At the outset, it is important to be clear about the scope of the implications of the claim that a patient lacks DMC in this context. Crucially, the mere fact that a patient lacks DMC does not entail that it is thereby permissible to treat that patient. First, there may be ways in which it would be possible to facilitate the patient's attaining the requisite DMC to provide valid consent.[1] However, even when it is not possible to enable a patient to acquire DMC for the material time at which the decision must be made, it may still not be permissible to initiate treatment in the absence of consent, because of other salient moral considerations. In particular, since non-consensual treatment can be a harrowing experience, and since some medical interventions may have only limited beneficial effects in the end of life context, a decision to refrain from providing non-consensual medical treatment may sometimes be grounded by considerations of well-being, rather than respect for autonomy per se.[2] Furthermore, patients may plausibly have a number of claim rights against bodily interference that do not depend on their status as autonomous agents.[3] Finally, there may also be

[1] Notably in this regard, one of the guiding principles of the MCA states that a patient should not be understood to lack capacity 'unless all practicable steps to help him to do so have been taken without success'. Mental Capacity Act 2005, 1(3). Furthermore, an individual is not to be precluded from DMC on the basis of inadequate understanding if he is able to understand an explanation of the treatment decision 'given to him in a way that is appropriate to his circumstances'. Mental Capacity Act 2005, 3(2).

[2] As Draper acknowledges, this is a particularly salient consideration in the context of anorexia nervosa. See Draper, 'Anorexia Nervosa and Respecting a Refusal of Life-Prolonging Therapy', 121. See also Geppert, 'Futility in Chronic Anorexia Nervosa'.

[3] Savulescu and Momeyer, 'Should Informed Consent Be Based on Rational Beliefs?' Rebecca Walker argues that we have moral reasons to abide by irrational choices made by competent individuals on the basis that a failure to abide by such choices would violate the rights held by these patients. Walker, 'Respect for Rational Autonomy', 356. Whilst I am sympathetic to the idea that unwaived rights claims may speak against involuntary treatment, I think Walker is mistaken to claim that this gives us a sufficient reason to abide by irrational choices. Part of the problem here is that, contrary to Walker's analysis, *non-competent* individuals also have a right to avoid unwanted and invasive bodily interference; and yet we believe it can be permissible to override this right. It is true that the Hohfeldian *incidents* incorporated into the right

Autonomy, Rationality, and Contemporary Bioethics. Jonathan Pugh, Oxford University Press (2020). © Jonathan Pugh.
DOI: 10.1093/oso/9780198858584.001.0001

societal and biopolitical considerations that enter into wise decision-making in this context.[4]

I shall explore many of these considerations in more detail in the following chapter when I turn to consider the value of autonomy. Here though, it suffices to note that the absence of DMC is not a sufficient condition of the permissibility of non-consensual medical treatment. Nonetheless, the fact that a patient lacks DMC has important moral implications in this context, since a patient's right to refuse medical treatment can be understood to be conditional on their having DMC to make an autonomous decision to refuse treatment, for reasons that I explored in the previous chapter.[5] If a patient has DMC, and exercises their right to refuse treatment, and that decision does not pose a direct harm to others (as it might in the context of public health) then it is thought that medical professionals are typically obligated to refrain from providing treatment.[6] Accordingly, establishing whether or not a patient has DMC thus has a crucial bearing on this strong form of protection that many patients are thought to enjoy.[7]

plausibly differ between competent and non-competent individuals. Whilst both enjoy a claim right against bodily interference, only the right of competent individuals incorporates the further power to waive that claim. Why should this be the case? To my mind, the most plausible explanation of the different elements of the rights of competent individuals is that we believe that waivers should only have normative authority if the decision to exercise this power is made autonomously. But, if this is right, then we should reject Walker's claim that we should abide by irrational choices of otherwise competent individuals on the basis of the rights we would violate if we failed to do so. Contrary to Walker's analysis, the fact that we would override an individual's rights in failing to abide by their treatment choice is often *not* sufficient to justify abiding by that choice. Indeed, we do not always abide by the choices of non-competent patients, despite their claim rights against bodily interference. In the case of non-competent patients, we abide by their choices if the benefits of failing to do so are insufficient to outweigh the interest protected by their claim. In contrast, the reason that we abide by the treatment choices of competent patients (even when the benefits of failing to do so would outweigh the harms) is that we acknowledge the normative authority of the individual's status as a competent individual by affording *them* the power to decide whether to waive their claims and to authorize treatment. However, if the authority of this decision to exercise this power is undermined by a lack of decisional autonomy, then it is unclear to me why this decision *must* be abided by in a manner that we would not similarly apply in the case of a non-competent individual. Walker herself implicitly acknowledges that we can have reasons to not abide by some choices of competent individuals, since she later claims that we should only abide by competent treatment refusals if they are 'freely made and informed'. Ibid., 358. But why only these refusals? Why rule out unfree or uninformed refusals if not because of the fact that they are not made autonomously? If one rules out these threats to autonomy, why not also rule out the threat posed by irrationality? Why suppose competence can have further moral force outside of its contribution to autonomy?

[4] Garasic, *Guantanamo and Other Cases of Enforced Medical Treatment*; Savulescu and Momeyer, 'Should Informed Consent Be Based on Rational Beliefs?'

[5] For an alternative view, see footnote 3.

[6] In England and Wales, the Mental Health Act is a counterexample to this, in so far as it permits the involuntary treatment of individuals with DMC who have been diagnosed with a mental disorder. UK Department of Health, Mental Health Act 1983 (Revised 2007). As others have argued, it is far from clear that this is ethically justified. Szmukler and Holloway, 'Mental Health Legislation Is Now a Harmful Anachronism'; Dawson and Szmukler, 'Fusion of Mental Health and Incapacity Legislation'; Bartlett, 'The United Nations Convention on the Rights of Persons with Disabilities and Mental Health Law'.

[7] Contrary to this analysis, Giordano argues that the moral force of autonomy is weakened in the specific context of anorexia nervosa, to the extent that we should not necessarily respect refusals of treatment by anorexic patients with DMC. For Giordano, the explanation for this is that the harms evinced by anorexia are distinctive, because the condition is reversible, and death from the condition is avoidable.

To recap the problem we face in this regard when adopting a rationalist conception of DMC: a plausible procedural account must accommodate the possibility that patients can make an autonomous treatment decision that others believe to be unwise. However, contrary to Lord Donaldson's claims analysed in the previous chapter, the rationalist approach denies that patients can make autonomous decisions on the basis of 'irrational reasons' or no 'reasons' at all. Rather, the challenge in this regard is how we can ascertain whether the patient is using and weighing the material information in a process of deliberation that is rational.

I shall begin my analysis with a straightforward example of how my rationalist approach is compatible with the claim that rational patients can make apparently 'unwise' choices. In the second half of the chapter, I shall consider the implications of my approach for more controversial cases concerning the rationality of treatment refusal on religious grounds, and treatment refusal in the context of anorexia nervosa. In doing so, I shall suggest that my rationalist approach is broadly compatible with the widely adopted view that (i) many religious believers who have DMC can refuse treatment forbidden by their religion and (ii) some anorexic patients can lack DMC to refuse treatment. However, my analysis shall suggest that we should take a much more nuanced approach to these cases than this generalized position implies, and which appears to be apparent in the standard view of autonomy's understanding of the implications of psychiatric disorders for decisional autonomy.

1. Rational DMC and 'Unwise' Decisions

Isobel is a 60-year-old woman who has developed pneumonia. She lives independently, but, after her husband died five years ago, has no surviving family or close friends. Isobel's physician tells her that pneumonia can be fatal, but that she has luckily been diagnosed very quickly. As such, her pneumonia can be treated with a short course of antibiotics, and she is expected to make a full recovery and live for at least another ten years. However, Isobel refuses consent; she says that she has had a 'good innings' but that she is now tired of life, and is ready to die.[8]

Death, typically, is something that we have a very strong self-interested reason to avoid, but can it ever be rational to prefer death to continued existence? In some cases, it seems quite uncontroversial to claim that this can be rational. To see why, we need to consider further why it is typically rational to prefer one's continued existence to death. In one sense, individuals can be understood to have a strong reason to avoid death, grounded by the fact that, in dying, we forgo any future

Giordano, *Understanding Eating Disorders*, 249–50. Whilst I agree that reversibility of the condition and the avoidability of death bear on the degree of harm at stake in treatment refusals in anorexia nervosa, far more argument is needed to establish that considerations of autonomy can be outweighed by harms that are worse in this sense. Further, contrary to Giordano's analysis, I am not convinced that anorexia nervosa is unique in this regard. As the example of Isobel below suggests, anorexia nervosa is not the only condition in which we might have to consider treatment refusals where the condition is reversible and death avoidable.

[8] For a case raising comparable but more complex issues, see Re B (Adult, refusal of medical treatment) 2, 449.

opportunity for well-being:[9] we will no longer have the opportunity to experience pleasurable mental states, to attempt to fulfil our desires, or to achieve objective goods.

Accordingly, we have a self-interested reason to safeguard the possibility of a future of value. However, if continued existence will only involve irrevocable pain and suffering, then such reasons may not apply; a person in this situation does not expect to experience a future of value, but rather one of disvalue. We can thus recognize, as David Hume did in his famous essay 'On Suicide',[10] that, despite our natural inclination to avoid death, life itself can become a burden of such disvalue, that our reasons to avoid that burden can outweigh both our natural inclinations and indeed our reasons to stave off our own non-existence. Indeed, the prospect that continued survival can become such a burden has been considerably enhanced by the development of medical technologies that afford us remarkable abilities to artificially sustain life.[11] Furthermore, we may note that we can plausibly value the exercise of our autonomy in shaping the end of our own existence, given the significant contribution that the end of life makes to the story of our life as a whole.

The rationality of preferring death to continued existence becomes more controversial as the expected value of one's future increases.[12] The above considerations suggest that it can be rational to prefer death to a future of disvalue, but can it be rational to prefer death to a future of some low, yet positive value? A key element of the theory that I have developed in this book is that rational agents can disagree about the relative weight that they attribute to their reasons to pursue different goods. Accordingly, even if we can construe someone as having a future that incorporates some valuable aspects, a rational agent can plausibly place greater weight on her reasons to avoid other aspects of that future that she disvalues.[13] Moreover, third parties lack epistemic access to other agents' own assessment of the comparative *strength* of certain reasons, and the truths regarding the comparative strength of our self-interested reasons are imprecise. Accordingly, whilst physicians may advocate the value and pursuit of health, and the reasons that patients have to pursue outcomes related to this good, this does not entail that it is irrational for a patient to choose otherwise, if that choice is demonstrably grounded in the patient's own broad evaluative framework.

Consider the implications that this has for Isobel. It is likely that her medical team would claim that, by forgoing treatment, Isobel is forgoing a future of value: after all, she is expected to make a full recovery from her pneumonia, she is living independently, and she is able to exercise her cognitive capacities in her day-to-day life. According to the standard account of autonomy and informed consent, in this

[9] For a developed hedonistic account of this point, see Bradley, *Well-Being and Death*.

[10] Hume, *On Suicide*.

[11] Garasic, *Guantanamo and Other Cases of Enforced Medical Treatment*, 11.

[12] Hedonic adaptation can raise a different kind of concern about the rationality of a patient's assessment of the expected value of their future. See Savulescu, 'Rational Desires and the Limitation of Life Sustaining Treatment'.

[13] This is one way in which the refusal of treatment may differ from voluntary passive euthanasia; the latter but not the former must be in the patient's best interests. For further discussion of this point, see Draper, 'Anorexia Nervosa and Respecting a Refusal of Life-Prolonging Therapy', 123–5.

situation, the medical team must ensure that Isobel understands (*inter alia*) the implications of forgoing treatment, that her decision is intentional, and that she is not deciding under controlling influences of the sort discussed in Chapters 4 and 5.

The account of rationalist autonomy and DMC that I am offering here demands something further; the medical team must try to establish that her decision is grounded by a personally endorsed preference, and that it is not grounded by irrational beliefs. What does this entail? Simply that the medical team investigates the reasons underlying her decision, and how these reasons are related to her other core values and beliefs. Recall that Isobel says she is 'tired of life'; part of investigating the rationality of her decision is to consider *why* this is the case. For instance, perhaps Isobel highly values social interaction, and her treatment decision might be the result of her experiencing social isolation following the death of her husband. Yet this is something that could be remedied in other ways; perhaps she could be entered into a befriending scheme, or a social group scheme run by local health authorities. Has she considered this alternative, and imagined what it might be like? If so, does she have reasons why she doesn't want to enrol in these schemes? Perhaps such reasons might be grounded by false beliefs about the schemes that the medical team could remedy.

This is not intended to be an exhaustive illustration of the kind of considerations that might be required in considering the rationality of Isobel's decision. The point of this brief illustration is that far from being elitist, rationalist DMC simply enjoins medical teams to make enquiries that represent a quite natural, caring response to a treatment decision of this kind. However, if after such enquiries, Isobel maintains her decision, and is able to give reasons for why she still wants to forgo treatment, grounded by her own values, then she should qualify as having DMC for that decision. Accordingly, respect for autonomy demands that the medical team should respect her decision to forgo treatment.

2. Religious Views and Psychiatric Disorder: A Justified Inconsistency in DMC?

Jack is a 32-year-old man who has been in a serious car accident and has lost a lot of blood. Still conscious, but bleeding heavily, he is rushed to A&E where doctors tell him that he urgently needs a blood transfusion or he will die. However, Jack refuses; he has been a life-long Jehovah's Witness, and he believes that he will not be permitted to enter the afterlife if he accepts the blood of another person.[14]

Keira is 43 years old and is a chronic sufferer of severe and enduring anorexia nervosa; although she is extremely malnourished, she refuses to eat. Moreover, repeated attempts at cognitive behavioural therapy have had no success in changing her eating behaviours. Her condition has deteriorated over time, and she is now at acute risk of organ failure if she does not receive nourishment soon. Keira is an intelligent and articulate woman, who recognizes that she is dangerously underweight, and that her refusal to eat is putting her life is at risk. However, she maintains her refusal to eat.[15]

[14] For a case raising comparable issues, see Re T (Adult: Refusal of Medical Treatment).

[15] For a case raising comparable issues, see Re E (Medical Treatment Anorexia) EWHC 1639 (COP).

Both of these cases involve choices that are likely to be understood as unwise from a medical perspective. However, this fact alone is not sufficient to demonstrate that these patients lack DMC on the approach that I am defending, nor on procedural approaches more generally.

These cases raise something of a puzzle for any theory of DMC. Jules Holroyd concisely diagnoses the issue as follows:

> As it stands, intuitions seem to pull in different directions: it appears intuitively plausible that over-valuing food avoidance or under-valuing continued existence thwarts the ability to weigh information relevant to treatment decisions. On the other hand it is less intuitively compelling to think that under-valuing the risk of death or disability due to a commitment to religious doctrine undermines decisional capacity (although anecdotally, intuitions seem to vary significantly on this).[16]

Contrary to Holroyd's analysis here, I shall suggest that our intuitions in these contexts may be influenced by considerations of theoretical as well as practical rationality. Here though, we may note that the Mental Capacity Act (MCA) to some extent reflects Holroyd's assessment of our intuitions in this area. Recall that an individual who lacks one of the abilities outlined in the functional test of DMC in the MCA will *not* qualify as lacking DMC unless their lacking this ability is also attributable to an impairment of, or a disturbance in the functioning of, the mind or brain. Accordingly, from the perspective of the MCA, Jack (or for that matter Isobel from the previous case) would not be found to lack capacity unless it could be established that his putative inability to use and weigh material information was due to an impairment of, or a disturbance in, the functioning of his mind or brain (rather than merely an upshot of his religious way of life).[17] In contrast, if one could establish that Keira lacks of one of the functional criteria of DMC due to her anorexia nervosa, then she could qualify as lacking DMC on the MCA.

It is difficult to see how this supplementary diagnostic criterion of mental capacity can be justified by philosophical considerations of autonomy. I argued in the previous chapter that the abilities that constitute DMC are the abilities that are necessary to making a particular decision autonomously. If an individual lacks one of these abilities, they cannot make that decision autonomously (or communicate it); the causal explanation for *why* the individual lacks the relevant ability thus seems to matter little for whether or not they are able to make an autonomous decision. This suggests that the diagnostic criterion requires an alternative justification. I lack the space to consider this particular issue here.[18] In the remainder of this chapter, I shall be concerned with the question of whether this discrepancy in widespread intuitions about these cases can be philosophically justified. I shall begin by focusing on Jack's case, and considering whether there may be philosophical grounds for claiming that Jack lacks DMC, contrary to the view outlined by Holroyd above.

[16] Holroyd, 'Clarifying Capacity', 12.

[17] Note that the impairment here need not be one grounded by pathology per se; for instance, temporary intoxication could disturb the functioning of the mind or brain in the relevant sense.

[18] Mirko Garasic makes some suggestive remarks in this regard in claiming that justifications for involuntary treatment are partly biopolitical rather than simply ethical. Garasic, *Guantanamo and Other Cases of Enforced Medical Treatment*, 12–16.

3. Jehovah's Witnesses, Theoretical Rationality, and the Doxastic Status of Faith

Jack holds true beliefs about the nature of the procedure he is declining, and his decision in this case is also practically rational; he makes his decision on the basis of a belief about the consequences which, if true, would give him a strongly decisive reason to refuse treatment. To see why, consider the belief in question and the values at stake for Jack. As a Jehovah's Witness (henceforth JW), Jack accepts the claim that the Bible prohibits blood transfusions and that accepting one would preclude him from blissful eternity in the afterlife. This is an outcome that Jack has a strongly decisive apparent reason to avoid; even if we assume that Jack would live a long (mortal) life with a high level of well-being following a transfusion, the value of this pales into comparison with the value of the life of eternal bliss that he would thereby forgo (or so he thinks).

Accordingly, it is difficult to argue that Jack is being practically irrational (although I shall consider one basis for this claim in my discussion of anorexia nervosa); he is deciding on the basis of what he believes he has strongly decisive reasons to do.[19] On this basis, we might claim that it is intuitively compelling that Jack can have DMC. However, although Jack appears to be practically rational, he might yet lack DMC on a rationalist conception, on the basis that he lacks theoretical rationality in holding what appear to be the operative beliefs in his decision-making process. Indeed, one might provocatively ask if there is anything that distinguishes religious beliefs from the sorts of delusional beliefs that uncontroversially undermine DMC.[20]

Savulescu and Momeyer come close to advocating this position; they claim that '... being autonomous requires that a person hold rational beliefs', and they argue that JWs' beliefs about blood transfusion and matters eschatological are theoretically irrational. Crucially, this argument does not rely on the premise that theism is true; rather, Savulescu and Momeyer argue that the relevant beliefs are theoretically irrational on the basis that those beliefs are not responsive to evidence, and that the interpretation of the scripture they imply lacks internal consistency.[21] Adrienne Martin has advanced the stronger claim that medical practice is committed to understanding JWs as lacking capacity on the basis that standard medical practice assumes these individuals have false (and not merely irrational) beliefs. Her explanation for this is that standard medical practical assumes that blood transfusions do

[19] Savulescu and Momeyer draw the same conclusion on this point at Savulescu and Momeyer, 'Should Informed Consent Be Based on Rational Beliefs?', 284.

[20] In the absence of a further philosophical argument to distinguish delusions grounded by a mental impairment and irrational beliefs held on religious grounds, it may be argued that their different treatment in mental capacity law amounts to discrimination. See Herring, *Medical Law and Ethics*, 157; Bartlett, 'The United Nations Convention on the Rights of Persons with Disabilities and Mental Health Law'. See also Fulford and Jackson, 'Spiritual Experience and Psychopathology' for a discussion of the difficulties in drawing this distinction.

[21] Savulescu and Momeyer, 'Should Informed Consent Be Based on Rational Beliefs?', 284.

not put patients at risk of eternal damnation, so JWs' beliefs prevent them from arriving at 'an even remotely accurate assessment of the risks of blood transfusion'.[22]

Despite these arguments, these authors nonetheless maintain that we should *not* treat JWs involuntarily. Savulescu and Momeyer advert to some of the competing moral considerations I outlined in the introduction to this chapter, whilst Martin argues that we should divorce considerations of DMC from the value of autonomy, and instead claim that patients lacking DMC can qualify as autonomous.[23] On such a view, autonomy has little to do with theoretical rationality, and instead concerns the consistency and coherence of one's values.[24] Once DMC has been separated from considerations of autonomy in this way, one can plausibly have autonomy-based reasons to respect the choices of patients lacking DMC.

It should be clear from my preceding arguments in this book that Martin's strategy here is incongruous with the position that I have developed. Theoretical rationality and the coherence and consistency of one's values *both* matter for autonomy; indeed, if the former did not, it is difficult to understand why it should be construed as a requirement of DMC to provide valid consent, a requirement Martin herself implicitly accepts. In contrast, Savulescu and Momeyer's conclusion that we should not treat JWs without consent even if their decision is not autonomous (on account of its theoretical irrationality) is compatible with the account that I have advanced.

In light of the MCA functionalist criterion, and what appear to be widespread intuitions about the autonomy and DMC of JWs, Savulescu and Momeyer's theory calls for a revisionist approach towards our understanding of the autonomy and DMC of JWs. However, contrary to their analysis, I shall argue that it is possible for a rationalist theory of autonomy to accommodate the thought that we should respect treatment refusals of JWs like Jack because they can be made autonomously (and not just because of the other moral considerations in favour of doing so). To do so, however, one must also embrace some further views in religious epistemology.

Martin, and Savulescu and Momeyer all accept that JWs *believe* that they will be precluded from eternal bliss if they accept a blood transfusion. Once this claim is in place, it is straightforward to argue that JWs are unable to decide autonomously on a rationalist approach, since these beliefs fail to meet the same standard of theoretical rationality to which we hold other beliefs. However, it is overly simplistic to view the operative cognitive states for many religious individuals simply as beliefs per se. Instead, they may be *items of faith*. Although items of faith may be conflated with beliefs in colloquial discussions, such conflation overlooks an important distinction, as I shall now explain.

[22] Martin, 'Tales Publicly Allowed', 36. Contrary to Martin's analysis, I contend that the fact that medical professionals act on the (rationally justified) assumption that a belief is false is not a sufficient epistemic basis for establishing the falsity of the belief in question. Indeed, on one prominent understanding, religious beliefs are unfalsifiable. See Flew, Hare, and Mitchell, 'Theology and Falsification'. Accordingly, I shall phrase my analysis in the weaker terms of theoretical rationality.

[23] Martin also proposes a second argument that we ought to respect the treatment wishes of religious believers in order to safeguard the valuable social institution of religion. Martin, 'Tales Publicly Allowed', 39–40. For a convincing rebuttal of this instrumentalist view, see Holroyd, 'Clarifying Capacity'.

[24] Martin, 'Tales Publicly Allowed', 38.

Bernard Williams famously argued that belief-formation is not under our voluntary control—call this thesis 'doxastic involuntarism'. Doxastic involuntarism is widely (though not universally) accepted, and part of one prominent defence of the thesis appeals to the underlying aim of beliefs. For instance, Williams claims that the goal of our beliefs it to aim at the truth, and notes that if 'deciding to believe' was under our voluntary control, then this would entail that one could decide to believe a proposition that one knew to be false. This, according to Williams, would be a necessarily bizarre state of affairs, given the aforementioned constitutive aim of beliefs (even if there might conceivably be some cases in which one could have non-truth based motives for believing such a proposition).[25]

This defence of doxastic involuntarism has been criticized but the details of this need not concern us here.[26] The important point to acknowledge is that even if we accept that doxastic involuntarism is true of beliefs *in general* (given their aims), it need not be true of all the cognitive states that individuals adopt with respect to items of faith. The aim of items of faith may not always be the same as beliefs; that is they may have aims other than that of merely capturing truth in the way that a typical belief does.

This is not to say that religious faith does not incorporate *any* beliefs. For instance, when one has what Robert Audi calls 'propositional faith' that *P* (that is, faith that some proposition *P* is true), this often implies that one also believes that *P* is true.[27] But faith can also incorporate a number of non-doxastic states that are not necessarily subject to the same epistemic norms as beliefs. Indeed, Audi explicitly identifies 'fiducial faith' as a form of non-doxastic propositional faith that does *not* connote or require the corresponding belief (much less a rational belief) that *P* is true.[28] Similarly, Andrei Buckareff suggests that items of religious faith may be understood as sub-doxastic pragmatic assumptions that an individual adopts in order to achieve a religious goal, namely forming a relationship with God.[29]

The thought here is that as well as not being subject to the same epistemic norms, or sharing the same aims as beliefs, agents can plausibly adopt sub-doxastic assumptions as items of faith on the basis of non-epistemic reasons, and as a voluntary act of will. That is, one can *choose* to have faith that *P*, in a way that one cannot choose to decide to believe *P*, even when there is little evidence for the truth of *P*. Moreover, this can be rational when the assumption of *P* is necessary to achieving a goal that one takes to be reason-giving.[30]

Whilst this is not the place to get into deep debates about religious epistemology, these somewhat cursory remarks reveal an avenue for understanding how JWs can be understood to make autonomous treatment decisions, despite the ostensible theoretical irrationality of their occurrent beliefs. As long as the operative cognitive states

[25] Williams, 'Deciding to Believe'.

[26] See Winters, 'Believing at Will'. For defences of doxastic involuntarism, see Buckareff, 'Deciding to Believe Redux'; Alston, *Epistemic Justification*; Levy and Mandelbaum, 'The Powers That Bind'.

[27] Audi, 'Belief, Faith, and Acceptance'. For defences of doxastic voluntarism, see Steup, 'Doxastic Voluntarism and Epistemic Deontology'; Weatherson, 'Deontology and Descartes's Demon'.

[28] Audi, 'Belief, Faith, and Acceptance'.

[29] Buckareff, 'Can Faith Be a Doxastic Venture?'

[30] Ibid.

here are not strictly beliefs (held in a manner that fails to meet standards of theoretical rationality), but rather items of faith, and as long as doxastic involuntarism does not apply to such items of faith, then JWs' accepting and abiding by the tenets of their faith can be understood to signify their choice to commit to a practice they take to be valuable. Their choice is to commit themselves to a number of sub-rational, sub-doxastic states, as a necessary element of a broader evaluative commitment to following a particular religious way of life.[31] The fact that this goal requires the endorsement of cognitive states that may be (mis)construed as simply theoretically irrational *beliefs* does not entail that these individuals lack autonomy. Rather, this feature of religious faith is broadly analogous to Odysseus tying himself to the mast. Whilst Odysseus forgoes local negative liberty in order to effectively pursue a broader goal he values, so too can the Jehovah's Witness forgo the requirements of theoretical rationality with regards to key cognitive states, as part of a rationally endorsed global commitment.[32]

The above considerations also suggest how we might distinguish religious beliefs from delusional states. According to the fifth edition of the *Diagnostic and Statistical Manual of Mental Disorders* (DSM 5), a delusional belief is:

> A false belief based on incorrect inference about external reality that is firmly held despite what almost everyone else believes and despite what constitutes incontrovertible and obvious proof or evidence to the contrary. The belief is not ordinarily accepted by other members of the person's culture or subculture (i.e., it is not an article of religious faith).[33]

The distinction that the DSM draws between delusions and religious belief is unsatisfying for a number of reasons. First, as I highlighted in previous chapters, this definition is incorrect to assume that a delusional belief must be false. Furthermore, it is unclear why the fact that a demonstrably false belief is widely held is sufficient to prevent it from being a delusion.[34] Certainly, whether or not such a false and theoretically irrational belief is 'ordinarily accepted by other members of the person's culture', does not appear to be directly relevant to the implications that the belief in question has for the individual's autonomy. However, my discussion above suggests that one thing that *can* matter for the individual's autonomy is whether the operant 'belief' in question is truly a theoretically irrational belief, or whether it is instead a sub-doxastic state to which the individual has voluntarily committed herself.

[31] Savulescu briefly alludes to this sort of strategy (amongst others) in his discussion. Savulescu, 'Rational Desires and the Limitation of Life Sustaining Treatment'. However, in his discussion of it, Savulescu assumes that the relevant belief is false. I have not made this assumption partly in view of the thought that religious beliefs of this sort are unfalsifiable for those who hold them.

[32] Dworkin similarly refers to JWs as tying 'themselves to the mast of their faith'. Dworkin, 'Autonomy and the Demented Self', 11. Dworkin is primarily concerned with whether we should prioritize past autonomous decisions over current non-autonomous decisions. In contrast, my discussion of faith highlights how religious beliefs can be incorporated into autonomous decision-making at all.

[33] American Psychiatric Association, *Diagnostic and Statistical Manual of Mental Disorders* (5th edition). For other criticisms see Bortolotti and Miyazono, 'Recent Work on the Nature and Development of Delusions'.

[34] Coltheart, 'The 33rd Sir Frederick Bartlett Lecture: Cognitive Neuropsychiatry and Delusional Belief'.

In accordance with the understanding of autonomy that I have developed here, voluntary commitment to the sub-doxastic states involved in some religious faith requires both (i) the understanding that one's item of faith amounts to adopting a sub-doxastic state that involves abandoning the norms of theoretical rationality and (ii) a rationale for doing so. That is, an individual who is to choose to commit to items of faith voluntarily must have insight into the fact that she lacks epistemic reasons that warrant *belief* in her item of faith, and that she must have practical reasons for maintaining this item of faith despite her lack of epistemic reasons. This is perhaps suggestive of one way in which delusional states, including religious delusional states, may come apart from sub-doxastic states that can be incorporated into religious faith.[35] If individuals suffering from delusional states lack this insight into the fact that they are not abiding by norms of theoretical rationality in holding their beliefs, then it is not clear that they consciously adopt or sustain these beliefs for any discernible practical reason.[36]

To conclude this discussion, let me briefly summarize its implications for the DMC of JWs. First, acknowledging that it is possible for JWs to decide autonomously about refusing blood transfusion on the basis of faith does not entail that they always do so. One particularly crucial question is whether their commitment to items of faith as part of a religious way of life is an autonomous one. There are of course a number of concerns about the voluntariness of an individual's adoption of a religious commitment, particularly amongst children who are vulnerable to what may amount to manipulative and coercive influence. At the individual level, we may note that in order for Jack's decision to refuse treatment to be a reflection of his autonomy, the operative belief about blood transfusions must be supported by a broader nexus of beliefs and values that serve to indicate that Jack is rationally committed to the life of a Jehovah's Witness. For instance, if Jack does not follow any other tenets of being a Witness, and lacks other relevant beliefs central to the religion, then it is less clear that his treatment choice is really a reflection of the sort of evaluative commitment that undergirds autonomous choice.[37] There is nothing elitist about the prescriptions of my rationalist theory here; in fact, these are precisely the sort of morally relevant

[35] One, but not the only difference. Bortolotti, quoting Siddle, suggests that religious delusions can be distinguished from religious beliefs because: (a) both the reported experience of the individual and her ensuing behaviour are accompanied by psychiatric symptoms; (b) other symptoms are observed in areas of the subject's experience or behaviour that are not necessarily related to the subject's religious beliefs; and (c) the individual's lifestyle after the event giving rise to the report indicates that the event has not been for the subject an enriching spiritual experience. Bortolotti, *Delusions and Other Irrational Beliefs*; Siddle et al., 'Religious Delusions in Patients Admitted to Hospital with Schizophrenia', 131.

[36] For difficulties distinguishing delusions from religious experience, see Fulford and Jackson, 'Spiritual Experience and Psychopathology'; Bortolotti, *Delusions and Other Irrational Beliefs*; Stephens and Graham, 'Reconceiving Delusion'. For a wide-ranging discussion of delusions, see Bortolotti, *Delusions and Other Irrational Beliefs*.

[37] Tellingly, in their discussion, Fulford and Jackson suggest that in order to distinguish between spiritual and pathological forms of psychotic phenomena, we must 'consider them as embedded in the structure of each individual's values and beliefs'. Fulford and Jackson, 'Spiritual Experience and Psychopathology', 60. My tentative suggestion is that the importance of this distinction is grounded by its implications for the voluntariness of the commitment to a sub-rational set of beliefs.

factors that have been taken into account by legal judgements in this area, including the judgement in the Re T case.[38]

Second, the approach that I have adopted is compatible with Savulescu and Momeyer's recommendation that physicians should draw attention to and seek to remedy any theoretical irrationality that JWs appear to evidence. More strikingly, it is also compatible with the fact that this strategy may succeed in changing the patient's mind. Savulescu and Momeyer suggest that many JWs would 'no doubt accept blood'[39] if they were to hold informed rational beliefs. On my approach, this may be true of those JWs whose propositional faith in the tenets of their religion is purely doxastic; that is, a JW who *believes* in the technical sense that a blood transfusion will rule them out of eternal bliss, a belief they aim to hold in accordance with the norms of theoretical rationality and which is thus sensitive to epistemic reasons. Such believers may respond to epistemic reasons to change their religious beliefs. However, the fact that some JWs would likely not change their minds, does not entail that they thereby lack autonomy on the approach I am outlining. The reason for this is that propositional faith can incorporate sub-doxastic elements that are less sensitive to epistemic considerations, and which can be voluntarily adopted.

4. Rationalist DMC in Anorexia Nervosa, Evaluative Delusions, and the Significance of Regret

It is sometimes claimed that there is an inextricable link between psychiatric disorders and irrationality.[40] In turn, this claim might lead one to conclude that individuals suffering from psychiatric disorders will always lack DMC. Indeed, it might be claimed that something like this assumption plays a role in the standard account of autonomy's stipulation that psychiatric disorders can amount to forms of controlling influence that undermine autonomous decision-making. However, irrationality is neither a necessary nor sufficient condition of psychiatric disorder. Individuals in non-clinical populations exhibit various forms of irrationality (undermining the claim that this is sufficient for psychiatric disorder), and some psychiatric disorders can obtain independently of manifestations of persistent irrationality.[41]

Furthermore, as Gavaghan notes in his discussion of depression and DMC, although depression *can* impact upon all of the standard elements of DMC (such as those identified in the MCA), '. . . to say that depression *can* result in these problems . . . is not to say that it invariably, or even usually, does so'.[42] Indeed, that a particular medical diagnosis (pertaining to mental disorder or otherwise) does not

[38] Re T (Adult: Refusal of Medical Treatment).

[39] Savulescu and Momeyer, 'Should Informed Consent Be Based on Rational Beliefs?', 286.

[40] For instance, see Edwards, 'Mental Health as Rational Autonomy'; Szasz, *Insanity*. For an excellent discussion of the relationship between rationality and psychiatric disorder, see Bortolotti, 'Rationality and Sanity'.

[41] Bortolotti, 'Rationality and Sanity'.

[42] Gavaghan, 'In Word, or Sigh, or Tear', 244; Giordano, *Understanding Eating Disorders*, 70; Garasic, *Guantanamo and Other Cases of Enforced Medical Treatment*, 26–7.

entail a lack of decision-making competence is explicitly recognized by the MCA.[43] In the context of clinical depression, this is supported by a burgeoning body of empirical data suggesting that sufferers of the disorder often qualify as competent on routinely employed competence assessment tests, and the observed phenomenon of depressive realism.[44]

Accordingly, in considering the DMC of patients suffering from psychiatric disorders, we cannot justifiably make generalized assumptions about the effects of 'psychiatric disorders' per se on DMC, and we cannot assume that a particular patient is irrational on the basis of their diagnosis alone.[45] Rather, in considering the DMC of patients suffering from psychiatric disorders, we must closely attend to the manner in which a particular disorder manifests itself in a particular individual, and whether this particular patient manifests either theoretical or practical irrationality in her treatment refusal. In short, we must go far beyond the standard account's stipulation than psychiatric disorders can amount to a form of controlling influence.

Whilst the most complex problems regarding DMC in the context of anorexia nervosa are grounded in concerns about the practical rationality of such patients, it should be acknowledged that these patients can also have deficits in theoretical rationality. According to DSM V, one necessary (but not sufficient) diagnostic criterion of anorexia nervosa is that the patient must display:

> Disturbance in the way one's body weight or shape is experienced, undue influence of body shape and weight on self-evaluation, or persistent lack of recognition of the seriousness of the current low body weight.[46]

Notice that this necessary diagnostic criterion is disjunctive, and also that the first and third clause may refer to *descriptive* beliefs that the anorexic patient holds. A patient's experience of body weight or shape could be disturbed in the sense that they believe (incorrectly) that they are overweight. Alternatively, a patient could persistently 'fail to recognize the seriousness of low body weight' in a descriptive sense, if she simply fails to recognize that her low body weight could have fatal implications. Accordingly, on this definition of the disorder, a patient may meet this necessary diagnostic condition because she *believes* that she is overweight despite being a dangerously low weight, or because she fails to *appreciate* that her low weight is likely to lead to serious health complications in *her* case.

However, other patients might only meet this criterion when the clauses are understood in an evaluatively laden sense. For example, it might be argued that a

[43] Mental Capacity Act 2005, s. 2 (3[b]). See also Re C (Adult: Refusal of Treatment) FD (1994), in which a patient suffering from a mental disorder was not deemed to lack capacity to make a treatment decision for a condition that was not related to their mental disorder.

[44] Okai et al., 'Mental Capacity in Psychiatric Patients'; Appelbaum and Grisso, 'The MacArthur Treatment Competence Study, I'; Hindmarch, Hotopf, and Owen, 'Depression and Decision Making Capacity for Treatment or Research'; Bortolotti, 'Rationality and Sanity'; Ackermann and DeRubeis, 'Is Depressive Realism Real?'; Radoilska, 'Depression, Decisional Capacity, and Personal Autonomy'.

[45] Whether or not the courts follow the MCA on this point is another question. See Kong, 'Beyond the Balancing Scales'.

[46] American Psychiatric Association, *Diagnostic and Statistical Manual of Mental Disorders* (5th edition).

patient fails to 'recognize the seriousness of her low body weight' not because of a failure to hold relevant descriptive beliefs, but rather because she does not attribute a *proportionate* degree of consideration to this point in deciding what to do. I shall return to this point below.

It seems that a strong case can be made for the claim that anorexic patients who satisfy the above diagnostic criterion in either of the first two ways just outlined lack DMC. Such patients lack the ability to understand and appreciate material information about their condition, and the reasons they have to increase their food intake. Indeed, some have argued that the beliefs held by patients suffering from anorexia nervosa can in some cases be near-delusional, although the DSM refrains from using the terminology of delusional beliefs in the context of anorexia nervosa.[47] Regardless of whether we classify such beliefs as delusional, they are not only held in a theoretically irrational manner, they are also clearly false, and inimical to adequate understanding of the sort that decisional autonomy requires. Moreover, it seems that these beliefs are not typically voluntarily adopted as pragmatic sub-doxastic states in the same way as religious items of faith may be.[48] As such both the standard account of autonomy and the rationalist account that I have developed may be invoked to support the claim that such patients lack DMC.

However, an individual can meet the diagnostic criteria of anorexia nervosa without holding these kinds of false or theoretically irrational descriptive beliefs. A patient may be aware that she is dangerously underweight, and realize that this will have drastic implications for her health, and yet still qualify as suffering from anorexia nervosa. She will do so if body shape and weight are construed as having an 'undue influence' on her self-evaluation. The case of Keira outlined at the beginning of this chapter is plausibly an example of such a patient; should we also claim that Keira lacks DMC?

The DSM criterion of these considerations having 'undue influence' is suggestive of the possibility that anorexia nervosa can involve what Fulford calls an evaluative delusion. As I discussed in previous chapters, such delusions involve maintaining theoretically irrational (but not necessarily false) evaluative beliefs.[49] It seems highly plausible that anorexic patients can be theoretically irrational with respect to their evaluation of thinness; there is, for example, evidence of rigidity in the thinking patterns of anorexic patients,[50] as well as reports of cognitive dissonance

[47] Steinglass et al., 'Is Anorexia Nervosa a Delusional Disorder?'

[48] Interestingly, there is a long-standing relation between self-starvation and religious asceticism. See Bemporad, 'Self-Starvation through the Ages'; Davis and Nguyen, 'A Case Study of Anorexia Nervosa Driven by Religious Sacrifice'; Bell, *Holy Anorexia*. This speaks against viewing anorexia nervosa as simply a disorder grounded by ideals of thinness and beauty alone. It also suggests that it may not be possible to draw a sharp distinction between treatment refusals based on religious belief and those based on pathological thinking patterns associated with a psychiatric disorder. Whilst I lack the space to consider this point in further detail, we may note that the implications of my theory for 'holy' anorexic patients depends largely on whether they voluntary commit themselves to irrational and demonstrably false beliefs about their weight and body shape. If they merely commit themselves to a particular evaluation of fasting, but not to other irrational descriptive beliefs per se that their condition may involve, then these irrational beliefs can be understood to undermine their autonomous decision-making.

[49] Fulford, 'Evaluative Delusions'.

[50] Elzakkers et al., 'Mental Capacity to Consent to Treatment in Anorexia Nervosa'.

(as I shall explore below) that belie a failure to adhere to basic norms of theoretical rationality concerning responsiveness to evidence and internal consistency.

However, it is important to be careful about how we demarcate the boundaries of evaluative delusions in this context, given that delusions are typically understood to undermine DMC. The claim that one dimension of a person's self-conception (in this case, body shape or weight) exerts 'undue influence' over the patient's decision-making, invites the thought that there is an objective standard of proportionate influence that different values *should* have on one's self-conception. On this understanding, it might be tempting to claim that an individual holds an evaluative delusion if their evaluative beliefs do not accord with this standard. However, there are a number of reasons to reject this approach. First, as I have already mentioned, standard delusional beliefs are not necessarily false beliefs, so it is unclear why we should suppose that evaluative delusions must be 'false' in the sense that they do not match up to a known, objectively correct, ranking of values. Second, this view is in tension with the claim that rational agents can place different weight on different goods. To put the problem more starkly, if we endorse the claim that anorexic patients simply fail to track objective truths about proportionate evaluative weightings, then it is not clear why we should not also make similar claims about Isobel. For instance, Isobel's negative evaluation of social isolation is arguably disproportionate given the value of independence, and the value of other goods she might plausibly pursue if she consents to life-saving treatment.

The boundaries of evaluative delusions are better demarcated by claiming that such delusions obtain when agents lack epistemic mechanisms for reliably tracking what evaluative truths about the good there may be, in the way that individuals who are deluded about descriptive matters similarly seem to lack epistemic mechanisms for reliably tracking truths about descriptive matters of fact. However, differences between the spheres of the evaluative and the descriptive, and their respective relationships to rationality, suggest that our understanding of evaluative delusions is likely to be far more vague than our understanding of descriptive delusions. There is widespread agreement on what constitutes the truth about descriptive matters of fact, so we can normally agree upon whether an individual is delusional with respect to such matters, and identify their defective epistemic mechanisms. Whilst the objectivist about practical reasons will agree that there are also truths about value in the same way that there are truths about descriptive matters of fact, this point is attended by the significant caveat that these truths about value are far less precise, and less well-understood than truths about descriptive matters of fact. Accordingly, even if one accepts the objectivist tenor of demarcating the boundaries of evaluative delusions by appealing to mechanisms for tracking truths about value and objectivist reasons, such an approach will allow for only a very blurry demarcation of the concept.

With these remarks about evaluative delusions in mind, let us return to a more direct consideration of the question of DMC in anorexia nervosa. Although I have suggested that Keira's psychiatric diagnosis is not alone sufficient to justify the claim that she lacks DMC, we might wonder if there is something about the particular kinds of desires that anorexic patients hold that makes them particularly problematic from the point of view of autonomy. In this vein, Tan et al. have claimed that anorexic patients can lack DMC to refuse treatment because their refusals are grounded by pathological values that are incorporated into the diagnostic criteria of their condition.[51]

However, it is not clear how much explanatory power this claim can have with regards to the question of whether such patients can decide autonomously. Of course, the mere fact that a particular behaviour is taken to be a constitutive element of a psychiatric disorder is not alone sufficient to establish that the behaviour is practically irrational. Irrationality is neither necessary nor sufficient for psychiatric disorder. More worryingly though, Tan et al.'s claim is problematically circular; the fact that the evaluative emphasis on low weight is part of the diagnostic criteria of the disorder we call anorexia nervosa is just to say that the evaluation is pathological.[52] However, this does not tell us anything about whether desires grounded by such pathological evaluations can be held autonomously.[53]

This is not to say that Tan et al.'s general conclusion that such patients lack DMC is incorrect; my point here is merely that the support offered for that view is not satisfactory. To support this claim, we would need some grounds for thinking that the values that are designated as pathological cannot ground autonomous decision-making. If there were a plausible story about how pathological desires bypassed or distorted rational reflection, then this would provide sufficient support for the claim; however, noting that a desire is pathological because it is incorporated into the diagnostic criteria of the condition under consideration does not provide us with this sort of explanatory story. To conclude that such desires cannot ground autonomous decisions in the absence of this explanation is thus to presume the very issue at stake.

The code of practice for the MCA offers a different rationale for suggesting that patients suffering from anorexia nervosa can lack DMC, even if they are able to understand relevant treatment information. According to this guidance, the problem in such cases is not that such a patient's values are pathological per se, but rather that their compulsion not to eat might be 'too strong for them to ignore'.[54]

Whilst this rationale is not circular, it too is unconvincing. Prima facie, we may find it appealing to claim that agents who decide on the basis of 'compulsions that they cannot ignore' are not autonomous with respect to those decisions. For instance, the example of Jane the unwilling addict in the introductory chapter seems to be a paradigm case of an individual who lacks autonomy in this way. Jane is compelled to act in ways that she does not rationally endorse because she finds her first-order desire to take drugs to be irresistible; there is a real sense in which she lacks a choice about how to act.[55]

[51] Tan et al., 'Competence to Make Treatment Decisions in Anorexia Nervosa'.

[52] Craigie, 'Competence, Practical Rationality and What a Patient Values'; Maslen, Pugh, and Savulescu, 'The Ethics of Deep Brain Stimulation for the Treatment of Anorexia Nervosa'.

[53] The problem of definitional circularity arising when competence assessments take into account diagnostic criteria also arises in the context of clinical depression, and the diagnostic criterion of suicidal ideation. See Gavaghan, 'In Word, or Sigh, or Tear', 253; McLean, *Assisted Dying*, 41.

[54] *Mental Capacity Act Code of Practice*, s 4.22.

[55] As Craigie and Davies note, this strong sense of compulsion is outlined in Foddy and Savulescu, 'Addiction and Autonomy'. Notably, the weakened sense of compulsion employed by the MCA code of

It may be that some sufferers of psychiatric disorders could be in a similar situation with respect to their pathological behaviour as Jane is to her drug-taking. That is, in some cases, sufferers of psychiatric disorders might be understood to engage in impulsive erratic episodic behaviours that they know to be incongruous with their evaluative judgements, such that these episodes of pathological behaviour can be appropriately designated as alien to the personality of the sufferer.[56] However, in many cases the situation is far more complex, because of the ego-synctonicity of some psychiatric disorders, whereby affected individuals identify with their pathological behaviours.[57] If such individuals are 'compelled', they are not compelled in the same way as Jane, who acknowledges the disparity between her actions and her values.

Indeed, the sense of compulsion that the MCA code of practice is interpreted to invoke with respect to anorexia nervosa is far broader than that which would be necessary to merely preclude individuals who are compelled in Jane's sense from qualifying for DMC. In their analysis of this feature of the MCA code of practice, Jillian Craigie and Alisa Davies write that:

> Where compulsion is given as grounds for incapacity due to anorexia, it is most often described in terms of extreme distortions and biases in the decision process, rather than the person being deprived of a choice.[58]

The relevant question in the present context then is thus whether this weaker sense of compulsion should be understood to be alone sufficient to undermine DMC.

It is telling that Craigie and Davies note that (weak) compulsions are typically taken as grounds for incapacity on the basis of something other than the fact that they are 'too strong to ignore'. This is important because this feature of (weak) compulsions alone is clearly not sufficient to undermine DMC. In fact, quite the opposite is true; rationality may often *require* that we ground our decisions on considerations that we cannot ignore, in the sense that they relate to facts that give us extremely strong reasons. For instance, suppose Sue suffers from very mild headaches once a year, so mild that she hardly notices them. A friend tells her about a highly experimental neurosurgical intervention that is being used in the treatment of life-threatening illnesses, which might cure her headaches, but which is extremely risky and dangerous, with a 90 per cent mortality rate. Sue has extremely strong reasons, ones that she plausibly cannot rationally ignore, to refuse to undergo the procedure. It would be absurd to deny that this sort of rational (weak)

practice would qualify as a form of coercive (rather than compulsive) influence on Feinberg's schema regarding the spectrum of force. Feinberg, *The Moral Limits of the Criminal Law*, 189. For discussion, see Bolton and Banner, 'Does Mental Disorder Involve Loss of Personal Autonomy?' However, in the case of chronic, non-episodic disorders such as anorexia nervosa, the questions are often more challenging, as patients' choices often cohere with their evaluative judgements, as I explore below.

[56] For further discussion of how episodic psychiatric disorders can undermine autonomy, see Bolton and Banner, 'Does Mental Disorder Involve Loss of Personal Autonomy?' Some evidence suggests that bulimia nervosa may begin as an impulsive disorder in this manner. See Pearson, Wonderlich, and Smith, 'A Risk and Maintenance Model for Bulimia Nervosa'.

[57] Tan et al., 'Competence to Make Treatment Decisions in Anorexia Nervosa'.

[58] Craigie and Davies, 'Problems of Control', 11.

compulsion is inimical to her making an autonomous decision to refuse treatment in this case.

Sue has a choice, but she is (weakly) compelled by considerations that she takes to imply very strong reasons. This distinguishes Sue from Jane the unwilling addict. However, it is not clear that it distinguishes Sue from Keira; Keira may also be understood to be (weakly) compelled by considerations that she takes to imply very strong reasons. Should we distinguish the two? The rationalist approach can offer two strategies here. First, in light of an objectivist account of reasons, one might claim that Sue's apparent reasons clearly track her real reasons, since Sue has a strongly decisive reason not to undergo the procedure. In contrast, Keira's apparent reasons do not similarly track what she has real reason to do. Whilst such a strategy allows us to distinguish the two cases, it relies on the claim that we have clear and precise understanding of the evaluative truths at stake in both of these contexts. Given the potential for doubt on this point, we might prefer a different rationalist strategy that does not rely on this objectivist claim, and instead appeals to internal deficiencies with the agent's practical rationality.

In fact, one may read the courts' interpretation of the MCA code of practice as adopting this latter strategy. As Craigie and Davies note in the quoted passage above, the courts' interpretation is typically grounded by the claim that anorexia nervosa appears to 'distort' or 'bias' the deliberation of sufferers. The focus here then is not on whether their decisions are grounded by considerations that sufferers cannot ignore, but rather on whether the disorder biases or distorts the considerations that sufferers take to imply reasons (of the sort that they cannot ignore).

Such bias and distortion would plausibly represent a morally significant difference between Sue and Keira with respect to their DMC for their treatment decision. However, if this strategy is to be a convincing proceduralist basis for claiming that sufferers of anorexia nervosa lack DMC, then we need an explanation for the manner in which anorexia distorts and biases practical decision-making. Given my discussion above, such an explanation cannot simply appeal to the notion of pathology alone, and it must serve to distinguish sufferers of anorexia from standard decision-makers.

A significant problem in attempting to account for the practical irrationality of anorexic patients is that in many cases such patients decide to refuse food in a manner that is rational *in light of their own values*. As Jillian Craigie notes, self-reports of recovered patients suggest a significant source of regret amongst such patients is:

> ... not that they failed to *do what they wanted to do* – on the contrary they pursued the goal of thinness very effectively. It seems more likely that the regret these people express has its source primarily in *what they valued*.[59]

So the question for a rationalist approach to this issue is whether we can plausibly have grounds for supposing that anorexia nervosa serves to distort or bias the patient's practical rationality despite the fact that patients choose in accordance with values that they may endorse as part of a coherent character system.

[59] Craigie, 'Competence, Practical Rationality and What a Patient Values', 331.

Craigie herself endorses a rationalist approach to DMC that broadly aligns with my arguments in this book, and suggests three reasons for thinking that a rationalist approach can answer this question affirmatively.[60] First, she suggests that consistent evidence of retrospective regret amongst survivors of anorexia nervosa about their earlier decision-making would give us grounds for doubting the practical rationality of anorexic patients. Second, some sufferers report cognitive dissonance with respect to their evaluation of thinness, and there is evidence that individuals with anorexia nervosa come to develop powerful internal conflicts due to their distorted affective states.[61] Finally, neuropsychological research suggests that anorexia is associated with impaired emotional arousal in decision-making, similar to impairments that have also been observed in patients who have suffered damage to the ventromedial cortex.[62] Although she acknowledges that none of these three strands is alone sufficient to justify the claim that anorexic patients may be prone to practical irrationality, Craigie concludes that they jointly begin to present a robust case.

I am broadly sympathetic to Craigie's approach, and agree that some of this evidence might plausibly give us reasons to suppose that the practical rationality of anorexic patients has been distorted by their disorder. However, I shall conclude by raising some doubts about the strength of the evidence that we can obtain in favour of this claim from observations of regret. Whilst this is only one strand of evidence that bears on considerations of practical rationality, it is a particularly salient form of evidence in Craigie's analysis. As well as suggesting that it could go some way to justifying a general claim about a lack of ability to recognize certain reasons amongst anorexic patients, Craigie notes that evidence of regret amongst JWs can provide us with sufficient reason to suggest that our policies of abiding by treatment refusals of such patients may deserve re-examination.[63]

In considering the significance of regret amongst survivors of anorexia nervosa, it is important to separate the empirical and the moral issue. The extent to which regret is experienced by anorexic patients is under-studied, and we should certainly be cautious in assuming that future regret will be experienced by all anorexic patients.[64] However, let us assume, perhaps counterfactually, that there is reasonably consistent empirical evidence of regret amongst survivors of anorexia nervosa.

With this assumption in place, what moral work can it do? The first thing to acknowledge is that the mere possibility that an individual may regret a decision is not sufficient grounds for claiming that they cannot make that decision in a practically rational manner. It is quite possible for a person to make an autonomous decision that they will later regret, and indeed, part of respecting an individual's

[60] For another discussion of how the autonomy of anorexic patients may be undermined by defects in their use of information, see Giordano, *Understanding Eating Disorders*, ch. 12.

[61] See also Charland, 'Ethical and Conceptual Issues in Eating Disorders'; Charland et al., 'Anorexia Nervosa as a Passion' on this point.

[62] Craigie, 'Competence, Practical Rationality and What a Patient Values', 332.

[63] Ibid., 333.

[64] Gavaghan makes a similar point in the context of depression in Gavaghan, 'In Word, or Sigh, or Tear', 250–1. Certainly, in considering only the regret of those who have *recovered* from the condition, there is a concern that the sample may be somewhat biased.

autonomy is that we allow them to make decisions that they could regret.[65] For instance, an individual can validly consent to having an inane tattoo as a 20-year-old that they are quite likely to regret when they are 50.

However, we might think that there are some exceptions to this general thought about the compatibility of autonomous decision-making and later regret. In some cases, our anticipation of another's future regret may be based on the fact that the individual lacks some crucial information. For instance, I might anticipate that Peter will regret deciding to cross a bridge to get to the other side of the river because I am (but he is not) aware that the bridge is about to collapse. In this case, the account of autonomy that I have developed here suggests that Peter may not make an autonomous decision about crossing the bridge, because of his failure to understand crucial features of the choice he is making.

Although we might plausibly deny DMC on the basis of anticipated regret when the latter is used a proxy for the individual's insufficient understanding at the time of their decision, it is not clear that this justification is applicable in the context of anorexia nervosa. Patients suffering from anorexia nervosa can (in some cases) have sufficient understanding of the implications of the choices that they make. In order for anticipated future regret to provide a plausible basis for denying DMC in such cases, we would need to have some basis for prioritizing the individual's future wishes over their (sufficiently informed) present wishes. As I explored above though, this runs contrary to how we think of DMC in standard cases, in which we respect the patient's present wishes, rather than the wishes we believe (even with good justification) that they will have in the future.

It might be argued that considering this question in the context of anorexia nervosa involves an obvious disanalogy with other contexts. When we are considering the present wishes of the anorexic patient, they are suffering from a psychiatric disorder, whilst the later regret we (might) observe amongst anorexic patients is expressed once they have recovered. Doesn't this give us reason to prioritize the later wishes over the earlier? However, given my discussion in this chapter, it should be clear that this argument is problematic. We would only have an autonomy-based reason to prioritize the individual's (anticipated) future wishes over their present wishes if we had some independent reason for believing that the individual's present wishes are not autonomous, but their future ones will be. For reasons I have discussed in this chapter, the individual's disease status alone does not provide this kind of reason, and nor does the content of their decision.

At best then, evidence of regret could only provide *supplementary* evidence of a lack of DMC amongst anorexic patients, once it has *already* been established that the individual's retrospective regret has greater agential authority than their past wishes had at the time of the decision. Although there is certainly also room for scepticism about the power of other strands of evidence that Craigie adverts to, it may be the case that further neuropsychological evidence and phenomenological evidence could help us to establish this. However, in the absence of another explanation for why we

[65] McQueen makes a similar point in his analysis of autonomy and regret. McQueen, 'Autonomy, Age and Sterilisation Requests'. See also Pugh, 'Legally Competent, But Too Young To Choose To Be Sterilized?'

should prioritize the individual's (anticipated) future wishes over their present wishes, appealing to considerations of regret as evidence of a lack of DMC is flawed. Furthermore, contrary to Craigie's suggestion, it is not sufficient to establish that JWs lack DMC, and there is danger in assuming that it would be alone sufficient in the case of anorexia nervosa. Such an assumption risks covertly basing claims about the absence of DMC on judgements about the individual's diagnostic status, or the content of the decision itself.

Perhaps more importantly though, even if we accept the claim that anorexic patients may be practically or theoretically irrational with respect to their pathological eating behaviours and beliefs, this does not entail that they lack DMC to refuse treatment. In order for that to be so, it must also be the case that it is these problematic beliefs and values that are primarily operative in the patient's decision-making process. Yet, this might not be the case. A chronically ill patient's refusal of treatment may be based on the quite rational belief that life-saving treatment is not in her long-term interests, by virtue of the suffering that living with a chronic and intractable disease can entail. In cases where there is a strong basis for claiming that the disorder is demonstrably intractable,[66] it seems that this decision could be rational, even if we deny that it would not be rational for a patient to refuse treatment on the basis of a distorted view that being thin is more important than survival.[67]

In view of the above limitations, where does this leave the rationalist approach to understanding DMC in anorexia nervosa? It certainly speaks in favour of clinicians compassionately seeking to investigate why the patient understands weight-loss or a particular body shape to be good in a reason-implying sense, and whether she takes her reasons to achieve this good to outweigh the strength of her reasons to pursue other incompatible goods. Investigation into these matters through the process of something like radical interpretation may sometimes reveal inconsistencies with other elements of that patient's character system, indicating that the patient does not in fact rationally endorse their overall commitment to this goal at a deep level.

However, suppose that for a particularly chronic sufferer of anorexia nervosa, such inconsistencies do not arise, and they are able to provide an account of why their goal is good in a reason-implying sense for them, and how it coheres with persisting elements of their character system without affective disturbance of the sort that might distort their practical rationality. Let us assume, perhaps contrary to clinical reality that such a patient could be presented as a hard case for a rationalist theory of autonomy. As I have suggested in outlining the strategies available to a rationalist account here, we are faced with a choice. First, we may concede that such a patient's decision can be rational if it is a reflection of the reason-giving facts in this context, such as those concerning the burden that both the disease and therapy have become

[66] Although for concerns about the concept of futility in this context, see Geppert, 'Futility in Chronic Anorexia Nervosa'.

[67] Giordano makes a similar point in observing that an anorexic patient's refusal may be grounded by beliefs about the quality of her life. See Giordano, *Understanding Eating Disorders*, 240–1. See also Draper, 'Anorexia Nervosa and Respecting a Refusal of Life-Prolonging Therapy', 122.

for the patient.[68] If it is rational in this way, then it ought to be respected. Such a strategy acknowledges both the lack of adequate explanatory support for the claim that the patient's 'pathological' desires undermine autonomy, the possibility that individuals can differ significantly on the weight they attribute to different goods, and the sad fact that continued existence can represent a significant burden for chronically ill patients.

The alternative is to maintain that such a decision can still be appropriately described as irrational, even if it does not appear to evidence distorted judgements or values that the individual does not recognize and accept as her own. How could such a claim be supported? On an objectivist approach, it might be argued that to claim that such a decision can be rational is to extend the tenet that 'individuals can attribute different weight to the pursuit of different goods' to a degree that stretches it beyond credulity. Although I have suggested that truths concerning the comparative strength of our self-interested reasons are often very imprecise, this is not to say that there are *no* circumstances in which we may say that someone is attributing disproportionate strength to a particular kind of reason.[69]

Which of these strategies should the rationalist adopt? The answer to this question depends on the deeper philosophical issue of just how imprecise the truths concerning the comparative strength of our self-interested reasons are. If we hold a strong version of this view, according to which these truths are so imprecise that we can rarely make an objective assessment of the relative strength of the reasons that others have to pursue different goals, then we should adopt the first strategy, and respect Keira's refusal. The question of the extent to which we can know these truths is thus a more fundamental epistemic barrier facing us when we attempt to make assessments of DMC in hard cases such as those presented here. On the second strategy, even allowing for variability in individual views about the comparative strength of reasons to pursue different goods (thus forestalling, to a considerable extent, the anti-paternalist objection against a rationalist criterion of DMC), we can claim that it is irrational to prefer certain goods (such as low weight) over others (such as survival). On this account, we may understand procedurally rational disagreements about the good to be possible only within broad substantive boundaries that outline the few 'known' truths regarding the comparative strength of different reasons, pertaining to goods at different ends of the spectrum with regards to their importance to well-being.

[68] Although we disagree on the semantics of the concept of rationality and how it features in DMC, the strategy I am outlining here coheres with Draper's practical conclusions. See Draper, 'Anorexia Nervosa and Respecting a Refusal of Life-Prolonging Therapy', 133.

[69] Culver and Gert similarly appeal to the importance of decisions being grounded by 'adequate reasons', where the notion of adequacy implicitly corresponds to an objective ranking of goods, and corresponding reasons. They write that 'A reason is an adequate reason when the harms avoided (or the goods gained) by suffering the harms of a contemplated act compensate for the harms caused by that act', and that 'a decision or action is irrational if the person making it knows (justifiably believes) or should know that its foreseeable results are that she will suffer any of the items on the following list: death, pain (either physical or mental), disabilities (physical, mental, or volitional), or loss of freedom, or loss of pleasure or be at increased risk of suffering any of these, and she has no adequate reason for her action or decision'. Culver and Gert, 'The Inadequacy of Incompetence', 630–1.

Which of these strategies we adopt will thus require substantial theoretical commitments in both the nature of well-being and epistemology. I confess to leaning towards the first strategy, but this requires far more defence than I can provide here. The difficulty of resolving this issue is, I suggest, precisely why we should find the case of Keira to be so complex. In this regard, it is worth contrasting the complexity that this approach raises with the problematic simplicity of the standard view of autonomy. In simply stipulating that psychiatric disorders can amount to a form of controlling influence that undermines autonomy, the standard account simply lacks the conceptual tools to adequately engage with this kind of hard case. In order to adequately assess DMC here, we must delve deeper into the decision-making procedure of such individuals, the nature of their beliefs, the reasons that they understand themselves to have, and these other deeper philosophical issues about the nature of well-being.

Finally, as my discussion here demonstrates, the rationalist can lend some theoretical support to widespread and diverging intuitions about DMC in cases of religious belief and psychiatry. Most importantly though, it shows that sound judgement on these cases requires a complex consideration of a wide range of factors, that we can ill-afford to leave to mere intuition alone.

9

The Prudential Value of Autonomy

The principle of respect for autonomy is undeniably afforded particular salience in Western bioethics, and accounts of autonomy should aim to give an explanation as to why that is the case.[1] However, as well as seeking to give an account of the nature of autonomy's value, one might also question whether we ought to value autonomy so much, and how it should be weighed against other values. Our understanding of these issues will have significant implications for the many bioethical issues in which considerations of autonomy are invoked.

In this book, I have outlined a broadly Millian understanding of the nature of autonomy and its relationship to rationality. One might raise the concern that a Millian account is going to have trouble offering a satisfactory justification for a stringent requirement to respect autonomy that is consistent with Mill's broader utilitarian moral framework.[2] I shall comment on this particular interpretation of Mill below, but notwithstanding this issue, it is quite possible to claim that a Millian conception of autonomy can be adopted into moral frameworks that do not perfectly align with Mill's own. As such, my primary concern in this chapter is not how we can reconcile the value of autonomy within a broader consequentialist understanding of morality, but rather with how we should understand the value of autonomy itself. I shall argue that autonomy should be understood as not only instrumentally valuable, but also valuable for its own sake. The argument that I make for this claim has important implications not only for how we should weigh the value of autonomy against other values in bioethics, but also for how we should understand the nature of well-being.

At the outset, it is important to delimit the scope of my claims about autonomy's value in this chapter. It is sometimes claimed that autonomy has *moral* value, and that autonomy undergirds the moral value of personhood.[3] On this approach, the principle of respect for autonomy can be understood as a particular instantiation of the more general moral principle of respect for persons. Modern statements of this view commonly find their source in Kant's moral philosophy, and his substantive account of autonomy.[4] The moral respect due to a person on this approach reflects

[1] Walker, 'Medical Ethics Needs a New View of Autonomy', 595. For non Western perspectives of autonomy's value, see Yang, 'Serve the People'; Kara, 'Applicability of the Principle of Respect for Autonomy'; Foster, *Choosing Life, Choosing Death*, 11.

[2] Walker, 'Medical Ethics Needs a New View of Autonomy', 603.

[3] Kant, *Groundwork for the Metaphysics of Morals*, 4:435.

[4] For some examples, see Velleman, 'A Right of Self-Termination?'; Darwall, 'The Value of Autonomy and Autonomy of the Will'; Habermas, *The Future of Human Nature*, particularly 37–44.

Autonomy, Rationality, and Contemporary Bioethics. Jonathan Pugh, Oxford University Press (2020). © Jonathan Pugh.
DOI: 10.1093/oso/9780198858584.001.0001

the high moral status that the person has as an autonomous agent, a being with intrinsic, non-exchangeable worth, or dignity that goes beyond mere price.[5]

As I pointed out in the introduction to this book, we may be sceptical about the extent to which this Kantian notion of autonomy is the sense that bioethicists typically intend to invoke in their discussions of autonomy. Whatever its merits, I shall not discuss it further here. As I have explained in previous chapters, my view of autonomy departs from Kant's substantive conception; accordingly, establishing that my procedural understanding of autonomy can provide a foundation for the moral value of personhood would require lengthy argument.[6] Further whilst it is widely held that the value of autonomy has an important role to play in justifying the exercise of political power in liberal societies, I shall not be directly concerned with this question here.[7] Instead, I shall focus my attention on whether autonomy bears prudential value; how, and to what extent does autonomy contribute to a person's well-being? I limit my discussion to this question in the hope that it has at least some bearing on other broader questions about the moral and political role of autonomy, on the assumption that the salient role of autonomy is at least partly attributable to its significant prudential value.

1. The Nature of Autonomy's Prudential Value

It is possible to distinguish two ways in which something can be prudentially valuable.[8] Consider first, 'final value'. Something bears final value if it is valuable as an end, or for its own sake; for instance, knowledge, happiness, and virtue, *inter alia*, might plausibly be understood as bearing final value. We can contrast final value with 'instrumental value'; something has merely instrumental value if it is only valuable for the sake of something else.[9] For instance, money has only instrumental value, in so far as it can be exchanged for other valuable goods.

Accordingly, if we are to claim that autonomy has instrumental value, we must also give an account of the valuable end to which autonomy serves as a means. Prima facie, one plausible candidate is well-being, broadly construed; a life lived

[5] Kant, *Groundwork for the Metaphysics of Morals*, 4:435.

[6] Jeff McMahan makes some remarks on this sort of project, and endorses the view that personal autonomy is a significant basis of the moral worth of persons. McMahan, *The Ethics of Killing*, 256–60. In a similar vein, Marilyn Friedman has argued that the first personal value of autonomy can provide reciprocity grounds for our moral obligations to others, and that personal autonomy is necessary for moral autonomy. Friedman, *Autonomy, Gender, Politics*, 60–7.

[7] For a selection of relevant discussions of this topic, see Friedman, *Autonomy, Gender, Politics*, 75; Christman, *The Politics of Persons*; Raz, *The Morality of Freedom*; Mill, *On Liberty*; Spector, *Autonomy and Rights*.

[8] For discussion of this distinction, see Korsgaard, 'Two Distinctions in Goodness'. Korsgaard's aim in this paper was to separate the distinction between final and instrumental value from the distinction between intrinsic and extrinsic value. The latter distinction pertains to whether or not something bears value in virtue of its intrinsic, non-relational properties, that is, 'in itself'. Although philosophers sometimes claim that autonomy has 'intrinsic' value, it seems that this is most naturally understood as the claim that autonomy has 'final' value. Whilst we may value autonomy as an end in itself, it is not clear that we value it by virtue of its non-relational properties. See Wall, *Liberalism, Perfectionism and Restraint*, 145 for discussion.

[9] Korsgaard, 'Two Distinctions in Goodness', 170.

autonomously, it might be claimed, is more likely to lead to the attainment of the goods that make a person's life prudentially better. Following Parfit, theories of well-being are commonly classified into one of the following three types, as schematized below:

> *Hedonistic Theories*—What would be best for someone is what would make their life happiest.
> *Desire-Fulfilment Theories*—What would be best for someone is what, throughout their life, would best fulfil their desires.
> *Objective List Theories*—Certain things are good or bad for us, whether or not we want to have the good things, or to avoid the bad things.[10]

We can also further distinguish *enumerative* theories of well-being from *explanatory* theories. The former sort of theory seeks to answer the question 'which things make someone's life go better for them?' In contrast *explanatory* theories of well-being seek to explain what it is about the things listed by enumerative theories of well-being that make them good for people.[11]

The claim that autonomy is *only* instrumentally valuable is perhaps most congruent with explanatory hedonism; on such a theory, it might be claimed that autonomy makes a life go better just because autonomy is conducive to happiness (understood in terms of the experience of pleasurable mental states), which is the only thing that has final value on this view.[12] This understanding of the value of autonomy is commonly, although perhaps mistakenly, attributed to Mill.[13] Such a reading of Mill might seem natural, given his insistence at the beginning of *On Liberty* that he regards utility as '... the ultimate appeal on all ethical questions' (a position that he defended in his *Utilitarianism*).[14] Moreover, this understanding might seem plausible in view of the fact that individuals are in a privileged epistemic position with regards to the question of what will make them happy. As Mill puts the point:

> With respect to his own feelings and circumstances, the most ordinary man/woman has means of knowledge immeasurably surpassing those that can be possessed by anyone else.[15]

[10] Parfit, *Reasons and Persons*, Appendix I. Although this tripartite classification is widely accepted, it has recently come under criticism, partly because it ignores Crisp's distinction between enumerative and explanatory theories. See Woodard, 'Classifying Theories of Welfare'. In the interests of clarity and space, I shall follow philosophical orthodoxy in discussing the tripartite classification, but I shall supplement this discussion with considerations pertaining to Crisp's distinction.

[11] Crisp, *Reasons and the Good*, 102–3.

[12] Happiness here is to be broadly understood in terms of the experience of pleasure (or desirable consciousness) and the absence of pain.

[13] Robert Young also makes this observation in Young, 'The Value of Autonomy', 36. For examples of this interpretation of Mill, see Berlin, 'John Stuart Mill and the Ends of Life' and Ladenson, 'Mill's Conception of Individuality'. The problem with this interpretation is that it fails to acknowledge the way in which Mill departed from Bentham's monistic conception of utility. Mill's view actually seems to be that autonomy is incorporated into his understanding of utility.

[14] Mill, *On Liberty*, 81; Mill, *Utilitarianism*.

[15] Mill, *On Liberty*, 74. For a similar observation, see Feinberg, 'The Child's Right to an Open Future', 91. On the basis of these epistemic considerations, Dworkin refers to this view of the relationship between autonomy and well-being as the evidentiary view. Dworkin, 'Autonomy and the Demented Self', 7–8.

However, even if autonomy can be instrumentally valuable in this way, it is problematic to claim that it is valuable *only* in so far as it is a means to happiness. First, individuals will often be mistaken about what will make them happy; they may in fact achieve *less* happiness if they are left to their own autonomous devices than they would have done otherwise.[16] To illustrate, we can imagine a young man who rejected his parent's advice and who autonomously decided that a career in finance would make him happy, but who comes to regret this decision in later life, when he realizes that he did not enjoy his career, and his choice meant forgoing a family life that he now believes his parents were right to suggest would have made him happy.

This observation alone is not an unimpeachable objection to the explanatory hedonist's claim that autonomy is only instrumentally valuable; perhaps most people *do* know what will make them happy, and counterexamples show only that there can be individuals whose autonomy lacks prudential value. In order to provide a stronger argument against the explanatory hedonist's claim, one would need to show that a life lived in the absence of autonomy could be *worse* than a life lived autonomously, even if the former life involved more happiness.

Consider an example in which this criterion is met. Would one believe that one's life would go better if one's affairs were to be determined by a wise and benevolent friend?[17] Notably, this is something that Mill explicitly denies:

> If a person possesses any tolerable amount of common sense and experience, his own mode of laying out his existence is the best not because it is the best, but because it is his own mode.[18]

More recently, James Griffin captures this Millian insight as follows:

> ... even if you convince me that, as my personal despot, you would produce more desirable consciousness for me than I do myself, I shall want to go on being my own master.[19]

Call the argument implicit in these observations the Personal Despot Argument (PDA). The thought underwriting the plausibility of the PDA is that autonomy has a special sort of value for us; there seems to be a value in *living a life of one's own* that is of central and fundamental importance to many of us.[20] Our rejection of even the wise and benevolent personal despot suggests that autonomy bears final value; we value autonomy for its own sake, and not just because we believe that being autonomous will lead to our attaining other prudentially valuable ends.[21] On this

[16] For a similar point, see Hart, *Law, Liberty and Morality*, 32; Dworkin, 'Autonomy and the Demented Self', 8; Hurka, 'Why Value Autonomy?', 364. Dworkin argues that Mill was also aware of this point. Dworkin, 'Paternalism', 73–4.

[17] Wall, *Liberalism, Perfectionism and Restraint*, 146.

[18] Mill, *On Liberty*, 131.

[19] Griffin, *Well-Being*, 9.

[20] See also Wall, *Liberalism, Perfectionism and Restraint*, 129–30; Glover, *Causing Death and Saving Lives*, 96; Sher, *Beyond Neutrality*, 176; Kymlicka, *Liberalism, Community and Culture*, 12. The value that we tend to place on living a life of one's own offers a further clue as to why it seems problematic to claim that it is good, in a reason-implying sense, to live in accordance with an essentialist conception of an authentic self from which one feels alienated. The problem is that an agent who lives in accordance with such an alienated self does not seem to be engaged in a project of living a life of her own; rather, she is living a life of a self that she has *dis*-owned.

[21] That the value here is *final* does not entail that it is not importantly related to other ends. For instance, Dworkin cashes out the value of autonomy by appealing to considerations of integrity. But the thought

approach, autonomy is at least partly *constitutive* of (rather than merely instrumental to) well-being.

I believe that the PDA captures an important truth, and I shall defend it in greater detail below. At this point though, we may observe that if the argument is indeed convincing, then it raises considerable problems for explanatory hedonism; however, both desire-fulfilment and objective list theories of well-being can accommodate our intuitive response to these examples, and allow for the view that autonomy has final value. Consider first desire-fulfilment theories; even if a personal despot could produce more happiness in your life, she would not be able to fulfil one's non-instrumental desire to live a life in which you make your own autonomous decisions. Alternatively, an objective list theory might simply claim that autonomy is an end that has final value. Indeed, many modern theorists have incorporated autonomy into their understanding of well-being in these ways.[22] For instance, the desire for autonomy is a central desire in Griffin's own informed desire account,[23] and Sumner claims that well-being consists in '...authentic happiness, the happiness of an informed and autonomous subject'.[24] In a similar vein, John Finnis' description of the good of 'practical reasonableness' included in his objective list account seems to bear a close relation to autonomy as I have understood it in this book.[25]

There are, however, important differences in how different theories of well-being account for the prudential value of autonomy. For instance, on enumerative *actual present* desire-fulfilment theories, autonomy is only incorporated into the good life for a particular person if they actually desire it. In contrast, on enumerative objective list theories that include autonomy, the final value of autonomy is not contingent upon the subject's desires in this way. I lack the space here to defend a full view of well-being. However, it should be acknowledged that the objectivist view of rational desires that I have defended in this book is based in part on a rejection of the view that our desires *simpliciter* can provide us with reasons. As such, the view of reasons, value, and autonomy that I have endorsed is incompatible with a purely desire-based *explanatory* account of well-being, since on such an account, the fact that something satisfies one of our desires makes that thing prudentially good for us; this sounds suspiciously like subjectivism about reasons of the sort that I rejected in Chapter 1. Accordingly, although the object-given view of reasons is compatible with a subjective desire-based account of well-being (as I discussed in Chapter 2), it is only so with respect to an *enumerative* desire-fulfilment account theory of well-being.

here is that living an autonomous life is constitutive of a living a life with integrity, rather than instrumental to it as a separate good.

[22] Notice that a further benefit of incorporating autonomy into one's theory of well-being is that such theories are able to explain why the satisfaction of adaptive preferences may not enhance well-being. Sen raises this point in Sen, *Resources, Values and Development*, 304. See Sumner, *Welfare, Happiness, and Ethics*, 166 for discussion.

[23] Griffin, *Well-Being*, Part One, particularly 33–6.

[24] Sumner, *Welfare, Happiness, and Ethics*, 172.

[25] Finnis, *Natural Law and Natural Rights*, 88–90. Savulescu acknowledges the possibility of incorporating autonomy into an objective list account at Savulescu, 'Rational Desires and the Limitation of Life Sustaining Treatment', 213.

In view of the failure of explanatory hedonism to adequately capture the value of autonomy, and the incompatibility of purely desire-based explanatory accounts with objectivism about reasons, how should we understand the claim that autonomy has final value? The most plausible remaining strategy is to endorse an explanatory theory of well-being that appeals to objective values, and to claim that autonomy is one of the things that have such objective, final value.

However, autonomy should not be understood to be the *only* good on this sort of theory; one reason for this is that the realization of some values may require the absence of autonomy.[26] Furthermore, an adequate theory of well-being should allow for the possibility that pleasurable experiences can contribute in some way to well-being, even if one is not autonomous with respect to the choice to experience them. For instance, suppose that your affairs were determined by a benevolent personal despot, and they were incredibly successful in leading you to do things that led you to experience highly pleasurable mental states. We can still make sense of the claim that the pleasurable mental states you would experience would have *some* prudential value, even if the prudential value of the life would be severely impoverished by the absence of autonomy.

One might advance two related further claims here; first that the final value of autonomy is conditional on other components of the good life, and second, that autonomy may lack value or even be detrimental to well-being if it is put to bad uses.[27] There is a degree of truth in the first claim; on the theory of autonomy that I have developed here, there is an inextricable link between autonomy and the agent's values. Autonomy itself (and not its value per se) is conditional on the agent's beliefs about what constitutes the good life, since autonomous choices must be grounded in part by these beliefs.

In fact, it is also plausible to claim that something like the reverse relationship outlined in the first claim is true. Although certain goods (such as pleasure) are possible in the absence of autonomy, autonomy may plausibly be construed as a condition of other goods having a particular kind of value for the agent. It is through achieving the various objective values that partly constitute well-being through the *autonomous* pursuit of our own goals that we can understand ourselves as living a life that is *ours*. Whilst this need not be understood as either a necessary foundation of all other values, or even as something that is in fact universally valued, living a life that is one's own is prudentially valuable for its own sake. Only in a life in which the agent is autonomous with respect to the sustainment of the fundamental commitments that guide her conduct, and in her achievement of other objective goods, is it the agent herself who can be said to meaningfully *realize* the values instantiated in that life. It is this that is sorely absent in the life determined by a personal despot. Autonomy can thus be construed as being conditional to a particular kind of contribution that other goods make to well-being, one that serves to amplify the contribution a good makes in abstraction: that of contributing to a life that is meaningfully the agent's own.

[26] Berofsky, *Liberation from Self*, 248.

[27] Wall, *Liberalism, Perfectionism and Restraint*, 130; Varelius, 'The Value of Autonomy in Medical Ethics', 381.

The above reflections might be understood to be in tension with the second claim outlined above. Can autonomy have value (or have this amplifying effect on other values) even if it is put to immoral uses? I believe that the answer is 'yes'; to suppose otherwise is to confuse judgements about the all things considered goodness of states of affairs, with an assessment of what is good *for a* person.

To illustrate, suppose that Paul takes a great deal of pleasure from non-consensually harming people, and his violent actions help him to cultivate a self-narrative of himself as a dominant and powerful individual, a project that he takes to define his purpose in life. It is undoubtedly a terrible state of affairs that Paul performs these harmful actions. We may even plausibly say that his performing these actions autonomously *exacerbates* the badness of this state of affairs, and renders him more blameworthy for the harms caused. Finally, we may also justifiably restrain Paul from performing these actions by appealing to moral considerations that outweigh the value of his autonomy. However, I do not see a compelling reason to claim that it is worse *for* Paul that he performs these actions autonomously rather than non-autonomously. These are, recall, actions that he enjoys, and which he takes to be central to his character and his projects. If his autonomy in performing these actions makes Paul prudentially worse off, then it would have to be true that the performance of blameworthy immoral actions is detrimental to well-being, perhaps on the basis of the Aristotelian claim that moral virtue is a necessary constituent of well-being. However, this is a highly controversial claim that requires defence quite independently from considerations about the value of autonomy.[28]

Another line of criticism to objective accounts of well-being that I have sketched here is that subjective attitudes seem to have an important influence on well-being, and it is not clear that objective accounts can accommodate this thought. All that matters for well-being on these theories is that objectively valuable things are incorporated into the agent's life; the agent's own subjective attitudes towards these goods are not important. Whilst there is considerable debate on the merits of this point, it suffices for my purposes here to say that if one finds this objection convincing, then it can be circumvented by adopting a hybrid account of well-being, according to which both the realization of objective values and one's holding subjective positive attitudes towards those objective values contribute to well-being. Such an account thus incorporates both objective and subjective elements.[29]

The plausibility of such an account stems from the fact that although we may have reason to doubt that a theory of well-being that completely ignores individual preferences and attitudes is mistaken, it also seems plausible to claim that we can have self-interested reasons to want certain things, such as pleasurable experiences, loving relationships, and knowledge, even if we do not believe (perhaps incorrectly) that they will cause us happiness, or even if we do not desire them. Moreover, as

[28] For two arguments against this moralistic view of well-being, see Hurka, *Perfectionism*, 19–20 and Hooker's argument from sympathy in Hooker, 'The Elements of Well-Being', 25–7.

[29] Brad Hooker has recently defended a hybrid account that incorporates autonomy, and addresses theoretical questions about the limits of (and trade-offs between) subjective and objective elements in Hooker, 'The Elements of Well-Being'. See also Adams, *Finite and Infinite Goods*, 95–101; Feldman, *Pleasure and the Good Life*.

I explained in Chapter 2, the account of rationality that I have appealed to in this book allows for a degree of subjectivity, in so far as it is compatible with there being a plurality of goods, and with the possibility that rational agents can disagree about the weight that should be attributed to these different goods. Such disagreements do not arise simply because one party is wrong, and the other is right. Rather it is because of the imprecise nature of the truths governing many value comparisons.

2. Defending the Personal Despot Argument

As I discussed above, one of the main arguments in defence of the claim that autonomy bears final value is the PDA. However, this argument has been criticized on the grounds that it conflates the value that we attach to making decisions for ourselves with '... the value we attach to having our decisions reflect our deepest goals and values'.[30] To illustrate this, Mikhail Valdman suggests a thought experiment in which you have the opportunity to cede your final decision-making authority about how to act to a Personal Expert Committee (PC); this committee is better than you are at determining how to accomplish your goals and how to live according to your values.[31] The PC, however crucially differs from the personal despot of the PDA. The PC does not determine your values; it only tells you how to live in accordance with them; the personal despot, on the other hand, might seek to increase your happiness by also harnessing control over your values.

Should we prefer the PC to self-government? Valdman suggests that we should, pointing out that we often cede decision-making authority in this way, such as in organizing our financial affairs.[32] He also takes care to pre-emptively respond to a number of objections to his arguments.[33] Whilst I do not believe that all of these responses are satisfactory, I shall not pursue them here. Rather I shall raise two new objections to the PC argument. The first objection calls into question the scope of the PC example; the second objection suggests that, rather than showing that self-government has no intrinsic value, the PC example merely indicates that different elements of autonomy can have different value.

Let us consider the PC in a little more detail. Although the PC would intervene when it detected flawed practical reasoning, it would always use the agent's own goals and values as the basis for its decisions. To illustrate, suppose that David has some prudential goal *X*, and has to choose between two possible acts *A* and *B*. Suppose that out of these two acts, only *A* would serve as a reliable means to David's achieving *X*; in this case, the PC would only intervene if David believed that he prudentially ought to *B*.

Valdman's model is not problematic when the value of the goal (*X*) is distinguishable from the acts that one must perform as a means to achieving that goal. However, it is problematic when this is not the case. Yet, the value of a number of goals is inextricably related to the way in which we achieve that goal. To illustrate, suppose that one valued being able to play a complex piece of music on the piano, say

[30] Valdman, 'Outsourcing Self-Government', 764. [31] Ibid., 770. [32] Ibid., 772.
[33] Ibid., 780–9.

Rachmaninov's second concerto. In a crude sense, in order to play this piece, one would simply need to hit certain combinations of keys, in a certain order, for a certain time. In order to play the piece in this crude sense, one would need to develop excellent motor skills and technique, normally through devoting hours to practising the requisite movements, and to learning the structure of the piece. Whilst it might be claimed that there is some value in the discipline and effort that this practice requires, the goal of being able to play Rachmaninov's concerto in the crude sense under consideration could retain its value for an agent, even if they achieved it via a more efficient means that did not involve effort or discipline; for example, instead of sitting through hours of lessons and practice sessions, suppose (somewhat fantastically) that one could simply 'download' the ability to play the right notes in the right order for the right amount of time.

In this crude sense of being able to play the piece, the value of the goal is distinguishable from the means that one takes to achieve it. However, consider now someone who has a more refined desire to be able to play the Rachmaninov piece; rather than valuing being able to simply 'play the right notes', this person values being able to play the piece according to their own interpretation of the music. This might involve, *inter alia*, their deciding which phrases of the piece need particular emphasis, and the strength they should exert in pressing the keys at particular points. Whilst the achievement of this goal requires the same abilities as the goal of playing the piece in the crude sense, it also requires something more, something like *creativity*; and because of this, it seems that the value of the goal is inextricably linked to the fact that the agent herself exercises *her own* creativity in its pursuit.

This is important, since on this understanding of the value of the goal, it does not make sense to say that one might be able to better achieve the goal by outsourcing to something like a PC. A PC, an expert tutor, or a futuristic downloadable music program could make you a better technical piano player; and this technical ability might be prerequisite for going on to exercise one's creativity in playing. However, completely relying on a PC to realize the goal of playing Rachmaninov's second concerto in a sophisticated sense would defeat the value of the goal itself.

The point that this example raises is that the relationship between the value of our goals and the means that we take to achieve them is not always as simple as the PC argument implies. Whilst Valdman is correct to point out that we often outsource decision-making authority, the examples he highlights are cases in which the value of the goal is clearly distinguishable from the manner in which the goal is achieved; for example, the value we attribute to achieving financial security is rarely taken away if we attain it by allowing a financial adviser to make our financial decisions for us.[34] However, in more complex cases, the value of some goals seems to be at least partly dependent on the fact that in achieving the goal, the agent herself makes her own mark in doing so. Rob Goodman captures a similar thought in his distinction between 'process goods' that pertain to excellence in the performance of an activity,

[34] Ibid., 772.

and 'outcome goods', that pertain to the benefits that an activity creates.[35] Playing Rachmaninov in the crude sense would qualify as an outcome good in my example, whilst playing the piece in the sophisticated sense would involve process goods.

The above considerations lend support to the claim that simply ensuring that an agent's goals are achieved may not facilitate their autonomy. The fact that some of our goals are process goods lends support to the claim that, at least in some cases, a '...crucial part of the notion of "self rule" is that it is *me* that achieves my goals'.[36] Although it seems that many of the goals that agents tend to have involve process goods, let us suppose that the PC would not intervene to ensure the achievement of process goods, and that the objection still stands in relation to a number of other goals that people tend to have. Even if we concede this point, the objection only shows that the value of different sorts of autonomy can come into conflict, not that autonomy lacks final value.

There are two central points undergirding this line of response. The first is that according to the PC argument, one may fail to be self-governing even when one is living in accordance with one's own goals and values. According to the terms of the argument, one will fail to be self-governing if it is the PC rather than the agent herself who ensures that they live in accordance with their goals and values. The second point concerns the distinction that I have drawn upon in this book between global and local autonomy. As I explained in the introduction, we can understand autonomy to be a property of agents in a particular time-slice, with respect to a particular decision. When we conceive of autonomy in this way, we are considering *local* autonomy. In contrast, we can also understand autonomy as a *global* property that agents can instantiate diachronically.

Notice that when the PC argument stipulates that one may fail to be self-governing even if one is living in accordance with one's own goals and values, the failure here is a failure of local, rather than global autonomy. After all, *ex hypothesi*, the PC would only govern you in accordance with your own deeply held commitments and values. As such, the PC will only intervene when one's own *local* decision-making is likely to prove counter-productive to one's pursuit of the long-term goals that may be understood to undergird one's *global* autonomy.

The reason that the PC argument may appear to be convincing is that it fails to adequately distinguish local and global autonomy. Although it might be true that there are cases in which we could have good reason to outsource our decision-making to experts, the strength of this reason is *itself* rooted in the value of being able to live what Valdman calls an 'acceptable' life, in accordance with one's own freely chosen goals and values;[37] however, this is simply what it is to be *globally* autonomous. Accordingly, the PC argument is only sufficient for proving that the value of local and global autonomy may sometimes be in conflict, and that we would

[35] Goodman, 'Cognitive Enhancement, Cheating, and Accomplishment', 146 and 152–4.

[36] Sandman and Munthe, 'Shared Decision Making, Paternalism and Patient Choice', 66. These authors make the strong claim that this is always true of respect for autonomy. However, I limit my endorsement of this claim, as my discussion below shall clarify.

[37] Valdman, 'Outsourcing Self-Government', 769.

often prioritize our global autonomy over our local autonomy. Yet, this is not a problematic conclusion for those who claim that autonomy bears final value.

3. The Value of Different Elements of Autonomy

The second response to the PC objection turns on the claim that it is possible for local autonomy to come into conflict with global autonomy. On some views of the relationship between local and global autonomy, this claim would be implausible. For instance, it would be implausible if one held the view that global autonomy is simply an aggregate of the instances of local autonomy over time.[38] However, in the introduction, I suggested an alternative understanding of the relationship, according to which an agent's global autonomy depends on the extent to which she lives in accordance with her own diachronic plans and commitments. Ronald Dworkin also implicitly acknowledges that the value of global autonomy is distinct from the value of individual decisions in outlining his integrity view of the value of autonomy as follows:

> [A]utonomy makes each of us responsible for shaping his own life according to some coherent and distinctive sense of character... This view of autonomy focuses not on individual decisions one by one, but the place of each decision in a more general program or picture of life the agent is creating...[39]

Despite this, in some cases, being able to make our own local choices *is* essential to the facilitation of our global autonomy. This is not simply because of our privileged epistemic access to knowing which goals we value; rather it is because the goals we aim to pursue in some cases are process, rather than outcome goods. Making local decisions about how one pursues such goals is inextricably linked to one's evaluation of the achievement of the goal itself.

However, when we consider the pursuit of outcome goods, conflicts between local and global autonomy become far more acute. In such cases, the value of one's goal can be distinguished from the value of making locally autonomous decisions about how to pursue it. Indeed, it may even be the case that we could better facilitate an agent's pursuit of the goal that undergirds their global autonomy by restricting their local autonomy. Which of these elements of autonomous agency should we prioritize?

In advocating the PC objection, Valdman himself implicitly highlights one possible explanation of why global autonomy might have precedence over local autonomy. As Valdman suggests, the deep commitments that one must live in accordance with to live an 'acceptable' life are central to our identity, on psychological understandings of that concept. This is not true of many of the short-term goals that our local decision-making concerns. These may sometimes be trivial, and in no way connected to any of our deep global commitments; I can, for instance, be locally

[38] Christman, 'Autonomy and Personal History', 18–19.

[39] Dworkin, 'Autonomy and the Demented Self', 8; see also Dworkin, *Life's Dominion*, 224. Interestingly, as Foster notes, judges invoked Dworkin's understanding of the value of autonomy in their judgement on *Chester v. Afshar*. See Foster, *Choosing Life, Choosing Death*, 84.

autonomous with respect to my decision about what to have for lunch. In contrast, the adoption of a long-term goal requires a far more significant kind of commitment; in making decisions about such commitments, we can clarify and shape the nexus of our judgements about what is valuable. As I discussed in Chapter 2, such judgements play a highly significant role in our character systems. As such, when the two sorts of autonomy cannot both be realized, concerns pertaining to our sense of identity, of defining who we are, may give us reason to prioritize our global autonomy over our local autonomy.

Accordingly, it should not be surprising that patients often believe that the best way to achieve their global commitments in a medical context is to sacrifice their local autonomy with respect to their treatment decisions by telling their doctor to 'do what you think would be best'. This should be viewed as an expression, rather than an abdication, of autonomy.[40] For instance, the patient might not trust herself to make a difficult local decision that is in harmony with her evaluative judgements, or she may not feel able to weigh the complex information involved in such a decision appropriately. Crucially, in light of my response to the PC objection, the amelioration of a patient's condition is typically most naturally understood as an outcome good, rather than a process good; as such, the patient may outsource her decision-making here without this undermining the value of her diachronic goal. Accordingly, an agent may retain her global autonomy in making this request if the patient believes that the doctor is more likely than she is to make a treatment decision that would best reflect her own evaluative judgement about what would be good for her in a reason-implying sense.

In light of this discussion of the significance of global autonomy, one might be tempted to ask why we should worry about locally autonomous decisions at all, rather than simply focusing on global autonomy alone. There are two reasons for why we should resist this temptation. First, as I discussed above, many of the goals that undergird our global autonomy are process goods. Second, as I explored in Chapter 6, an individual's local autonomous decisions can have considerable moral significance when they concern whether the agent wishes to exercise their power to waive a claim right. Although I argued that local autonomy has some role to play in our understanding and justification of rights such as these, the interest they serve to protect may crucially not be best understood in terms of their contribution to an individual's global autonomy. To take Archard's example again, if one violates another's right to bodily integrity by non-consensually inserting a painless mouth-swab, the wrong done here is not plausibly construed as one of subverting the victim's ability to lead her life as she chooses.[41]

It is far from clear that considerations of the agent's own global autonomy are sufficient to justify the infringement in this case.[42] More broadly, an autonomous

[40] In view of my discussion here, we should not view the empirical data concerning patient behaviour that Foster presents on this point as undermining the significance of autonomy in the manner that he intimates. See Foster, *Choosing Life, Choosing Death*, 97.

[41] Archard, 'Informed Consent', 22.

[42] For more on the distinction between right violation and infringement, see Thomson, *The Realm of Rights*, 82–104.

agent can plausibly wish to exercise her autonomy by refusing to waive a right against some interference, even when that interference would facilitate the pursuit of goals that undergird her global autonomy. The interest it protects may, in some cases, have greater reason-giving strength for an individual.

Despite these caveats, we should not be blind to the cases in which there can be conflicts between global and local autonomy in which considerations of global autonomy might plausibly win out. When the goals in question concern outcome goods, and facilitating the agent's pursuit of those goals would not require interference of the sort that would violate a powerful claim right, we might plausibly be justified in prioritizing the agent's global autonomy over her local autonomy. To unreflectively assume that appropriate respect for autonomy *always* demands that we should respect locally autonomous decisions that will certainly undermine the agent's pursuit of what we know to be the goals that undergird her global autonomy, is to fetishize one kind of autonomy over another, in a manner that does not reflect the prudential value of these different kinds of autonomy. Respect for autonomy should thus consider both global and local understandings of that which is being respected.

The above considerations lend an autonomy-based justification of weak paternalism. According to weak paternalism it is legitimate to interfere with the *means* that agents choose to achieve their ends, if those means are likely to defeat their own ends. For example, suppose Fred is overweight and autonomously wants to lose weight; however, he chooses means to this end that will not be effective, buying unproven weight-loss products he finds on the internet, continuing to eat unhealthy food that hinders his ability to lose weight, and refusing to exercise. The weak paternalist would claim that we could intervene in order to ensure that David will choose a more effective means of reaching his goal, perhaps by restricting the availability of unhealthy foods. On the autonomy-based approach I am outlining, weak paternalist measures could be justifiable in such cases if the goal in question is an outcome good, and the measures would not infringe upon a claim right that David has not waived. Similarly, the above considerations offer the most plausible prospect of a broadly autonomy-based justification of nudges that undermine local autonomy. Such a justification would qualify as a weak form of paternalism outlined above.[43]

Weak paternalism can be contrasted with strong paternalism, which states that it is legitimate to interfere to prevent people from achieving those ends that they are mistaken in believing to be good for them.[44] For instance, suppose that Grant is overweight but believes that this is not something he ought to worry about; in fact, Grant values the experience of gastronomic pleasures over his health, and accepts the health risks that his lifestyle involves. A strong paternalist might potentially claim that Grant is weighing his values incorrectly here, and that it may be permissible to somehow restrict Grant's intake of unhealthy foods. Whilst strong paternalism requires a particular kind of beneficence-based justification (as I shall explore below), weak paternalism may be justified by an appeal to the precedence of global

[43] For a similar strategy in favour of limiting informed consent procedures, see Levy, 'Forced to Be Free?'

[44] Dworkin, 'Paternalism'.

over local autonomy, in so far as it calls for the safeguarding of the agent's ability to effectively pursue their own ends, over their freedom to make locally autonomous decisions about the means to take to their end.

It might be claimed that in advocating weak paternalism, I am betraying my above comments about the prudential value of autonomy; indeed, Sarah Conly's recent book defending a broadly similar strategy was titled *Against Autonomy*.[45] I cannot deny that there is a sense in which the approach that I am outlining here is 'against autonomy'. However, the point of this discussion has been that because local and global autonomy can come into conflict, we *have to* be against autonomy in one of these senses if we are to reconcile these conflicts. My argument has been that we should prioritize the kind of autonomy that often plausibly holds more significant prudential value, and it is a mistake to believe that this will always be local autonomy.

However, a key point underlying this justification is that the use of weak paternalism must be limited to cases in which it will promote what we know to be the values and goals undergirding the target's global autonomy. Given epistemological barriers to knowing that this will be the case,[46] the blunt nature of most proposed paternalist interventions, and the fact that reasonable agents can disagree about the weight they attribute to different goods, the scope of justifiable paternalist strategies on this approach will be extremely limited. Indeed, as I have argued elsewhere, we should be concerned about the possibility that these features of the justification might be overlooked, and the back-door perfectionism that could be ushered in under the guise of such weak paternalist justifications of manipulative interferences.[47] This would amount to considerations of beneficence (narrowly conceived in the sense that I discuss below) being dressed up in the language of (global) autonomy.

To conclude the discussion of the value of different elements of autonomy, could the decisional and practical dimensions of autonomy be valuable to different degrees? I have argued that the decisional element of autonomy is theoretically prior to the practical dimension. This analysis might tempt one to claim that whilst the decisional element of autonomy might bear final value, the practical dimension of autonomy might bear only instrumental value.[48] However, this thought should be resisted, since it fails to adequately capture the point that the way in which we value autonomy for its own sake is, as I suggested above, inextricably related to our fundamental interest in *living* a life that is our own, in acting on the basis of our autonomous decisions. Even if it were possible to separate the two dimensions of autonomy into discrete categories (which, I argued in Chapter 5, is doubtful) neither dimension alone seems sufficient for the project of living a life of one's own. This point is perhaps clearest with respect to practical autonomy; the fact that an agent is able to act effectively in pursuit of an end that she does *not* autonomously desire does not seem to be valuable

[45] Conly, *Against Autonomy*.

[46] For this reason, the relationship that the individual performing a weakly paternalistic intervention bears to its recipient can have considerable implications for its permissibility. For the significance of relationships to understanding permissible manipulative interference, see Blumenthal-Barby, 'A Framework for Assessing the Moral Status of "Manipulation"'.

[47] Pugh, 'Coercive Paternalism and Back-Door Perfectionism'.

[48] In a similar vein, Taylor claims that increasing an agent's freedoms does not increase her autonomy, but rather increases the value of her autonomy. Taylor, *Practical Autonomy and Bioethics*, 6.

in the same way as the ability to act in pursuit of an end that one autonomously desires;[49] only then can this freedom be said to be integral to the agent's ability to lay out her own mode of existence.

The value of decisional autonomy is also to a considerable extent conditional on the presence of practical autonomy, although this point is perhaps less immediately obvious. The reason for this is that it is difficult to imagine cases in which an agent lacks *all* freedoms that are relevant to their practical autonomy. To illustrate, reconsider the case of the slave philosopher Epictetus. Despite his being enslaved, and thus seemingly lacking *any* freedom, one might claim that Epictetus nonetheless represents the epitome of autonomy, in so far as he defied his lack of freedom by spending his life in the pursuit of a self-determined goal; namely the pursuit of philosophical truth. However, this example does not demonstrate that decisional autonomy *alone* is valuable for its own sake. Although Epictetus lacked many practical freedoms, he crucially retained the freedom to act effectively in pursuit of his goal of philosophizing; to this extent, he had both decisional and practical autonomy.

Therefore we should reject the claim that one dimension of autonomy is more prudentially valuable than the other. Neither dimension of autonomy in abstraction from the other is prudentially valuable for its own sake. Rather, we should understand the conjunction of the two dimensions of autonomy to form an organic whole which is prudentially valuable for its own sake, and whose value is derived from fundamental value in the exercise of laying out our own mode of existence, of living a life that is our own. It is not enough to be autonomous in our practical deliberations; we must also be able to act on the basis of those deliberations. This, I take it, is part of what John Harris means to capture in his bold claim (quoted in Chapter 5), that 'without agency, decision-making is ... both morally and practically barren'.[50]

4. Autonomy and Conflicting Values in Bioethics

Prior to outlining the sorts of values with which autonomy might come into conflict, it is crucial to first establish that autonomy can conceptually come into conflict with other values at all. On some views, autonomy cannot come into conflict with other values, because autonomy itself is understood to be the source of all other values.[51]

I mention this so-called 'autonomism' view only to reject it. I do so for the following reasons: First, there are some values to which autonomy cannot plausibly serve as a source, because their very possibility presupposes the absence of autonomy. For instance, certain values such as familial unity and dignity can be found in

[49] For this reason, I am less concerned than Berlin about unavoidable conflicts between his conceptions of positive and negative liberty, although I similarly acknowledge the potential for abuse of the prospect of constraining negative liberty in the name of positive liberty. See Berlin, 'Two Concepts of Liberty', 44–5. Further, I am not denying that practical freedoms can have other forms of instrumental value; the effective pursuit of non-autonomously endorsed goals could lead to other goods such as pleasure. Contrary to what I have claimed here, Feinberg has argued that freedom has intrinsic value. See Feinberg, *The Moral Limits of the Criminal Law*, 211–12. For a comprehensive rebuttal of these arguments see Haworth, *Autonomy*, 139–47. See also Griffin, *Well-Being*, 237.

[50] Harris, '"...How Narrow the Strait!"', 249.

[51] Haworth, *Autonomy*, 7 and 184.

communities that eschew autonomy, and the presence of these values in such communities is '...in part a function of the very absence of individual autonomy'.[52] Second, it seems that we can make sense of a life incorporating prudential value even if it lacks autonomy. As I argued above, whilst we may disagree with the hedonist's claim that we should hand over control of our lives to a benevolent personal despot if we had the chance, this does not entail that such a life would lack *any* prudential value; *ex hypothesi*, it would contain a great deal of pleasure. It seems implausible to claim that this pleasure would count for *nothing* simply because the agent in question lacked autonomy. Finally, we will clearly need further moral principles to guide us in cases of competing autonomy claims, when satisfying the autonomous preference of an individual requires frustrating the autonomous preferences of another.

It would thus be 'absurdly simplistic'[53] to understand autonomy to be the sole value governing medical ethics. However, the truth in autonomism is that autonomy seems to be related to a particular sort of value that we understand to be salient; in section 1, I described this as the value of 'living a life of one's own'. For this reason, although autonomy can conceptually come into conflict with other values in bioethics, one might maintain that autonomy is likely to win out in such conflicts. Indeed, one might worry that this understanding of the value of autonomy lends support to what Onora O'Neill disparagingly calls the 'consumerist view' of autonomy, according to which considerations of respect for autonomy serve as both necessary and sufficient conditions for the moral justification of some course of action.[54] In the following discussion, I shall explain that this view is neither reflected in medical law, nor a corollary of the understanding of the value autonomy I have outlined here.

According to the widely invoked four principles approach to biomedical ethics, our ethical decision-making should be governed by four ethical principles; namely, the principle of beneficence, the principle of non-maleficence, the principle of autonomy, and the principle of justice.[55] In outlining these principles, Beauchamp and Childress explicitly claim that none of these principles takes priority over any of the others; as such, it would be a mistake to assume that autonomy should trump these other values.[56]

One of the clearest examples of where the consumerist understanding of autonomy fails is in the context of health resource allocation, where considerations of autonomy and justice will often conflict. Since the demand for many health resources (such as organs for transplantation and hospital ward space) far outstrips supply, it is not the case that the autonomous wishes of all the patients who wish to use these

[52] See Berofsky, *Liberation from Self*, 248. Oshana also posits 'security' as a value that can conflict with autonomy. See Oshana, 'How Much Should We Value Autonomy?', 113–14.

[53] Foster, *Choosing Life, Choosing Death*, 9.

[54] O'Neill, *Autonomy and Trust in Bioethics*, 2.7 particularly p. 47.

[55] Beauchamp and Childress, *Principles of Biomedical Ethics*. In his discussion, Foster suggests that medical law and ethics should also consider principles relating to professional integrity and rights and duties of doctors and patients. See Foster, *Choosing Life, Choosing Death*, ch. 2.

[56] See Beauchamp and Childress, *Principles of Biomedical Ethics*, especially 57 and 177. However, it is questionable whether all those who invoke the four principles approach abide by this dictum; see Gillon, 'Ethics Needs Principles—Four Can Encompass the Rest—and Respect for Autonomy Should Be "First among Equals"'.

resources can be respected. Indeed, when societies have to make decisions about health resource allocation, considerations of distributive justice will unavoidably take precedence over considerations of individual autonomy, since it is simply not possible to satisfy the autonomous preferences of each person to have access to the scarce resource.[57] Since individual patients cannot generally be said to have a positive claim right to a scarce medical resource, an autonomous request for treatment generates a much weaker moral reason than a patient's autonomous decision not to waive negative rights that she does enjoy, when she refuses medical treatment.[58] In any case, contrary to what the consumerist view implies, reasons of autonomy are often not sufficient to justify actions, including the allocation of a scarce resource to an individual, given the implications that such actions can have for others.

This is quite compatible with the claims I have advanced in this chapter. Even if we accept the view that autonomy is fundamental to an individual's well-being, this is compatible with the claim that moral reasons generated by the well-being (and indeed the autonomy) of *others* can be sufficient to outweigh our reasons to respect the autonomy of the individual herself. Despite his staunch defence of liberty and individuality, even Mill claimed that considerations of justice can override the individual's right to liberty in this way. This thought is apparent in his 'Harm Principle', according to which:

> The only purpose for which power can be rightfully exercised over any member of a civilized community, against his will, is to prevent harm to others.[59]

Strikingly, the Harm Principle allows for the possibility that an individual's negative rights can, in some cases, be permissibly infringed by Mill's own lights; respect for autonomy then is not necessary for the moral justification of some actions, contrary to the consumerist view. Of course, one broadly autonomy-based reason that might justify a restriction of liberty against an individual's (occurrent) will is if the individual can be understood to have implicitly consented to a particular infringement, on the basis that doing so is a condition of the social contract that affords them a number of other strong and important protections. For instance, one might plausibly explain why one may justifiably prevent a would-be thief from robbing a bank in this way, even if one believes that the thief's autonomy would be best served by both affording him these protections *and* the freedom to rob the bank.

However, other restrictions of liberty might be justified by the need to safeguard the interests of others. Infectious disease control is an example where one might plausibly exercise power over another person against their will in a manner that is

[57] Pugh, 'Navigating Individual and Collective Interests in Medical Ethics'.

[58] If individuals have a positive claim right to a particular medical treatment, this would entail that physicians have a duty to provide it. We may also note that this might generate reasons that speak against an autonomy-based positive right to treatment. For instance, one might contend that such a right would compete with doctors' right to conscientious objection. Foster, *Choosing Life, Choosing Death*, ch. 8; Schuklenk and Smalling, 'Why Medical Professionals Have No Moral Claim to Conscientious Objection Accommodation in Liberal Democracies'; Cowley, 'Conscientious Objection in Healthcare and the Duty to Refer'; Wicclair, 'Justifying Conscience Clauses'. Alternatively, one might hold that doctors do not have a duty to perform treatments that violate unwaivable claim rights.

[59] Mill, *On Liberty*, 80.

morally permissible by the lights of the Harm Principle. Suppose a person infected with the Ebola virus refused to enter isolation voluntarily, and thus risked spreading the virus to other members of his community; it seems plausible to claim that public health authorities would be ethically justified in enforcing compulsory isolation on such an individual. In England and Wales, the right of the state to impose compulsory isolation in this sort of situation is legally enshrined in the Health and Social Care Act 2008.[60]

Contrary to the consumerist view, respecting autonomy thus does not serve as a necessary condition of all kinds of permissible medical intervention. However, simply invoking the language of autonomy alone to understand the forms of protection that are owed to individuals in public health contexts is perhaps too blunt an instrument; depending on one's overall approach to ethics, we may also need to take into account the degree of harm that an intervention will cause (on broadly consequentialist approaches) or the kinds of rights it would violate (on broadly deontological approaches). To illustrate the importance of this, suppose that instead of refusing isolation, an individual refused to undergo an invasive medical injection that was necessary to prevent him from spreading a deadly infectious disease to others. It is less straightforwardly clear that it would be permissible to impose this treatment; indeed, in England and Wales, the law allowing the imposition of quarantine explicitly rules out the imposition of non-consensual treatment, including vaccinations.[61] However, in both cases, we may presume that the moral reasons generated by considerations of public safety are held constant.

In order to make sense of the intuition that the individual has a stronger claim against the imposition of a medical treatment than he does against the imposition of quarantine, it seems that one would have to supplement considerations of the individual autonomy of the quarantined individual and harm to others with considerations of the quarantined individual's rights, or the harms that non-consensual quarantine will do to them. For instance, on a rights-based approach, it might be claimed that whilst quarantine violates the individual's right to freedom of movement and association, non-consensual medical treatment violates the recipient's right to bodily integrity. It might then be argued that the latter is a more robust right.[62] Alternatively, it might be claimed that bodily invasive interventions cause greater harms than placing restrictions on an individual's freedom of movement and association.

As I suggested in previous chapters, it is a mistake to think that the justification of claim rights that incorporate a power to waive the claim can be entirely divorced from considerations of autonomy. In a similar vein, we may note that the harmfulness of an intervention may plausibly turn to some degree on the strength of the individual's autonomous preference to avoid that interference. So these considerations are importantly related to autonomy. However, in order to adequately capture

[60] Health and Social Care Act 2008, Part 2A, 45.

[61] Ibid. Although see Herring, *Medical Law and Ethics*, 169 for discussion of courts' reluctance to preclude the permissibility of non-consensual treatment of competent individuals to save others.

[62] The UK Health and Social Care Act implicitly seems to endorse this view, in so far as it permits non-consensual quarantine, but prohibits non-consensual medical treatment.

the nuances of whether public safety should outweigh considerations of autonomy, we should also take into account these further considerations. The issue cannot be settled just by establishing whether the agent has or has not autonomously consented to the intervention itself.

Furthermore, the nature and degree of the harms that we can expect to *prevent* by violating the individual's autonomy should also factor into our overall weighting of these competing values. In the case of preventing the spread of a deadly pandemic, we might claim that we may be permitted to impose a very invasive non-consensual intervention that would prevent the spread of disease, given the number of lives at stake; in contrast, many find abhorrent the possibility that it might be permissible to carry out non-consensual interventions in order to save very few lives. Consider for instance the permissibility of carrying out a Caesarean section that is necessary to save an unborn child's life on a non-consenting competent woman in labour.[63]

The Harm Principle claims that it can be permissible to intervene on an individual's liberty to prevent the non-consensual imposition of harms to third parties that might otherwise occur. However, it also states that this is the *only* justification for such an intrusion on the individual; indeed, the main thrust of the Harm Principle is that the principle of autonomy trumps considerations of individual beneficence. This asymmetry between the moral weight of harm to others and harm to self in conflicts with autonomy may be understood to be a reflection of the fact that the individual herself may be understood to tacitly consent to harm when they autonomously choose to engage in self-harming behaviour, whilst third parties do not similarly consent to being harmed.[64]

Mill himself limited the application of the principle to those 'human beings who are in the maturity of their faculties'.[65] So, the fact that it can be lawful to perform unwanted beneficial medical procedures on patients who lack decision-making capacity is quite compatible with the principle. However, even observing this feature of Mill's thought, the salience attributed to autonomy on the Millian approach is only *partially* reflected in medical law. Contrary to those who perceive a consumerist view of autonomy at work in modern bioethics, elements of medical law are quite difficult to reconcile with the Millian understanding of the competing values of autonomy and well-being. As I explored in Chapter 6, consent cannot serve as a sufficient defence for certain kinds of intervention; accordingly, it seems that individuals may plausibly be said to enjoy certain negative claim rights that are *not* attended by the second-order power to waive those claims. Since such powers significantly demarcate the individual's sphere of autonomy in the law, it seems that the absence

[63] For discussion, see Savulescu, 'Future People, Involuntary Medical Treatment in Pregnancy and the Duty of Easy Rescue'; Herring, *Medical Law and Ethics*, 169. I have discussed the justification of non-consensual medical interventions in criminal justice in Pugh and Douglas, 'Justifications for Non-Consensual Medical Intervention'.

[64] Eyal hints at something similar in Eyal, 'Paternalism, French Fries and the Weak-Willed Witness'.

[65] Mill, *On Liberty*, 81.

of such powers with regard to some claims is best justified by appealing to the strength of the interest that the claims protect.[66]

Accordingly, even with regards to primarily self-regarding action, autonomy is not understood in the law to serve as a sufficient basis for the moral justification of any such action, as the consumerist view of autonomy would hold. In order to assess whether the law should delimit the scope of this individualistic aspect of the harm principle, we need to consider the relationship between beneficence and autonomy in more detail.

In the medical context, the principle of beneficence is sometimes understood in an extremely narrow sense to pertain only to medical benefits, that is, benefits concerning the end of healing.[67] On this interpretation, the goal of healing does not merely take precedence over other goods; it is the *only* good to which the principle of beneficence pertains. This interpretation is implausibly narrow; the reason for this is that we commonly use biomedical technologies in order to pursue ends that go beyond mere healing, and it can clearly be in our interests to do so. Although much depends on how widely we define the concept of health in our understanding of the narrow interpretation, vision enhancement surgery, or cosmetic procedures are examples of such interventions that can indisputably go beyond mere healing, but that are still plausibly in the individual's interests.

In view of this inadequacy, we need to refine the narrow interpretation of beneficence. Even if we maintain that medical interests should play a particularly salient role in a narrow understanding of the principle of beneficence in medical ethics, a plausible understanding of the principle should allow it to incorporate a broader range of benefits. As such, I suggest that we should understand the narrow interpretation of the principle of beneficence to be making the more plausible claim that medical benefits should override other kinds of benefit that might contribute to well-being. This allows for the possibility that interventions that do not aim at healing can still benefit the patient, whilst still affording a particularly salient role to health benefits in this conception of beneficence.

We can contrast these narrow interpretations of the principle, to a broad conception of beneficence, according to which the principle can be taken to pertain to *any* prudential benefits, without assigning any particular weight to a specific category of those benefits. To illustrate the difference, on the narrow interpretation of the scope of beneficence, it is difficult to see how death could ever be in a person's interests; such a choice is clearly contrary to the ends of healing, and this end takes precedence over other prudential goods on a narrow conception of beneficence. However, as I explained in my discussion of Isobel's case in the previous chapter, it seems possible for one to have a future life of prudential disvalue. In such cases, the broader conception might claim that death can be in a person's interests.

The extent to which the principles of beneficence and autonomy come into conflict depends significantly on our understanding of the scope of the principle of

[66] For instance, on similar matters, Foster writes: 'There will often be countervailing interests so powerful that they will outweigh autonomy interests. No one's autonomy right entitles them to be given poison, for instance'. Foster, *Choosing Life, Choosing Death*, 89.

[67] Pellegrino, *For the Patient's Good.*

beneficence. According to a commonly endorsed view that implicitly endorses something like the refined narrow conception that I illustrated above, the concepts of autonomy and beneficence are understood to represent two distinct domains; the question of what is in a patient's best interests is understood to be a conceptually different question to the question of what a patient autonomously desires. For instance, in introducing the concept of beneficence, Beauchamp and Childress point out that '[m]orality requires not only that we treat persons autonomously... but also that we contribute to their welfare'.[68]

I shall argue that we should reject the narrow interpretation of beneficence that the commonly endorsed view relies upon. I have already suggested that we should understand the principle of beneficence to encompass goods beyond the ends of healing, and to pertain to prudential goods more broadly. In doing so though, we should also acknowledge the point that I have defended in this chapter, namely that autonomy plays an important role in a person's well-being. Thus, contrary to the commonly endorsed view, treating persons autonomously and contributing to their welfare should not be understood as distinct requirements; in order to adequately contribute to a person's welfare, we must take into account the agent's own autonomous preferences.

The problem with even the refined narrow conception is that it relies on an overly objective account of what is in a person's interests. Recall that on purely objective accounts of well-being, there are certain things that are intrinsically good or bad, that all agents have impersonal self-interested reasons to either want or avoid, regardless of their own attitudes towards these outcomes. The narrow interpretation of the principle of beneficence in medical ethics takes the end of healing to be the primary objective good of concern here. However, such a view is unattractive. This claim may seem somewhat surprising, since in section 1, I endorsed an explanatory account of well-being that appeals to objective values. However, what is problematic about the view that I am considering here is not that it relies upon the claim that there are objective elements of well-being. Rather, the problem with the view that I am considering here is that it implicitly assumes that there is an objective *ranking* of the different objective elements of well-being.

This assumption is problematic because the decisions that we make in medical contexts concern a far greater range of goods than those that are adequately captured by the end of healing. Our choices in this domain can have implications for pursuing the various other goods we may value in our life, and it is a mistake to assume that rationality requires that we must prioritize health over the promotion of these other goods. Indeed, whilst the interpretation of 'best interests' in medical law traditionally endorsed the narrow interpretation outlined above, this has shifted towards a broader conception of beneficence. For instance, best interests assessments under the MCA incorporate consideration of non-medical issues such as 'the person's past and present wishes and feelings' and also the 'beliefs and values that would be likely to influence his decision if he had capacity'.[69] This is an example of the way in which

[68] Beauchamp and Childress, *Principles of Biomedical Ethics*, 202.

[69] Mental Capacity Act 2005, 4(6). *Aintree University Hospitals NHS Foundation Trust v. James*, paragraph 24. Herring et al. argue that this interpretation of best interests is also echoed in the

the requirements of beneficence are not neatly separated from considerations of autonomy in medical law.

Even on theories of well-being that incorporate *only* objective elements, agents can still rationally disagree about the relative strengths of the self-interested reasons that different objective goods imply; I have suggested that truths concerning the comparative strength of such reasons are often very imprecise. Thus, even if we accept a purely objective list theory of well-being, we need not accept the claim implicit in the narrow interpretation of beneficence, that the goods in this list must have a set impartial degree of goodness, or that there is a supreme value that overrides others on the list. This point is all the more powerful if we endorse a hybrid view of the sort that I sketched at the end of section 1, which incorporates both objective and subjective elements of well-being.

On some objective views of well-being, such as that which is endorsed by the narrow interpretation of the principle of beneficence, conflicts between the principle of autonomy and the principle of beneficence will typically arise whenever an agent's autonomous desires conflict with the objective ranking of values that the view may stipulate. Such views of well-being naturally lend support to two types of paternalism; first, what Feinberg terms 'hard paternalism', and second, the sense of 'strong paternalism' that I explained above. According to hard paternalism, a third party may permissibly interfere with even an agent's voluntary choices in order to protect them from the harmful consequences of those choices; by way of contrast, soft paternalism only permits a third party to interfere with an agent's involuntary choices.[70] We may note that hard and strong paternalism are not necessarily co-extensive. For example, Sarah Conly's so-called 'coercive paternalism' is hard but weak, in so far as it allows the state to force people to act (or refrain from acting) in certain ways and impose actions on them that they would not choose (even if properly informed), but only in order to ensure that individuals are better able to achieve their own autonomously chosen goals.[71] For instance, Conly argues in favour of banning cigarettes on the basis that doing so would be likely to advance individuals' effective pursuit of their long-term goal of better health.[72]

The objection that I have raised against the narrow interpretation of beneficence, and the arguments that I have raised in favour of the final value of autonomy speak against both hard and strong forms of paternalism. First, contrary to strong paternalism, we seldom have warrant for assuming that rational agents should prioritize a particular goal, such that we would be warranted in determining that they pursue that end over other goods. The truths governing the relative weights of objective goods are imprecise, and rational agents can disagree about the relative weight they assign to the goods (such as health and pleasure) that are mutually incompatible in a particular context. Second, with respect to hard paternalism, if we believe that autonomy has final prudential value, then it may be a mistake to claim that overriding our autonomous choices is actually in our interests. Autonomy makes a

Montgomery judgement, which I considered in an earlier chapter. See Herring et al., 'Elbow Room for Best Practice?', 9.

70 Feinberg, *The Moral Limits of the Criminal Law*, 12–13.

71 Conly, *Against Autonomy*, particularly 45.

72 Ibid., 169–72.

particular kind of contribution to well-being that cannot be replicated by the imposition of other good things. This is precisely the insight of the PDA.

The claim that autonomy has final prudential value entails that there is a great deal of overlap between the values of autonomy and beneficence. This in turn lends support to the Harm Principle's contention that considerations of an individual's well-being cannot outweigh those of their autonomy. For this reason, many of the conflicts that are ostensibly conflicts between the two are more aptly construed as conflicts between different elements of well-being. This provides a philosophical basis for criticizing those elements of the law that appear to prioritize strong welfare interests over individual autonomy. Naturally, considerations of autonomy lend little support to claim rights that are not attended by the power of a waiver. More strikingly though, given the role of autonomy in well-being, we can also coherently challenge whether such rights are sufficiently supported by considerations of individual well-being. The claim that the law should safeguard unwaivable claim rights against *inter alia* sado-masochistic interactions or unusual body piercings, on the basis of the strength of the interests they protect, is to adopt an impoverished view of well-being that does not adequately capture the particular contribution that autonomy makes not only to a good life itself, but also to the nature of the contribution that other goods in that life can make to a person's well-being.

On the view that I am outlining, conflicts between autonomy and beneficence will be less commonplace; as long as an individual's choice is autonomous, that should give us at least a *pro tanto* reason to believe that respecting that choice will benefit that person, not because the choice is likely to lead to greater happiness (as the explanatory hedonist might claim), but rather because on this view there is prudential value to directing the course of one's life in accordance with one's own beliefs about what is of value, and with one's own beliefs about which values should take precedence.

However, the view that I endorse does not entail that there *cannot* be conflicts between autonomy and beneficence. Rather, I have suggested here that our analysis of cases in which there appears to be such a conflict should be more nuanced. Contrary to the overly objectivist account that the narrow view of beneficence implies, the fact that an agent has an autonomous preference is a fact that is relevant to our assessment of what is in their best interests. If an individual harbours an autonomous preference to engage in a behaviour that they believe they have reason to perform but that also endangers their life, such as the base-jumping thrill-seeker, or the gourmand who eats to the point of morbid obesity, there is a sense in which that behaviour is in their interests. However, whether that behaviour is in their *best* interests depends on the strength of their self-interested reasons to refrain from that behaviour, and the weight that we ascribe to autonomy in our general account of well-being.

One might worry that the principle of beneficence becomes superfluous on this approach, since it seems to have been subsumed by the principle of autonomy.[73] One

[73] Buchanan raises this sort of concern about this approach. See Buchanan, 'The Physician's Knowledge and the Patient's Best Interest', 94.

response to this worry is to interpret the principle of beneficence in a purely negative sense, by understanding it as '. . . an admonition to the physician not to allow the interests of others . . . to compromise his or her commitment to the patient'.[74] However, this reading seems to give the principle too narrow an interpretation, especially given that it may need to be operative in cases where we must consider the positive care of an individual who lacks autonomy.[75] Yet, the principle of beneficence can still have substance on the understanding of well-being and autonomy that I have outlined in this chapter, because it does not entail that the realization of autonomous choices *exhausts* the concept of well-being. The concept of 'beneficence' can incorporate both the patient's autonomous choices, and other goods that agents have impersonal self-interested reasons to want. On this understanding, conflicts will arise when the agent's autonomous choice is not co-extensive with what they have an impersonal self-interested reason to want. To resolve the conflict, we must compare the strength of these impersonal self-interested reasons, with the reasons we have to safeguard the agent's autonomy by respecting their own assessment of what is in their best interests.

That the principle of beneficence still has substance on this understanding becomes further apparent when we consider cases in which a patient has not and cannot make their choices clear to their physician. For example, considering what agents have impersonal self-interested reasons to want can give physicians guidance when they are dealing with incompetent patients who lack a surrogate decision-maker or when asking for a competent patient's consent would be too time-consuming in an emergency situation. Moreover, as Buchanan suggests, physicians need to have their own understanding of the patient's best interests when deciding which courses of treatment to provide as viable choices for a particular patient and when making a recommendation to patients.[76]

Conclusion

I have argued that whilst autonomy may often bear instrumental prudential value, it is primarily prudentially valuable for its own sake. I have also claimed that this implies that we should broaden our understanding of what is in an agent's best interests. However, it should be acknowledged that I have not attempted to assign a particular definite value to autonomy. I have simply suggested that autonomy represents a special type of value for us, one that serves to amplify the contribution of other goods to well-being, in so far as there is a particular value in living a life that is our own. Yet, I have left open the possibility that this value can have different weight in different people's conceptions of the good life. The extent to which autonomy will contribute to a person's welfare will depend in part on the extent to which autonomy conflicts with other outcomes that the agent has reasons to pursue.

These claims are compatible with rejecting a consumerist view of autonomy that understands autonomy to be both necessary for and sufficient to the moral justification of medical interventions. I have argued that the view of autonomy's value that

[74] Ibid., 95. [75] Ibid. [76] Ibid., 95–6.

I have presented here does not entail the consumerist view. At most, the view of autonomy's value that I have presented suggests that respect for autonomy, broadly conceived, is very often necessary to the justification of permissible medical interventions that are purely self-regarding. Given the central role that autonomy plays in well-being, narrowly construed beneficence-based justifications of non-consensual interventions are likely to come undone. For this reason, although the consumerist view should be rejected, autonomy still has a considerable bearing on our understanding of permissible self-regarding decisions in bioethical contexts.

Concluding Remarks

In the introduction to this book, I outlined my intention to provide an account of personal autonomy that can usefully be applied to issues in contemporary bioethics, and that clarifies its ambiguous relationship with rationality. At the most fundamental level, I understood the concept of autonomy to denote a particular capacity to which we seem to attribute prudential value in bioethical contexts, namely, a capacity that we invoke to capture concerns pertaining to an agent's ability to both:

(i) Make their own decisions about what to do
And
(ii) To act on the basis of those decisions.

In accordance with this understanding, I suggested that the concept of personal autonomy incorporates two corresponding dimensions: a decisional dimension, and a practical dimension.

The theory of autonomy that I have described as the standard view of autonomy in bioethics is a theory of the decisional dimension of autonomy. On this account an agent is autonomous with respect a particular decision if it is made:

(1) Intentionally,
(2) With understanding,
and
(3) Without controlling influences that determine their action.

In delineating this theory in the introduction, I suggested that it implicitly bases its understanding of decisional autonomy on two senses of voluntariness, identified by Aristotle in book III of *The Nicomachean Ethics*. Conditions (1) and (3) capture the Aristotelian sense of voluntariness that pertains to acts that are motivated by forces that are in some sense internal rather than external to the agent. In contrast, condition (2) captures the Aristotelian sense of voluntariness that pertains to actions that are not performed from reasons of ignorance.

I argued that the standard account of decisional autonomy fails to provide an adequate account of what it is for an agent to make their own decisions, due to an inadequate conception of the first Aristotelian sense of voluntariness identified above. I argued that in order to offer a unified, non-stipulative explanation of why the controlling influences that the standard account appeals to (in condition (3) above) undermine decisional autonomy, an adequate conception of this sense of voluntariness requires a broader understanding of forces that can be 'external to the self'.

Autonomy, Rationality, and Contemporary Bioethics. Jonathan Pugh, Oxford University Press (2020).
DOI: 10.1093/oso/9780198858584.001.0001

The concept of rationality can help in this regard. By attending to different features of rationality, and how they relate to our beliefs and values, I sought to clarify some important misunderstandings of the relationship between rationality and autonomy, and to develop a rationalist account of decisional autonomy. I argued for the following supplementary rationalist conditions of autonomy:

Theoretical Rationality: Decisional autonomy is precluded by theoretically irrational beliefs about information that is material to one's decisions.

Practical Rationality: The autonomous agent's motivating desires must be rational in the following sense. They must:

(a) Be endorsed by preferences that are sustained on the basis of the agent's holding (rational) beliefs that, if true, would give the agent reason to pursue the object of the desire.
And
(b) These preferences must cohere with other elements of the agent's character system.

The rationalist model I have developed provides a deeper explanation of why rationality plays such an integral role in autonomy. It sought to provide an answer to the question of why we should trust that this aspect of our agency is the right place for the 'buck to stop' with regards to autonomous decision-making. In the case of practical rationality, the answer to this question is that our evaluative judgements play a particularly central role in our character systems. Practical rationality thus facilitates our ability to decide in accordance with elements of our character that should be understood to have agential authority. In the case of theoretical rationality, the answer to this question lay in the role that rationality plays in developing the sort of understanding that decisional autonomy requires.

This rationalist account allows for a more nuanced understanding of the sorts of controlling influence that serve to undermine decisional autonomy than the understanding outlined in the standard account of autonomy. It also highlighted the role that an interpersonal sense of voluntariness can play in our judgements about what constitutes 'controlling influence'. Furthermore, by tying a rationalist theory of decisional autonomy to an analysis of the oft-overlooked practical dimension of autonomy, I suggested a new way of understanding the role of true beliefs in autonomous agency, and why some beliefs might appropriately be deemed to be decisionally necessary, as the cognitive dimension of decisional autonomy implies.

Partly on this basis, I defended the claim that the requirements of informed consent can be justified by considerations of personal autonomy, a claim also endorsed by the standard view of autonomy. However, I suggested that a rationalist account of decisional autonomy suggests that we should reform our understanding of what informed consent requires. In Chapter 6, I began to make this claim by further investigating the cognitive element of decisional autonomy, before going on to consider the implications of this investigation for standards of information disclosure and tests of materiality. I concluded this analysis by applauding the spirit, although not the letter, of the recent Montgomery judgement concerning medical negligence, in its apparent attempt to further the cause of patient autonomy in clinical decision-making.

The most controversial aspect of understanding autonomy in a rationalist sense concerns its implications for our understanding of decision-making capacity. Contrary to the anti-rationalist tenor of many philosophical treatments of the issue, I explained that existing medical law implicitly incorporates a number of considerations pertaining to the rationality of a patient's decisions. I also defended the view that a rationalist conception of decisional autonomy would not unduly restrict the boundaries of decision-making capacity. To further illustrate this point, I explained how my rationalist approach could be brought to bear on three different cases of end of life decision-making. In particular, I suggested that a rationalist approach calls for a more nuanced understanding of whether we should respect treatment refusals of psychiatric patients, and refusals based on religious beliefs.

By virtue of the objectivist approach to rationalist autonomy that I incorporated into my understanding of decisional autonomy, and my agreement with the Millian claim that we have a fundamental prudential interest in 'laying out our own mode of our existence', I claimed that there is an important relationship between personal autonomy and individual well-being on the approach that I have defended. In Chapter 9, I sought to explicate the nature of this relationship, explaining how autonomy could be understood to bear final prudential value, whilst acknowledging the possibility that we might have prudential reasons to prioritize global autonomy over local autonomy in some cases. I also suggested that my understanding of the relationship between autonomy and well-being spoke in favour of reconceptualizing the nature of beneficence and its conflict with autonomy, a move that is at least partly reflected in the evolving understanding of 'best interests' employed in medical law.

I shall conclude with two rather more general theoretical observations about what we may broadly conclude from this study. As well as developing an account of autonomy that avoids the flaws of the standard account of autonomy in bioethics, I have also been wary of the flaws attending many of the alternative philosophical accounts of this dimension of autonomy that are often invoked in bioethical contexts. However, over the course of developing this account of autonomy, I have attempted to somewhat bridge the gap between philosophical discussions of the concept of autonomy, and the way in which the concept is invoked in bioethics in other ways. It is no doubt true that our discussions of autonomy in bioethics, and the related notions of capacity, consent, and freedom, can of course be enriched by a philosophically informed understanding of autonomy. However, I also believe that the way in which the concept of autonomy is invoked in contemporary bioethical issues suggests some important insights for our philosophical understanding of autonomy. In particular, the importance of acknowledging both what I have called the practical dimension of autonomy, and the cognitive element of decisional autonomy in bioethical discussions should also be extended to our philosophical discussions of autonomy more generally. Philosophical approaches to the concept of autonomy should branch out from their somewhat myopic focus on the reflective element of decisional autonomy, because the different dimensions of autonomy that I have appealed to here are not just useful for understanding bioethical issues; an adequate understanding of the nature of autonomy must recognize the influence that each of these elements of autonomy can have.

Second, there is no 'moral danger' that understanding autonomy in the rationalist sense that I have outlined here would unduly restrict the boundaries of what would qualify as an autonomous decision. If there is any moral danger in adopting this approach, it lies in the highly ambiguous ways in which the concepts of rationality, autonomy, and value have frequently been treated in bioethical discussions, and the potential that this raises for misinterpretation and conflict. My hope is that this book has at the least shed some light on these ambiguities and, perhaps, offered a coherent way of thinking about these concepts that can help us navigate the various bioethical issues in which considerations of autonomy are salient.

Bibliography

Ackermann, Ruby, and Robert J. DeRubeis. 'Is Depressive Realism Real?' *Clinical Psychology Review* 11, no. 5 (1991): 565–84.

Adams, Robert Merrihew. *Finite and Infinite Goods: A Framework for Ethics*. New York and Oxford: Oxford University Press, 1999.

Aintree University Hospitals NHS Foundation Trust v. James (UKSC 67 2013).

Alston, William P. *Epistemic Justification: Essays in the Theory of Knowledge*. Ithaca and London: Cornell University Press, 1989.

American Psychiatric Association. *Diagnostic and Statistical Manual of Mental Disorders*, 5th edition. Washington, DC: American Psychiatric Association.

Anderson, Joel, and Axel Honneth. 'Autonomy, Vulnerability, Recognition, and Justice'. In *Autonomy and the Challenges to Liberalism: New Essays*, edited by John Christman and Joel Anderson, 127–49. Cambridge: Cambridge University Press 2005.

Anderson, Scott. 'Coercion'. In *The Stanford Encyclopedia of Philosophy*, edited by Edward N. Zalta, Winter 2011. http://plato.stanford.edu/archives/win2011/entries/coercion/.

Andorno, R. 'The Right Not to Know: An Autonomy Based Approach'. *Journal of Medical Ethics* 30, no. 5 (2004): 435–9.

Annas, George J. 'Life, Liberty, and the Pursuit of Organ Sales'. *The Hastings Center Report* 14, no. 1 (1984): 22–3.

Appelbaum, P. S., and T. Grisso. 'Assessing Patients' Capacities to Consent to Treatment'. *The New England Journal of Medicine* 319, no. 25 (1988): 1635–8.

Appelbaum, Paul S., and Thomas Grisso. 'The MacArthur Treatment Competence Study, I: Mental Illness and Competence to Consent to Treatment'. *Law and Human Behavior* 19, no. 2 (1995): 105–26.

Appelbaum, Paul S., Thomas Grisso, Ellen Frank, Sandra Donnell, and David Kupfer. 'Competence of Depressed Patients for Consent to Research'. *American Journal of Psychiatry* 156, no. 9 (1999): 1380–4.

Appelbaum, Paul S., Charles W. Lidz, and Robert Klitzman. 'Voluntariness of Consent to Research: A Conceptual Model'. *The Hastings Center Report* 39, no. 1 (2009): 30–9.

Appleton v. Garrett, 5 PIQR, P1 (1996).

Archard, David. 'Informed Consent: Autonomy and Self-Ownership'. *Journal of Applied Philosophy* 25, no. 1 (2008): 19–34.

Aristotle. *Nicomachean Ethics*, 2nd edition. Cambridge Texts in the History of Philosophy. Cambridge: Cambridge University Press, 2014.

Arpaly, Nomy. 'On Acting Rationally against One's Best Judgment'. *Ethics* 110, no. 3 (2000): 488–513.

Arpaly, Nomy. 'Responsibility, Applied Ethics, and Complex Autonomy Theories'. In *Personal Autonomy: New Essays on Personal Autonomy and Its Role in Contemporary Moral Philosophy*, edited by James Stacey Taylor, 162–80. Cambridge: Cambridge University Press, 2005.

Arpaly, Nomy. *Unprincipled Virtue: An Inquiry into Moral Agency*. New York and Oxford: Oxford University Press, 2003.

Ashcroft, Richard E. 'Law and the Perils of Philosophical Grafts'. *Journal of Medical Ethics* 44, no. 1 (2018): 72. https://doi.org/10.1136/medethics-2017-104319.

Athanassoulis, Nafsika. 'The Role of Consent in Sado-Masochistic Practices'. *Res Publica* 8, no. 2 (2002): 141–55.

Audi, Robert. 'Belief, Faith, and Acceptance'. *International Journal for Philosophy of Religion* 63, no. 1 (2008): 87–102.

Axelrod, Lawrence J., and Darrin R. Lehman. 'Responding to Environmental Concerns: What Factors Guide Individual Action?' *Journal of Environmental Psychology* 13, no. 2 (1993): 149–59.

Baergen, Ralph. 'Assessing the Competence Assessment Tool'. *Journal of Clinical Ethics* 13, no. 2 (2002): 160–4.

Bakhurst, David. 'On Lying and Deceiving'. *Journal of Medical Ethics* 18, no. 2 (1992): 63–6.

Bandura, Albert. 'Perceived Self-Efficacy in the Exercise of Personal Agency'. *Journal of Applied Sport Psychology* 2, no. 2 (1990): 128–63.

Bandura, Albert, Claudio Barbaranelli, Gian Vittorio Caprara, and Concetta Pastorelli. 'Self-Efficacy Beliefs as Shapers of Children's Aspirations and Career Trajectories'. *Child Development* 72, no. 1 (2001): 187–206.

Banner, Natalie F., and George Szmukler. '"Radical Interpretation" and the Assessment of Decision-Making Capacity'. *Journal of Applied Philosophy* 30, no. 4 (2013): 379–94.

Barnhill, Anne. 'What Is Manipulation?' In *Manipulation: Theory and Practice*, edited by Christian Coons and Michael Weber, 51–72. New York: Oxford University Press, 2014.

Barnhill, Anne, and Katherine F. King. 'Ethical Agreement and Disagreement about Obesity Prevention Policy in the United States'. *International Journal of Health Policy and Management* 1, no. 2 (2013): 117–20.

Baron, Jonathan. *Rationality and Intelligence*. Cambridge: Cambridge University Press, 1985.

Bartlett, Peter. *Blackstone's Guide to the Mental Capacity Act 2005*, 2nd edition. Oxford and New York: Oxford University Press, 2008.

Bartlett, Peter. 'The United Nations Convention on the Rights of Persons with Disabilities and Mental Health Law'. *The Modern Law Review* 75, no. 5 (2012): 752–78.

Bayles, Michael. 'A Concept of Coercion'. In *Nomos XIV: Coercion*, edited by James Pennock and John Chapman, 16–29. Chicago: Aldine-Atherton, 1972.

Beauchamp, T. L. 'Viewpoint: Why Our Conceptions of Research and Practice May Not Serve the Best Interest of Patients and Subjects'. *Journal of Internal Medicine* 269, no. 4 (2011): 383–7.

Beauchamp, Tom L., and James F. Childress. *Principles of Biomedical Ethics*. Oxford: Oxford University Press, 1979.

Beauchamp, Tom L., and James F. Childress. *Principles of Biomedical Ethics*, 7th edition. Oxford: Oxford University Press, 2013.

Beck, Aaron T. *Depression: Clinical, Experimental, and Theoretical Aspects*. Philadelphia: University of Pennsylvania Press, 1967.

Bell, Rudolph M. *Holy Anorexia*. Chicago and London: University of Chicago Press, 1987.

Bemporad, Jules R. 'Self-Starvation through the Ages: Reflections on the Pre-History of Anorexia Nervosa'. *The International Journal of Eating Disorders* 19, no. 3 (1996): 217–37.

Benn, Piers. 'Medicine, Lies and Deceptions'. *Journal of Medical Ethics* 27, no. 2 (2001): 130–4.

Benson, Paul. 'Autonomy and Oppressive Socialization'. *Social Theory and Practice* 17, no. 3 (1991): 385–408.

Benson, Paul. 'Feminist Intuitions and the Normative Substance of Autonomy'. In *Personal Autonomy: New Essays on Personal Autonomy and Its Role in Contemporary Moral Philosophy*, edited by James Stacey Taylor, 124–42. Cambridge: Cambridge University Press, 2005.

Benson, Paul. 'Freedom and Value'. *The Journal of Philosophy* 84, no. 9 (1987): 465–86.

Berlin, Isaiah. 'John Stuart Mill and the Ends of Life'. In *On Liberty in Focus*, edited by John Gray and G. W. Smith, 131–61. London: Routledge, 1991.

Berlin, Isaiah. 'Two Concepts of Liberty'. In *The Liberty Reader*, edited by David Miller, 33–57. Edinburgh: Edinburgh University Press, 2006.

Berofsky, Bernard. *Liberation from Self: A Theory of Personal Autonomy*. Cambridge: Cambridge University Press, 1995.

Blumenthal, Susanna. 'The Default Legal Person'. *UCLA Law Review* 54, no. 5 (2007): 1135–265.

Blumenthal-Barby, J. S. 'A Framework for Assessing the Moral Status of "Manipulation"'. In *Manipulation: Theory and Practice*, edited by Christian Coons and Michael Weber, 120–34. Oxford: Oxford University Press, 2014.

Blumenthal-Barby, J. S., and Hadley Burroughs. 'Seeking Better Health Care Outcomes: The Ethics of Using the "Nudge"'. *The American Journal of Bioethics* 12, no. 2 (2012): 1–10.

Blumenthal-Barby, J. S., and Aanand D. Naik. 'In Defense of Nudge-Autonomy Compatibility'. *The American Journal of Bioethics* 15, no. 10 (2015): 45–7.

Bok, Sissela. *Lying: Moral Choice in Public and Private Life*. New York: Vintage Books, 1989.

Bolam v. Friern Hospital Management Committee (1975).

Bolton, Derek, and Natalie Banner. 'Does Mental Disorder Involve Loss of Personal Autonomy?' In *Autonomy and Mental Disorder*, edited by Lubomira Radoilska, 77–99. Oxford: Oxford University Press, 2012.

Bolton, Helen. 'The Montgomery Ruling Extends Patient Autonomy'. *BJOG: An International Journal of Obstetrics & Gynaecology* 122, no. 9 (2015): 1273. https://doi.org/10.1111/1471-0528.13467.

Bortolotti, Lisa. *Delusions and Other Irrational Beliefs*. International Perspectives in Philosophy and Psychiatry. Oxford: Oxford University Press, 2010.

Bortolotti, Lisa. 'Rationality and Sanity: The Role of Rationality Judgements in Understanding Psychiatric Disorders'. In *The Oxford Handbook of Philosophy and Psychiatry*, edited by K. M. W. Fulford, Martin Davies, Richard Gipps, George Graham, John Sadler, Giovanni Stanghellini, and Tim Thornton, 480–96. Oxford: Oxford University Press, 2013.

Bortolotti, Lisa, Rochelle Cox, Matthew Broome, and Matteo Mameli. 'Rationality and Self-Knowledge in Delusion and Confabulation: Implications for Autonomy as Self-Governance'. In *Autonomy and Mental Disorder*, edited by Lubomira Radoilska, 100–22. Oxford: Oxford University Press, 2012.

Bortolotti, Lisa, and Kengo Miyazono. 'Recent Work on the Nature and Development of Delusions'. *Philosophy Compass* 10, no. 9 (2015): 636–45.

Bostrom, Nick. 'In Defense of Posthuman Dignity'. *Bioethics* 19, no. 3 (2005): 202–14.

Bostrom, Nick, and Anders Sandberg. 'Cognitive Enhancement: Methods, Ethics, Regulatory Challenges'. *Science and Engineering Ethics* 15, no. 3 (2009): 311–41.

Bradley, Ben. *Well-Being and Death*. Oxford: Oxford University Press, 2011.

Bratman, Michael E. 'Identification, Decision, and Treating as a Reason'. *Philosophical Topics* 24, no. 2 (1996): 1–18.

Bratman, Michael E. 'Planning Agency, Autonomous Agency'. In *Personal Autonomy: New Essays on Personal Autonomy and Its Role in Contemporary Moral Philosophy*, edited by James Stacey Taylor, 33–57. Cambridge: Cambridge University Press, 2005.

Bratman, Michael E. 'Reflection, Planning, and Temporally Extended Agency'. In *Structures of Agency: Essays*, 21–46. Oxford: Oxford University Press, 2007.

Bratman, Michael E. 'Valuing and the Will'. In *Structures of Agency: Essays*, 47–67. Oxford: Oxford University Press, 2007.

Brazier, Margaret. 'Patient Autonomy and Consent to Treatment: The Role of the Law?' *Legal Studies* 7, no. 2 (1987): 169–93.

Brazier, M., and J. Miola. 'Bye-Bye Bolam: A Medical Litigation Revolution?' *Medical Law Review* 8, no. 1 (2000): 85–114.

Brewer, Talbot. 'The Real Problem with Internalism About Reasons'. *Canadian Journal of Philosophy* 32, no. 4 (2002): 443–73.

Brock, Dan W. *Life and Death: Philosophical Essays in Biomedical Ethics*. Cambridge: Cambridge University Press, 1993.

Brock, Dan W. ' Patient Competence and Surrogate Decision-Making'. In *The Blackwell Guide to Medical Ethics*, edited by Rosamond Rhodes, Leslie P. Francis, and Anita Silvers, 128–41. Malden, MA: Blackwell, 2007.

Brock, Dan W. ' Voluntary Active Euthanasia'. *The Hastings Center Report* 22, no. 2 (1992): 10–22.

Bromwich, Danielle. 'Understanding, Interests and Informed Consent: A Reply to Sreenivasan'. *Journal of Medical Ethics* 41, no. 4 (2015): 327–31.

Bromwich, Danielle, and Joseph Millum. 'Disclosure and Consent to Medical Research Participation'. *Journal of Moral Philosophy* 10, no. 4 (2013): 195–219.

Bublitz, Jan Christoph. 'Crimes Against Minds: On Mental Manipulations, Harms and a Human Right to Mental Self-Determination'. *Criminal Law and Philosophy* 8, no. 1 (2014): 51–77.

Bublitz, Jan Christoph, and Reinhard Merkel. 'Autonomy and Authenticity of Enhanced Personality Traits'. *Bioethics* 23, no. 6 (2009): 360–74.

Buchanan, Alec. 'Mental Capacity, Legal Competence and Consent to Treatment'. *Journal of the Royal Society of Medicine* 97, no. 9 (2004): 415–20.

Buchanan, Alec. 'The Physician's Knowledge and the Patient's Best Interest'. In *Ethics, Trust, and the Professions: Philosophical and Cultural Aspects*, edited by Edmund Pellegrino, Robert Veatch, and John Langan, 93–112. Washington, DC: Georgetown University Press, 1991.

Buchanan, Allen E., and Dan W. Brock. *Deciding for Others: The Ethics of Surrogate Decision Making*. Cambridge: Cambridge University Press, 1989.

Buckareff, Andrei A. 'Can Faith Be a Doxastic Venture?' *Religious Studies* 41, no. 4 (2005): 435–45.

Buckareff, Andrei A. 'Deciding to Believe Redux'. In *The Ethics of Belief: Individual and Social*, edited by Jonathan Matheson and Rico Vitz, 33–50. Oxford: Oxford University Press, 2014.

Canterbury v. Spence (464 F.2d 772) 1972.

Caplan, Arthur L. *Am I My Brother's Keeper? The Ethical Frontiers of Biomedicine*. Bloomington: Indiana University Press, 1997.

Carter, Ian. 'Respect and the Basis of Equality'. *Ethics* 121, no. 3 (2011): 538–71.

Chan, Sarah W., Ed Tulloch, E. Sarah Cooper, Andrew Smith, Wojtek Wojcik, and Jane E. Norman. 'Montgomery and Informed Consent: Where Are We Now?' *British Medical Journal* 357 (2017): j2224. https://doi.org/10.1136/bmj.j2224.

Chandler, Jennifer A. 'Autonomy and the Unintended Legal Consequences of Emerging Neurotherapies'. *Neuroethics* 6, no. 2 (2013): 249–63.

Chang, Ruth. 'Hard Choices'. *Journal of the American Philosophical Association* 3, no. 1 (2017): 1–21.

Charland, Louis C. 'Anorexia and the MacCAT-T Test for Mental Competence: Validity, Value, and Emotion'. *Philosophy, Psychiatry, & Psychology* 13, no. 4 (2007): 283–7.

Charland, Louis C. 'Ethical and Conceptual Issues in Eating Disorders'. *Current Opinion in Psychiatry* 26, no. 6 (2013): 562–5.

Charland, Louis C., Tony Hope, Anne Stewart, and Jacinta Tan. 'Anorexia Nervosa as a Passion'. *Philosophy, Psychiatry, & Psychology* 20, no. 4 (2013): 353–65.

Chatterton v. Gerson (1981) 1 All ER.

Chester v. Afshar (2004) 3 WLR 927 House of Lords.
Christman, John. 'Autonomy and Personal History'. *Canadian Journal of Philosophy* 21, no. 1 (1991): 1–24.
Christman, John. *The Politics of Persons: Individual Autonomy and Socio-Historical Selves*. Cambridge: Cambridge University Press, 2011.
Christman, John. 'Relational Autonomy, Liberal Individualism, and the Social Constitution of Selves'. *Philosophical Studies* 117, no. 1 (2004): 143–64.
Ciurria, Michelle. 'A Virtue Ethical Approach to Decisional Capacity and Mental Health'. *Philosophical Psychology* 29, no. 3 (2016): 462–75.
Clarke, Steve. 'The Neuroscience of Decision Making and Our Standards for Assessing Competence to Consent'. *Neuroethics* 6, no. 1 (2013): 189–96.
Coggon, John, and José Miola. 'Autonomy, Liberty, and Medical Decision-Making'. *The Cambridge Law Journal* 70, no. 3 (2011): 523–47.
Cohen, Shlomo. 'The Gettier Problem in Informed Consent'. *Journal of Medical Ethics* 37, no. 11 (2011): 642–5.
Cohen, Shlomo. 'Nudging and Informed Consent'. *The American Journal of Bioethics* 13, no. 6 (2013): 3–11.
Cohen, Shlomo. 'A Philosophical Misunderstanding at the Basis of Opposition to Nudging'. *The American Journal of Bioethics* 15, no. 10 (2015): 39–41.
Colburn, Ben. 'Autonomy and Adaptive Preferences'. *Utilitas* 23, no. 1 (2011): 52–71.
Coltheart, Max. 'The 33rd Sir Frederick Bartlett Lecture: Cognitive Neuropsychiatry and Delusional Belief'. *Quarterly Journal of Experimental Psychology* 60, no. 8 (2007): 1041–62.
Conly, Sarah. *Against Autonomy: Justifying Coercive Paternalism*. Cambridge: Cambridge University Press, 2013.
Consent Form/Patient Information Sheet. A Phase-I, Single-Centre, Double-Blind, Randomised, Placebo-Controlled, Single Escalating-Dose Study to Assess the Safety, Pharmacokinetics, Pharmacodynamics and Immunogenicity of TGN1412 Administered Intravenously to Healthy Volunteers. Protocol Number: TGN1412. Parexel Project Number: 68419. Version: 02 Final (2006). http://www.circare.org/foia5/tgn1412_consentform.pdf.
Convention on the Rights of Persons with Disabilities (CRPD). https://www.un.org/development/desa/disabilities/convention-on-the-rights-of-persons-with-disabilities.html.
Cowley, Christopher. 'Conscientious Objection in Healthcare and the Duty to Refer'. *Journal of Medical Ethics: The Journal of the Institute of Medical Ethics* 43, no. 4 (2017): 207–12.
Cox, Caitriona L., and Zoe Fritz. 'Should Non-Disclosures Be Considered as Morally Equivalent to Lies within the Doctor–Patient Relationship?' *Journal of Medical Ethics* 42, no. 10 (2016): 632–5.
Craigie, Jillian. 'Competence, Practical Rationality and What a Patient Values'. *Bioethics* 25, no. 6 (2011): 326–33.
Craigie, Jillian, and Ailsa Davies. 'Problems of Control: Alcohol Dependence, Anorexia Nervosa, and the Flexible Interpretation of Mental Incapacity Tests'. *Medical Law Review* 27, no. 2 (2019): 215–41.
Crisp, Roger. *Reasons and the Good*. Oxford: Oxford University Press, 2006.
Culver, Charles, and Bernard Gert. 'The Inadequacy of Incompetence'. *The Milbank Quarterly* 68, no. 4 (1990): 619–43.
Darwall, Stephen. 'The Value of Autonomy and Autonomy of the Will'. *Ethics* 116, no. 2 (2006): 263–84.
Darwall, Stephen. *Welfare and Rational Care*. Princeton, NJ: Princeton University Press, 2004.
Davis, Amelia A., and Mathew Nguyen. 'A Case Study of Anorexia Nervosa Driven by Religious Sacrifice'. *Case Reports in Psychiatry* (2014). https://doi.org/10.1155/2014/512764.

Davis, Dena S. 'Genetic Dilemmas and the Child's Right to an Open Future'. *The Hastings Center Report* 27, no. 2 (1997): 7–15.

Dawson, John, and George Szmukler. 'Fusion of Mental Health and Incapacity Legislation'. *The British Journal of Psychiatry* 188, no. 6 (2006): 504–9.

DeGrazia, David. *Human Identity and Bioethics*. Cambridge: Cambridge University Press, 2005.

Dickenson, D. 'Ethical Issues in Long-Term Psychiatric Management'. *Journal of Medical Ethics* 23, no. 5 (1997): 300–4.

Dive, Lisa, and Ainsley J. Newson. 'Reconceptualizing Autonomy for Bioethics'. *Kennedy Institute of Ethics Journal* 28, no. 2 (2018): 171–203.

Dodds, Susan. 'Choice and Control in Feminist Bioethics'. In *Relational Autonomy: Feminist Perspectives on Automony, Agency, and the Social Self*, edited by Catriona Mackenzie and Natalie Stoljar, 213–35. Oxford: Oxford University Press, 2000.

Donagan, Alan. 'Informed Consent in Therapy and Experimentation'. *Journal of Medicine and Philosophy* 2, no. 4 (1977): 307–29.

Doorn, Neelke. 'Mental Competence or Capacity to Form a Will: An Anthropological Approach'. *Philosophy, Psychiatry, & Psychology* 18, no. 2 (2011): 135–45.

Double, Richard. 'Two Types of Autonomy Accounts'. *Canadian Journal of Philosophy* 22, no. 1 (1992): 65–80.

Douglas, Thomas. 'Criminal Rehabilitation Through Medical Intervention: Moral Liability and the Right to Bodily Integrity'. *The Journal of Ethics* 18, no. 2 (2014): 101–22.

Douglas, Thomas. 'Neural and Environmental Modulation of Motivation: What's the Moral Difference?' In *Treatment for Crime*, edited by David Birks and Thomas Douglas, 208–24. Oxford: Oxford University Press, 2018.

Douglas, Thomas, Pieter Bonte, Farah Focquaert, Katrien Devolder, and Sigrid Sterckx. 'Coercion, Incarceration, and Chemical Castration: An Argument from Autonomy'. *Journal of Bioethical Inquiry* 10, no. 3 (2013): 393–405.

Drane, J. F. 'The Many Faces of Competency'. *The Hastings Center Report* 15, no. 2 (1985): 17–21.

Draper, Heather. 'Anorexia Nervosa and Respecting a Refusal of Life-Prolonging Therapy: A Limited Justification'. *Bioethics* 14, no. 2 (2000): 120–33.

Dunn, Michael, K. W. M. Fulford, Jonathan Herring, and Ashok Handa. 'Between the Reasonable and the Particular: Deflating Autonomy in the Legal Regulation of Informed Consent to Medical Treatment'. *Health Care Analysis*, 30 June 2018, 1–18. https://doi.org/10.1007/s10728-018-0358-x.

Dworkin, Gerald. 'Paternalsim'. In *The Stanford Encyclopedia of Philosophy*, edited by Edward N. Zalta, 2010. http://plato.stanford.edu/entries/paternalism/#ConIss.

Dworkin, Gerald. *The Theory and Practice of Autonomy*. Cambridge: Cambridge University Press, 1988.

Dworkin, Ronald. 'Autonomy and the Demented Self'. *The Milbank Quarterly* 64, Suppl. 2 (1986): 4–16.

Dworkin, Ronald. *Life's Dominion: An Argument about Abortion and Euthanasia*. London: HarperCollins, 1993.

Dworkin, Ronald. 'Rights as Trumps'. In *Theories of Rights*, edited by Jeremy Waldron, 153–67. Oxford: Oxford University Press, 1984.

Eastman, Nigel L. G., and R. A. Hope. 'The Ethics of Enforced Medical Treatment: The Balance Model'. *Journal of Applied Philosophy* 5, no. 1 (1988): 49–59.

Edozien, Leroy C. 'UK Law on Consent Finally Embraces the Prudent Patient Standard'. *British Medical Journal* 350 (2015): h2877. https://doi.org/10.1136/bmj.h2877.

Edwards, Rem. 'Mental Health as Rational Autonomy'. *The Journal of Medicine and Philosophy* 6, no. 3 (1981): 309–22.
Ekstrom, Laura Waddell. 'A Coherence Theory of Autonomy'. *Philosophy and Phenomenological Research* 53, no. 3 (1993): 599–616.
Elster, Jon. *Sour Grapes: Studies in the Subversion of Rationality*. Cambridge: Cambridge University Press, 1983.
Elzakkers, Isis F. F. M., Unna N. Danner, Hans W. Hoek, and Annemarie A. van Elburg. 'Mental Capacity to Consent to Treatment in Anorexia Nervosa: Explorative Study'. *BJPsych Open* 2, no. 2 (2016): 147–53. https://doi.org/10.1192/bjpo.bp.115.002485.
Emanuel, Ezekiel J., and Franklin G. Miller. 'Money and Distorted Ethical Judgments about Research: Ethical Assessment of the TeGenero TGN1412 Trial'. *The American Journal of Bioethics* 7, no. 2 (2007): 76–81.
Erler, Alexandre, and Tony Hope. 'Mental Disorder and the Concept of Authenticity'. *Philosophy, Psychiatry, & Psychology* 21, no. 3 (2015): 219–32.
Evans, David. 'Parexel Misled Subjects Sickened in London Study, Ethicists Say'. *Bloomberg*, April 2006. http://www.sskrplaw.com/parexel-misled-subjects-sickened-in-london-study-ethicists-say.html.
Eyal, Nir. 'Paternalism, French Fries and the Weak-Willed Witness'. *Journal of Medical Ethics* 40, no. 5 (2014): 353–4.
Eyal, Nir. 'Using Informed Consent to Save Trust'. *Journal of Medical Ethics* 40, no. 7 (2014): 437–44.
Faden, Ruth R., and Tom L. Beauchamp. *A History and Theory of Informed Consent*. New York: Oxford University Press, 1986.
Family Law Reform Act. Text, 1969. http://www.legislation.gov.uk/ukpga/1969/46.
Farrell, Anne Maree, and Margaret Brazier. 'Not so New Directions in the Law of Consent? Examining Montgomery v Lanarkshire Health Board'. *Journal of Medical Ethics* 42, no. 2 (2016): 85. https://doi.org/10.1136/medethics-2015-102861.
Feinberg, Joel. 'The Child's Right to an Open Future'. In *Freedom and Fulfillment: Philosophical Essays*, 76–97. Princeton, NJ: Princeton University Press, 1992.
Feinberg, Joel. *Freedom and Fulfillment: Philosophical Essays*. Princeton, NJ: Princeton University Press, 1992.
Feinberg, Joel. *The Moral Limits of the Criminal Law*, Volume 3: *Harm to Self*. New York: Oxford University Press, 1989.
Feldman, Fred. *Pleasure and the Good Life: Concerning the Nature, Varieties and Plausibility of Hedonism*. Oxford: Clarendon Press, 2004.
Feldman, Fred. 'What Is the Rational Care Theory of Welfare?' *Philosophical Studies: An International Journal for Philosophy in the Analytic Tradition* 130, no. 3 (2006): 585–601.
Finnis, John. *Natural Law and Natural Rights*, 2nd edition. Oxford: Oxford University Press, 2011.
Fischer, John Martin. 'Recent Work on Moral Responsibility'. *Ethics* 110, no. 1 (1999): 93–139.
Fischer, John Martin, and Mark Ravizza. *Responsibility and Control: A Theory of Moral Responsibility*. Cambridge: Cambridge University Press, 1998.
Flew, Antony, R. M. Hare, and Basil Mitchell. 'Theology and Falsification: The University Discussion'. In *New Essays in Philosophical Theology*, edited by Antony Flew. New York: Macmillan, 1964.
Flory, James, and Ezekiel Emanuel. 'Interventions to Improve Research Participants' Understanding in Informed Consent for Research: A Systematic Review'. *JAMA* 292, no. 13 (2004): 1593–601.
Foddy, Bennett, and Julian Savulescu. 'Addiction and Autonomy: Can Addicted People Consent to the Prescription of Their Drug of Addiction?' *Bioethics* 20, no. 1 (2006): 1–15.

Foddy, Bennett, and Julian Savulescu. 'A Liberal Account of Addiction'. *Philosophy, Psychiatry, & Psychology* 17, no. 1 (2010): 1–22.

Foot, Philippa. *Virtues and Vices*. Oxford: Oxford University Press, 2002.

Forsberg, Lisa, and Thomas Douglas. 'Anti-Libidinal Interventions in Sex Offenders: Medical or Correctional?' *Medical Law Review* 24, no. 4 (2016): 453–73.

Foster, Charles. *Choosing Life, Choosing Death: The Tyranny of Autonomy in Medical Ethics and Law*. Bloomsbury Collections. Oxford: Hart Publishing, 2009.

Frankfurt, Harry G. 'Alternate Possibilities and Moral Responsibility'. *The Journal of Philosophy* 66, no. 23 (1969): 829–39.

Frankfurt, Harry G. 'Freedom of the Will and the Concept of a Person'. *The Journal of Philosophy* 68, no. 1 (1971): 5–20.

Frankfurt, Harry G. *The Importance of What We Care About: Philosophical Essays*. Cambridge: Cambridge University Press, 1988.

Frankfurt, Harry G. *Necessity, Volition, and Love*. Cambridge: Cambridge University Press, 1999.

Friedman, Marilyn. *Autonomy, Gender, Politics: Studies in Feminist Philosophy*. Oxford and New York: Oxford University Press, 2003.

Fulford, K. W. 'Evaluative Delusions: Their Significance for Philosophy and Psychiatry'. *The British Journal of Psychiatry*. Suppl. 14 (November 1991): 108–12.

Fulford, K. W. M., and Mike Jackson. 'Spiritual Experience and Psychopathology'. *Philosophy, Psychiatry, & Psychology* 4, no. 1 (1997): 41–65.

Fulford, K. W. M. (Bill), and Lubomira Radoilska. 'Three Challenges from Delusion for Theories of Autonomy'. In *Autonomy and Mental Disorder*, edited by Lubomira Radoilska, 44–74. Oxford: Oxford University Press, 2012.

Garasic, Mirko Daniel. *Guantanamo and Other Cases of Enforced Medical Treatment: A Biopolitical Analysis*. Cham: Springer, 2015.

Garcia, Frederico D., and Florence Thibaut. 'Current Concepts in the Pharmacotherapy of Paraphilias'. *Drugs* 71, no. 6 (2011): 771–90.

Gardner, John. 'The Many Faces of the Reasonable Person'. *Law Quarterly Review* 131 (2015): 563–84.

Gavaghan, Colin. 'In Word, or Sigh, or Tear: Depression and End of Life Choices'. In *Inspiring a Medico-Legal Revolution*, edited by G. Laurie and P. Ferguson, 231–53. London: Routledge, 2015.

General Medical Council. 'Ethical Guidance for Doctors, Part 1', 2008. https://www.gmc-uk.org/ethical-guidance/ethical-guidance-for-doctors/consent/part-1-principles.

Geppert, Cynthia M. A. 'Futility in Chronic Anorexia Nervosa: A Concept Whose Time Has Not Yet Come'. *The American Journal of Bioethics* 15, no. 7 (2015): 34–43.

Gilbert, Frederic, J. N. M. Viaña, and C. Ineichen. 'Deflating the "DBS Causes Personality Changes" Bubble'. *Neuroethics* (19 June 2018): 1–17. https://doi.org/10.1007/s12152-018-9373-8.

Gillick v. West Norfolk and Wisbech Area Health Authority and Department of Health and Social Security, HL 17 October 1985 (1985).

Gillon, R. 'Ethics Needs Principles—Four Can Encompass the Rest—and Respect for Autonomy Should Be "First among Equals"'. *Journal of Medical Ethics* 29, no. 5 (2003): 307–12.

Gillon, R. 'Is There an Important Moral Distinction for Medical Ethics between Lying and Other Forms of Deception?' *Journal of Medical Ethics* 19, no. 3 (1993): 131–2.

Giordano, Simona. *Understanding Eating Disorders: Conceptual and Ethical Issues in the Treatment of Anorexia and Bulimia Nervosa*. Issues in Biomedical Ethics. Oxford: Oxford University Press, 2005.

Glover, Jonathan. *Causing Death and Saving Lives*. Harmondsworth: Penguin, 1977.
Goldman, Alan H. 'Desire Based Reasons and Reasons for Desires'. *Southern Journal of Philosophy* 44, no. 3 (2006): 469–88.
Goodin, Robert E. *Manipulatory Politics*. New Haven: Yale University Press, 1980.
Goodman, Rob. 'Cognitive Enhancement, Cheating, and Accomplishment'. *Kennedy Institute of Ethics Journal* 20, no. 2 (2010): 145–60.
Goold, Imogen, and Hannah Maslen. 'Must the Surgeon Take the Pill? Negligence Duty in the Context of Cognitive Enhancement'. *The Modern Law Review* 77, no. 1 (2014): 60–86.
Green, Rebecca. 'The Ethics of Sin Taxes'. *Public Health Nursing* (Boston, MA) 28, no. 1 (2011): 68–77.
Green, William. 'Depo-Provera, Castration, and the Probation of Rape Offenders: Statutory and Constitutional Issues'. *University of Dayton Law Review* 12, no. 1 (1986): 1–26.
Grice, H. P. *Studies in the Way of Words*. Cambridge, MA: Harvard University Press, 1989.
Griffin, James. 'Darwall on Welfare as Rational Care'. *Utilitas* 18, no. 4 (2006): 427–33.
Griffin, James. *Well-Being: Its Meaning, Measurement and Moral Importance*. Oxford: Clarendon Press, 1986.
Griffiths, Morwenna. *Feminisms and the Self: The Web of Identity*. London: Routledge, 1995.
Grisso, Thomas, and Paul S. Appelbaum. *Assessing Competence to Consent to Treatment: A Guide for Physicians and Other Health Professionals*. Oxford: Oxford University Press, 1998.
Grisso, T., P. S. Appelbaum, and C. Hill-Fotouhi. 'The MacCAT-T: A Clinical Tool to Assess Patients' Capacities to Make Treatment Decisions'. *Psychiatric Services* (Washington, DC) 48, no. 11 (1997): 1415–19. https://doi.org/10.1176/ps.48.11.1415.
Grzybowski, Andrzej, Rafal K. Patryn, Jaroslaw Sak, and Anna Zagaja. 'Vaccination Refusal: Autonomy and Permitted Coercion'. *Pathogens and Global Health* 111, no. 4 (2017): 200–5.
Haan, Sanneke de, Erik Rietveld, Martin Stokhof, and Damiaan Denys. 'Becoming More Oneself? Changes in Personality Following DBS Treatment for Psychiatric Disorders: Experiences of OCD Patients and General Considerations'. *PLoS ONE* 12, no. 4 (20 April 2017): e0175748. https://doi.org/10.1371/journal.pone.0175748.
Habermas, Jürgen. *The Future of Human Nature*. Cambridge: Polity Press, 2003.
Haji, Ishtiyaque. *Moral Appraisability: Puzzles, Proposals and Perplexities*. Oxford: Oxford University Press, 1998.
Harris, John. '". . . How Narrow the Strait!"' *Cambridge Quarterly of Healthcare Ethics* 23, no. 3 (2014): 247–60.
Harris, John, and Kirsty Keywood. 'Ignorance, Information and Autonomy'. *Theoretical Medicine and Bioethics* 22, no. 5 (2001): 415–36.
Hart, H. L. A. *Law, Liberty and Morality*. London: Oxford University Press, 1963.
Hausman, Daniel M., and Brynn Welch. 'Debate: To Nudge or Not to Nudge'. *Journal of Political Philosophy* 18, no. 1 (2010): 123–36.
Haworth, Lawrence. *Autonomy: An Essay in Philosophical Psychology and Ethics*. New Haven: Yale University Press, 1986.
Heathwood, C. 'Review of Rational Care and Welfare'. *Australasian Journal of Philosophy* 81, no. 4 (2003): 615–17.
Henderson, Gail E., Larry R. Churchill, Arlene M. Davis, Michele M. Easter, Christine Grady, Steven Joffe, Nancy Kass, et al. 'Clinical Trials and Medical Care: Defining the Therapeutic Misconception'. *PLoS Medicine* 4, no. 11 (2007). https://doi.org/10.1371/journal.pmed.0040324.
Herman, Barbara. *The Practice of Moral Judgment*. Cambridge, MA: Harvard University Press, 1993.

Herring, Jonathan. *Medical Law and Ethics*, 7th edition. Oxford: Oxford University Press, 2018.

Herring, Jonathan, K. M. W. Fulford, Michael Dunn, and Ashok I. Handa. 'Elbow Room for Best Practice? Montgomery, Patients' Values, and Balanced Decision-Making in Person-Centred Clinical Care'. *Medical Law Review* 25, no. 4 (2017): 582–603.

Herring, Jonathan, and Jesse Wall. 'Autonomy, Capacity and Vulnerable Adults: Filling the Gaps in the Mental Capacity Act'. *Legal Studies* 35, no. 4 (2015): 698–719.

Heywood, Rob. 'R.I.P. Sidaway: Patient-Oriented Disclosure – A Standard Worth Waiting For? Montgomery v Lanarkshire Health Board 2015 UKSC 11'. *Medical Law Review* 23, no. 3 (2015): 455–66.

Hill, Thomas E. *Autonomy and Self-Respect*. Cambridge: Cambridge University Press, 1991.

Hindmarch, Thomas, Matthew Hotopf, and Gareth S. Owen. 'Depression and Decision-Making Capacity for Treatment or Research: A Systematic Review'. *BMC Medical Ethics* 14 (2013): 54. https://doi.org/10.1186/1472-6939-14-54.

Hobbes, Thomas. *Leviathan*. Oxford World's Classics. Oxford: Oxford University Press, 1998.

Holroyd, Jules. 'Clarifying Capacity: Value and Reasons'. In *Autonomy and Mental Disorder*, edited by Lubomira Radoilska, 145–69. Oxford: Oxford University Press, 2012.

Hooker, Brad. 'The Elements of Well-Being'. *Journal of Practical Ethics* 3, no. 1 (2015): 15–35.

Hope, R. A., Julian Savulescu, and Judith Hendrick. *Medical Ethics and Law: The Core Curriculum*, 2nd edition. Edinburgh: Churchill Livingstone Elsevier, 2008.

Hughes, P. M. 'Ambivalence, Autonomy, and Organ Sales'. *Southern Journal of Philosophy* 44, no. 2 (2006): 237–51.

Humberstone, I. L. 'Direction of Fit'. *Mind* 101, no. 401 (1992): 59–83.

Hume, David. *On Suicide*. London: Penguin, 2005.

Hume, David. *A Treatise of Human Nature*, 2nd edition with text revised and variant readings by P. H. Nidditch. Oxford: Clarendon Press, 1978.

Hurd, Heidi M. 'The Moral Magic of Consent'. *Legal Theory* 2, no. 2 (1996): 121–46.

Hurka, Thomas. *Perfectionism*. Oxford Ethics Series. Oxford: Oxford University Press, 1993.

Hurka, Thomas. 'Why Value Autonomy?' *Social Theory and Practice* 13, no. 3 (1987): 361–82.

Hyun, Insoo. 'Authentic Values and Individual Autonomy'. *The Journal of Value Inquiry* 35, no. 2 (2001): 195–208.

Ingelfinger, F. J. 'Informed (but Uneducated) Consent'. *The New England Journal of Medicine* 287, no. 9 (1972): 465–6.

Jackson, Jennifer. 'Telling the Truth'. *Journal of Medical Ethics* 17, no. 1 (1991): 5–9.

Jaworska, A. 'Caring, Minimal Autonomy, and the Limits of Liberalism'. In *Naturalized Bioethics: Toward Responsible Knowing and Practice*, edited by Hilde Lindemann, Marian Verkek, and Margaret Walker, 80–105. New York: Cambridge University Press, 2009.

Jaycox, Michael P. 'Coercion, Autonomy, and the Preferential Option for the Poor in the Ethics of Organ Transplantation'. *Developing World Bioethics* 12, no. 3 (2012): 135–47.

Jennings, Bruce. 'Reconceptualizing Autonomy: A Relational Turn in Bioethics'. *The Hastings Center Report* 46, no. 3 (2016): 11–16.

Jones, Ma. 'Informed Consent and Other Fairy Stories'. *Medical Law Review* 7, no. 2 (1999): 103–34.

Joussemet, Mireille, Renée Landry, and Richard Koestner. 'A Self-Determination Theory Perspective on Parenting'. *Canadian Psychology/Psychologie Canadienne* 49, no. 3 (2008): 194–200.

Joyce, Richard. *The Myth of Morality*. Cambridge Studies in Philosophy. Cambridge: Cambridge University Press, 2001.

Juth, Niklas. 'Enhancement, Autonomy, and Authenticity'. In *Enhancing Human Capacities*, edited by Julian Savulescu, Ruud ter Meulen, and Guy Kahane, 34–48. Chichester: Wiley-Blackwell, 2011.

Kant, Immanuel. *Groundwork for the Metaphysics of Morals*, translated by Allen W. Wood and J. B. Schneewind. New Haven: Yale University Press, 2002.

Kara, M. A. 'Applicability of the Principle of Respect for Autonomy: The Perspective of Turkey'. *Journal of Medical Ethics* 33, no. 11 (2007): 627–30.

Kennedy, Ian. 'The Patient on the Clapham Omnibus'. *The Modern Law Review* 47, no. 4 (1984): 454–71.

Kenny, Anthony. *The Self.* Milwaukee: Marquette University Press, 1988.

Kihlbom, U. 'Autonomy and Negatively Informed Consent'. *Journal of Medical Ethics* 34, no. 3 (2008): 146–9.

Killmister, Suzy. 'Autonomy and False Beliefs'. *Philosophical Studies* 164, no. 2 (2013): 513–31.

Killmister, Suzy. 'The Woody Allen Puzzle: How "Authentic Alienation" Complicates Autonomy'. *Noûs* 49, no. 4 (2015): 729–47.

Kim, Scott Y. H. 'When Does Decisional Impairment Become Decisional Incompetence? Ethical and Methodological Issues in Capacity Research in Schizophrenia'. *Schizophrenia Bulletin* 32, no. 1 (2006): 92–7.

Kleinig, John. 'The Nature of Consent'. In *The Ethics of Consent*, edited by Franklin G. Miller and Alan Wertheimer, 3–24. Oxford: Oxford University Press, 2010.

Kong, Camillia. 'Beyond the Balancing Scales: The Importance of Prejudice and Dialogue in a Local Authority v E and Others'. *Child and Family Law Quarterly* 26 (2014): 216–36.

Kong, Camillia. *Mental Capacity in Relationship: Decision-Making, Dialogue, and Autonomy.* Cambridge: Cambridge University Press, 2017.

Korsgaard, Christine M. *The Sources of Normativity.* Cambridge: Cambridge University Press, 1996.

Korsgaard, Christine M. 'Two Distinctions in Goodness'. *The Philosophical Review* 92, no. 2 (1983): 169–95.

Kraemer, Felicitas. 'Authenticity or Autonomy? When Deep Brain Stimulation Causes a Dilemma'. *Journal of Medical Ethics* 39, no. 12 (2013): 757–60.

Krueger, Norris, and Peter R. Dickson. 'How Believing in Ourselves Increases Risk Taking: Perceived Self-Efficacy and Opportunity Recognition'. *Decision Sciences* 25, no. 3 (1994): 385–400.

Kukla, Rebecca. 'How Do Patients Know?' *The Hastings Center Report* 37, no. 5 (2007): 27–35.

Kymlicka, Will. *Liberalism, Community and Culture.* Oxford: Clarendon Press, 1989.

Ladenson, Robert F. 'Mill's Conception of Individuality'. *Social Theory and Practice* 4, no. 2 (1977): 167–82.

Lamond, Graint. 'Coercion, Threats, and the Puzzle of Blackmail'. In *Harm and Culpability*, edited by A. P. Simester and A. T. H. Smith, 215–38. Oxford: Clarendon Press, 1996.

Largent, Emily, Christine Grady, Franklin G. Miller, and Alan Wertheimer. 'Misconceptions about Coercion and Undue Influence: Reflections on the Views of IRB Members'. *Bioethics* 27, no. 9 (2013): 500–7.

Levy, Neil. 'Autonomy and Addiction'. *Canadian Journal of Philosophy* 36, no. 3 (2006): 427–47.

Levy, Neil. 'Enhancing Authenticity'. *Journal of Applied Philosophy* 28, no. 3 (2011): 308–18.

Levy, Neil. 'Forced to Be Free? Increasing Patient Autonomy by Constraining It'. *Journal of Medical Ethics* 40, no. 5 (2012): 293–300.

Levy, Neil. *Hard Luck: How Luck Undermines Free Will and Moral Responsibility.* Oxford: Oxford University Press, 2011.

Levy, Neil, and Eric Mandelbaum. 'The Powers That Bind: Doxastic Voluntarism and Epistemic Obligation'. In *The Ethics of Belief: Individual and Social*, edited by Jonathan Matheson and Rico Vitz, 15–33. Oxford: Oxford University Press, 2014.

Locke, John. *An Essay on Human Understanding*. Ware: Wordsworth Editions, 1998.

Lovett, Francis N. 'Domination: A Preliminary Analysis'. *The Monist* 84, no. 1 (2001): 98–112.

MacCallum Jr, Gerald C. 'Negative and Positive Freedom'. In *The Liberty Reader*, edited by David Miller, 100–22. Edinburgh: Edinburgh University Press, 2006.

McKenna, Michael. 'The Relationship between Autonomous and Morally Responsible Agency'. In *Personal Autonomy: New Essays on Personal Autonomy and Its Role in Contemporary Moral Philosophy*, edited by James Stacey Taylor, 205–34. Cambridge: Cambridge University Press, 2005.

McKenna, Michael. 'Responsibility and Globally Manipulated Agents'. *Philosophical Topics* 32, no. 1/2 (2004): 169–92.

Mackenzie, Catriona. 'Three Dimensions of Autonomy'. In *Autonomy, Oppression and Gender*, edited by Andrea Veltman and Mark Piper, 15–41. Oxford: Oxford University Press, 2014.

Mackenzie, Catriona, and Susan Sherwin. 'Relational Autonomy, Self-Trust, and Health Care for Patients Who Are Oppressed'. In *Relational Autonomy: Feminist Perspectives on Automony, Agency, and the Social Self*, edited by Catriona Mackenzie and Natalie Stoljar, 259–79. New York: Oxford University Press, 2000.

Mackenzie, Catriona, and Natalie Stoljar. 'Autonomy Reconfigured'. In *Relational Autonomy: Feminist Perspectives on Autonomy, Agency, and the Social Self*, edited by Catriona Mackenzie and Natalie Stoljar, 3–31. New York: Oxford University Press, 2000.

Mackenzie, Catriona, and Natalie Stoljar, eds. *Relational Autonomy: Feminist Perspectives on Autonomy, Agency, and the Social Self*. New York: Oxford University Press, 2000.

Macklin, Ruth. 'The Paradoxical Case of Payment as Benefit to Research Subjects'. *IRB: Ethics & Human Research* 11, no. 6 (1989): 1–3.

Maclean, Alasdair R. 'The Doctrine of Informed Consent: Does It Exist and Has It Crossed the Atlantic?' *Legal Studies* 24, no. 3 (2004): 386–413.

McLean, Sheila. *Assisted Dying: Reflections on the Need for Law Reform*. Abingdon: Routledge-Cavendish, 2007.

McMahan, Jeff. *The Ethics of Killing: Problems at the Margins of Life*. Oxford: Oxford University Press, 2002.

McMillan, John. 'The Kindest Cut? Surgical Castration, Sex Offenders and Coercive Offers'. *Journal of Medical Ethics* 40, no. 9 (2014): 583–90.

McQueen, Paddy. 'Autonomy, Age and Sterilisation Requests'. *Journal of Medical Ethics* 43, no. 5 (2017): 310–13.

Malinow, M. Rene, David L. McGarry, and Kerry Kuehl. 'Is Exercise Testing Indicated for Asymptomatic Active People?' *Journal of Cardiac Rehabilitation* 4, no. 9 (1984): 376–8.

Malmqvist, Erik. 'Reprogenetics and the "Parents Have Always Done It" Argument'. *The Hastings Center Report* 41, no. 1 (2011): 43–9.

Manne, Kate. 'Internalism about Reasons: Sad but True?' *Philosophical Studies: An International Journal for Philosophy in the Analytic Tradition* 167, no. 1 (2014): 89–117.

Manson, Neil C., and Onora O'Neill. *Rethinking Informed Consent in Bioethics*. Cambridge: Cambridge University Press, 2007.

Maron, Barry J. 'The Paradox of Exercise'. *New England Journal of Medicine* 343, no. 19 (2000): 1409–11.

Martin, Adrienne M. 'Tales Publicly Allowed: Competence, Capacity, and Religious Belief'. *The Hastings Center Report* 37, no. 1 (2007): 33–40.

Maslen, Hannah, Brian D. Earp, Roi Cohen Kadosh, and Julian Savulescu. 'Brain Stimulation for Treatment and Enhancement in Children: An Ethical Analysis'. *Frontiers in Human Neuroscience* 8 (2014). https://doi.org/10.3389/fnhum.2014.00953.

Maslen, Hannah, Nadira Faulmüller, and Julian Savulescu. 'Pharmacological Cognitive Enhancement—How Neuroscientific Research Could Advance Ethical Debate'. *Frontiers in Systems Neuroscience* 8 (2014). https://doi.org/10.3389/fnsys.2014.00107.

Maslen, Hannah, Jonathan Pugh, and Julian Savulescu. 'The Ethics of Deep Brain Stimulation for the Treatment of Anorexia Nervosa'. *Neuroethics* 8, no. 3 (2015): 215–30.

Mason, Elinor. 'Coercion and Integrity'. In *Oxford Studies in Normative Ethics, Volume 2*, edited by Mark Timmons, 180–205. Oxford: Oxford University Press, 2012.

Mele, Alfred R. *Autonomous Agents: From Self-Control to Autonomy*. Oxford: Oxford University Press, 1995.

Mele, Alfred R. 'Fischer and Ravizza on Moral Responsibility'. *The Journal of Ethics* 10, no. 3 (2006): 283–94.

Mele, Alfred R. *Free Will and Luck*. Oxford: Oxford University Press, 2006.

Mental Capacity Act 2005. Text. http://www.legislation.gov.uk/ukpga/2005/9.

Mental Capacity Act Code of Practice. London: The Stationery Office, 2007. https://www.gov.uk/government/publications/mental-capacity-act-code-of-practice.

Mertes, Heidi. 'The Role of Anticipated Decision Regret and the Patient's Best Interest in Sterilisation and Medically Assisted Reproduction'. *Journal of Medical Ethics* 43, no. 5 (2017): 314–18.

Meyer, Susan S. 'Aristotle on the Voluntary'. In *The Blackwell Guide to Aristotle's Nicomachean Ethics*, edited by Richard Kraut, 137–57. Oxford: Blackwell, 2006.

Meyers, Diana T. 'The Feminist Debate Over Values in Autonomy Theory'. In *Autonomy, Oppression, and Gender*, edited by Mark Piper and Andrea Veltman, 114–40. Oxford: Oxford University Press, 2014.

Meyers, Diana T. *Self, Society, and Personal Choice*. New York: Columbia University Press, 1989.

Meynen, Gerben. 'Depression, Possibilities, and Competence: A Phenomenological Perspective'. *Theoretical Medicine and Bioethics* 32, no. 3 (2011): 181–93.

Mill, John Stuart. *On Liberty*, edited by David Bromwich and George Kateb. New Haven: Yale University Press, 2003.

Mill, John Stuart. *Utilitarianism*, 12th edition. London: George Routledge & Sons, 1895.

Miller, A. D., and R. Perry. 'The Reasonable Person'. *NYU Law Review* 87 (2012): 323–92.

Miller, David. 'Introduction'. In *The Liberty Reader*, edited by David Miller. Edinburgh: Edinburgh University Press, 2006.

Miller, Franklin G., and Howard Brody. 'Clinical Equipoise and the Incoherence of Research Ethics'. *The Journal of Medicine and Philosophy* 32, no. 2 (2007): 151–65.

Miller, Franklin G., and Alan Wertheimer, eds. *The Ethics of Consent: Theory and Practice*. Oxford: Oxford University Press, 2010.

Miller, Paul, and N. Fagley. 'The Effects of Framing, Problem Variations, and Providing Rationale on Choice'. *Personality and Social Psychology Bulletin* 17, no. 5 (1991): 517–22.

Mills, Claudia. 'The Child's Right to an Open Future?' *Journal of Social Philosophy* 34, no. 4 (2003): 499–509.

Miola, José. 'On the Materiality of Risk: Paper Tigers and Panaceas'. *Medical Law Review* 17, no. 1 (2009): 76–108.

Montgomery (Appellant) v. Lanarkshire Health Board (Respondent) (Scotland) (UK Supreme Court, 3 November 2015).

Mullin, Amy. 'Children, Paternalism and the Development of Autonomy'. *Ethical Theory and Moral Practice* 17, no. 3 (2014): 413–26.

Nedelsky, Jennifer. 'Reconceiving Autonomy: Sources, Thoughts and Possibilities'. *Yale Journal of Law & Feminism* 1, no. 1 (1989): 7–36.

Nelson, Robert M., Tom Beauchamp, Victoria A. Miller, William Reynolds, Richard F. Ittenbach, and Mary Frances Luce. 'The Concept of Voluntary Consent'. *The American Journal of Bioethics: AJOB* 11, no. 8 (2011): 6–16.

NHS – 'Female Sterilisation', 21 December 2017. https://www.nhs.uk/conditions/contraception/female-sterilisation/.

NHS – 'Vasectomy (Male Sterilisation)', 21 December 2017. https://www.nhs.uk/conditions/contraception/vasectomy-male-sterilisation/.

Noggle, Robert. 'Autonomy and the Paradox of Self-Creation: Infinite Regresses, Finite Selves, and the Limits of Authenticity'. In *Personal Autonomy: New Essays on Personal Autonomy and Its Role in Contemporary Moral Philosophy*, edited by James Stacey Taylor, 87–108. Cambridge: Cambridge University Press, 2005.

Nordenfelt, Lennart. *Rationality and Compulsion: Applying Action Theory to Psychiatry*. International Perspectives in Philosophy and Psychiatry. Oxford: Oxford University Press, 2007.

Nozick, Robert. *Anarchy, State and Utopia*. New York: Basic Books, 1974.

Nozick, Robert. 'Coercion'. In *Philosophy, Science, and Method: Essays in Honor of Ernest Nagel*, edited by Sidney Morgenbesser, Patrick Suppes, and Morton White, 440–72. New York: St. Martin's Press, 1969.

Nussbaum, Martha Craven. *Women and Human Development: The Capabilities Approach*. Cambridge: Cambridge University Press, 2000.

O'Connor, Annette M., Alaa Rostom, Valerie Fiset, Jacqueline Tetroe, Vikki Entwistle, Hilary Llewellyn-Thomas, Margaret Holmes-Rovner, Michael Barry, and Jean Jones. 'Decision Aids for Patients Facing Health Treatment or Screening Decisions: Systematic Review'. *British Medical Journal* 319, no. 7212 (1999): 731–4.

O'Neill, Onora. *Autonomy and Trust in Bioethics: The Gifford Lectures, University of Edinburgh, 2001*. Cambridge: Cambridge University Press, 2002.

Okai, David, Gareth Owen, Hugh McGuire, Swaran Singh, Rachel Churchill, and Matthew Hotopf. 'Mental Capacity in Psychiatric Patients'. *The British Journal of Psychiatry* 191, no. 4 (2007): 291–7.

Olsaretti, Serena. 'Freedom, Force and Choice: Against the Rights-Based Definition of Voluntariness'. *Journal of Political Philosophy* 6, no. 1 (1998): 53–78.

Olson, Eric T. 'There Is No Problem of the Self'. *Journal of Consciousness Studies* 5, no. 5–6 (1998): 645–57.

Oshana, Marina. 'How Much Should We Value Autonomy?' *Social Philosophy and Policy* 20, no. 2 (2003): 99–126.

Oshana, Marina. 'The Misguided Marriage of Responsibility and Autonomy'. *The Journal of Ethics* 6, no. 3 (2002): 261–80.

Oshana, Marina. 'Personal Autonomy and Society'. *Journal of Social Philosophy* 29, no. 1 (1998): 81–102.

Parfit, Derek. *On What Matters*. Oxford: Oxford University Press, 2011.

Parfit, Derek. *Reasons and Persons*. Oxford: Clarendon Press, 1984.

Pearson, Carolyn M., Stephen A. Wonderlich, and Gregory T. Smith. 'A Risk and Maintenance Model for Bulimia Nervosa: From Impulsive Action to Compulsive Behavior'. *Psychological Review* 122, no. 3 (2015): 516–35.

Pellegrino, Edmund D. *For the Patient's Good: The Restoration of Beneficence in Health Care*. Oxford: Oxford University Press, 1988.

Persson, Ingmar. *The Retreat of Reason: A Dilemma in the Philosophy of Life*. Oxford: Clarendon Press, 2005.

Peterson, Andrew. 'Should Neuroscience Inform Judgements of Decision-Making Capacity?' *Neuroethics* 12, no. 2 (2019): 133–51.
Pettit, Philip. 'Freedom as Antipower'. *Ethics* 106, no. 3 (1996): 576–604.
Pettit, Philip. *Republicanism: A Theory of Freedom and Government*. Oxford: Oxford University Press, 1999.
Pettit, Philip, and Michael Smith. 'Backgrounding Desire'. *The Philosophical Review* 99, no. 4 (1990): 565–92.
Pitkin, Hanna Fenichel. 'Are Freedom and Liberty Twins?' *Political Theory* 16, no. 4 (1988): 523–52.
Platts, Mark de Bretton. *Ways of Meaning: An Introduction to a Philosophy of Language*. London: Routledge & Kegan Paul, 1979.
Ploug, Thomas, and Søren Holm. 'Doctors, Patients, and Nudging in the Clinical Context—Four Views on Nudging and Informed Consent'. *American Journal of Bioethics* 15, no. 10 (2015): 28–38.
Ploug, Thomas, and Søren Holm. 'Informed Consent, Libertarian Paternalism, and Nudging: A Response'. *American Journal of Bioethics* 15, no. 12 (2015): 10–13.
Pritchard, Duncan. 'Risk'. *Metaphilosophy* 46, no. 3 (2015): 436–61.
Pugh, Jonathan. 'Autonomy, Natality and Freedom: A Liberal Re-Examination of Habermas in the Enhancement Debate'. *Bioethics* 29, no. 3 (2015): 145–52.
Pugh, Jonathan. 'Coercion and the Neurocorrective Offer'. In *Treatment for Crime*, edited by David Birks and Thomas Douglas, 94–114. Oxford: Oxford University Press, 2018.
Pugh, Jonathan. 'Coercive Paternalism and Back-Door Perfectionism'. *Journal of Medical Ethics* 40, no. 5 (2014): 350–1.
Pugh, Jonathan. 'Legally Competent, But Too Young To Choose To Be Sterilized? Practical Ethics'. Practical Ethics Blog (blog), May 2015. http://blog.practicalethics.ox.ac.uk/2015/05/legally-competent-but-too-young-to-choose-to-be-sterilized/.
Pugh, Jonathan. 'Moral Bio-Enhancement, Freedom, Value and the Parity Principle'. *Topoi*, 12 April 2017, 1–14. https://doi.org/10.1007/s11245-017-9482-8.
Pugh, Jonathan. 'Navigating Individual and Collective Interests in Medical Ethics'. *Journal of Medical Ethics* 44, no. 1 (2018): 1–2.
Pugh, Jonathan, and Thomas Douglas. 'Justifications for Non-Consensual Medical Intervention: From Infectious Disease Control to Criminal Rehabilitation'. *Criminal Justice Ethics* 35, no. 3 (2016): 205–29.
Pugh, Jonathan, Guy Kahane, Hannah Maslen, and Julian Savulescu. 'Lay Attitudes toward Deception in Medicine: Theoretical Considerations and Empirical Evidence'. *AJOB Empirical Bioethics* 7, no. 1 (2016): 31–8.
Pugh, Jonathan, Hannah Maslen, and Julian Savulescu. 'Deep Brain Stimulation, Authenticity and Value'. *Cambridge Quarterly of Healthcare Ethics* 26, no. 4 (2017): 640–57.
Pugh, Jonathan, Christopher Pugh, and Julian Savulescu. 'Exercise Prescription and the Doctor's Duty of Non-Maleficence'. *British Journal of Sports Medicine* 51, no. 21 (2017). https://doi.org/10.1136/bjsports-2016-097388.
Pugh, Jonathan, Laurie Pycroft, Anders Sandberg, Tipu Aziz, and Julian Savulescu. 'Brainjacking in Deep Brain Stimulation and Autonomy'. *Ethics and Information Technology* 20, no. 3 (2018): 219–32.
Quill, T. E., and H. Brody. 'Physician Recommendations and Patient Autonomy: Finding a Balance between Physician Power and Patient Choice'. *Annals of Internal Medicine* 125, no. 9 (1996): 763–9.
Radoilska, Lubomira. *Aristotle and the Moral Philosophy of Today* (*L'Actualité d'Aristote en Morale*). Paris: Presses Universitaires de France, 2007.

Radoilska, Lubomira. 'Autonomy and Ulysses Arrangements'. In *Autonomy and Mental Disorder*, edited by Lubomira Radoilska, 252–80. Oxford: Oxford University Press, 2012.

Radoilska, Lubomira. 'Depression, Decisional Capacity, and Personal Autonomy'. In *The Oxford Handbook of Philosophy and Psychiatry*, edited by K. M. W. Fulford, Martin Davies, Richard Gipps, George Graham, John Sadler, Giovanni Stanghellini, and Tim Thornton, 1155–70. Oxford University Press, 2013.

Raz, Joseph. *Engaging Reason: On the Theory of Value and Action*. Oxford: Oxford University Press, 1999.

Raz, Joseph. *The Morality of Freedom*. Oxford: Clarendon Press, 1986.

Raz, Joseph. *Practical Reason and Norms*. London: Hutchinson, 1975.

Re B (Adult, Refusal of Medical Treatment) 2, 449 (All ER 2002).

Re C (Adult: Refusal of Treatment) FD 1994 (1994).

Re E (Medical Treatment Anorexia) EWHC 1639 (COP) (2012).

Re SB (EWHC 1417 (COP) 2013).

Re T (Adult: Refusal of Medical Treatment) (All ER 1992).

Richards, Janet Radcliffe. *The Ethics of Transplants: Why Careless Thought Costs Lives*. Oxford: Oxford University Press, 2012.

Rippon, Simon. 'Imposing Options on People in Poverty: The Harm of a Live Donor Organ Market'. *Journal of Medical Ethics* 40, no. 3 (2014): 145–50.

Robinson v. Bleicher (559 N.W.2d 473) 1997.

Rudnick, A. 'Depression and Competence to Refuse Psychiatric Treatment'. *Journal of Medical Ethics* 28, no. 3 (2002): 151–5.

Rulli, Tina, and Joseph Millum. 'Rescuing the Duty to Rescue'. *Journal of Medical Ethics* 42, no. 4 (2016): 260–4.

Sachs, Benjamin. 'Why Coercion Is Wrong When It's Wrong'. *Australasian Journal of Philosophy* 91, no. 1 (2013): 63–82.

Saghai, Yashar. 'Salvaging the Concept of Nudge'. *Journal of Medical Ethics* 39, no. 8 (2013): 487–93.

Sandman, Lars, and Christian Munthe. 'Shared Decision Making, Paternalism and Patient Choice'. *Health Care Analysis: HCA: Journal of Health Philosophy and Policy* 18, no. 1 (2010): 60–84.

Savulescu, Julian. 'Future People, Involuntary Medical Treatment in Pregnancy and the Duty of Easy Rescue'. *Utilitas* 19, no. 1 (2007): 1–20.

Savulescu, Julian. 'Liberal Rationalism and Medical Decision-Making'. *Bioethics* 11, no. 2 (1997): 115–29.

Savulescu, Julian. 'Rational Desires and the Limitation of Life Sustaining Treatment'. *Bioethics* 8, no. 3 (1994): 191–222.

Savulescu, Julian. 'Rational Non-Interventional Paternalism: Why Doctors Ought to Make Judgments of What Is Best for Their Patients'. *Journal of Medical Ethics* 21, no. 6 (1995): 321–37.

Savulescu, J., and R. W. Momeyer. 'Should Informed Consent Be Based on Rational Beliefs?' *Journal of Medical Ethics* 23, no. 5 (1997): 282–8.

Savulescu, Julian, and Ingmar Persson. 'Moral Enhancement, Freedom, and the God Machine'. *The Monist* 95, no. 3 (2012): 399–421.

Schonfeld, Toby, Bruce Gordon, Jean Amoura, and Joseph Spencer Brown. 'Money Matters'. *The American Journal of Bioethics* 7, no. 2 (2007): 86–8.

Schuklenk, Udo, and Ricardo Smalling. 'Why Medical Professionals Have No Moral Claim to Conscientious Objection Accommodation in Liberal Democracies'. *Journal of Medical Ethics: The Journal of the Institute of Medical Ethics* 43, no. 4 (2017): 234–40.

Schwartz, Barry. *The Paradox of Choice: Why More Is Less*, revised edition. New York: Ecco, 2016.

Scottish Government. Mental Health (Care and Treatment) (Scotland) Act 2003 (2003). https://www.legislation.gov.uk/asp/2003/13/contents.

Secker, B. 'The Appearance of Kant's Deontology in Contemporary Kantianism: Concepts of Patient Autonomy in Bioethics'. *The Journal of Medicine and Philosophy* 24, no. 1 (1999): 43–66.

Sen, Amartya. *Development as Freedom*. Oxford: Oxford University Press, 2001.

Sen, Amartya. *Resources, Values and Development*. Oxford: Basil Blackwell, 1984.

Sharp, Daniel, and David Wasserman. 'Deep Brain Stimulation, Historicism, and Moral Responsibility'. *Neuroethics* 9, no. 2 (2016): 173–85.

Shaw, Elizabeth. 'Offering Castration to Sex Offenders: The Significance of the State's Intentions'. *Journal of Medical Ethics* 40, no. 9 (2014): 594–5.

Sher, George. *Beyond Neutrality: Perfectionism and Politics*. Cambridge: Cambridge University Press, 1997.

Sher, George. 'Liberal Neutrality and the Value of Autonomy'. *Social Philosophy and Policy* 12, no. 1 (1995): 136–59.

Sherwin, Susan, and Katie Stockdale. 'Whither Bioethics Now? The Promise of Relational Theory'. *Ijfab: International Journal of Feminist Approaches to Bioethics* 10, no. 1 (2017): 7–29.

Shiffrin, Seana Valentine. *Speech Matters: On Lying, Morality, and the Law*. Carl G. Hempel Lecture Series. Princeton, NJ: Princeton University Press, 2014.

Sibley, Amanda, Mark Sheehan, and Andrew J. Pollard. 'Assent Is Not Consent'. *Journal of Medical Ethics* 38, no. 1 (2012): 3.

Sidaway v. Board of Governors of the Bethlem Royal Hospital [1985] (UK House of Lords, 21 February 1985).

Siddle, Ronald, Gillian Haddock, Nicholas Tarrier, and E. Brian Faragher. 'Religious Delusions in Patients Admitted to Hospital with Schizophrenia'. *Social Psychiatry and Psychiatric Epidemiology* 37, no. 3 (2002): 130–8.

Skinner, Quentin. *Liberty before Liberalism*. Cambridge: Cambridge University Press, 1998.

Smith, Janet. 'The Pre-Eminence of Autonomy in Bioethics'. In *Human Lives: Critical Essays in Consequentialist Bioethics*, edited by David Oderberg and J. A. Laing, 182–95. New York: St. Martin's Press, 1997.

Smith, Michael. *The Moral Problem*. Oxford: Blackwell, 1994.

Smith, Michael. 'Parfit's Mistaken Meta-Ethics'. In *Does Anything Really Matter? Essays on Parfit on Objectivity*, edited by Peter Singer, 99–120. Oxford: Oxford University Press, 2017.

Sneddon, Andrew. 'What's Wrong with Selling Yourself Into Slavery? Paternalism and Deep Autonomy'. *Critica* 33, no. 98 (2001): 97–121.

Sobel, David. 'Parfit's Case Against Subjectivism'. In *Oxford Studies in Metaethics*, Volume 6, edited by Russ Shafer-Landau, 52–78. Oxford: Oxford University Press, 2011.

Sobel, David. 'Subjective Accounts of Reasons for Action'. *Ethics* 111, no. 3 (2001): 461–92.

Sparrow, Robert. 'Better Living Through Chemistry? A Reply to Savulescu and Persson on "Moral Enhancement"'. *Journal of Applied Philosophy* 31, no. 1 (2014): 23–32.

Spector, Horacio. *Autonomy and Rights: The Moral Foundations of Liberalism*. Oxford: Oxford University Press, 2007.

Sreenivasan, Gopal. 'Does Informed Consent to Research Require Comprehension?' *Lancet* 362, no. 9400 (2003): 2016–18.

Srivastava, Ranjana. 'My Patient Swapped Chemotherapy for Essential Oils. Arguing Is a Fool's Errand', Opinion, *The Guardian*. https://www.theguardian.com/commentisfree/2019/feb/14/my-patient-swapped-chemotherapy-for-essential-oils-arguing-is-a-fools-errand.

Stalnaker, Robert C. 'A Theory of Conditionals'. *American Philosophical Quarterly*, Monograph Series 2 (1968): 98–112.

Steinglass, Joanna E., Jane L. Eisen, Evelyn Attia, Laurel Mayer, and B. Timothy Walsh. 'Is Anorexia Nervosa a Delusional Disorder? An Assessment of Eating Beliefs in Anorexia Nervosa'. *Journal of Psychiatric Practice* 13, no. 2 (2007): 65–71.

Stephens, G. Lynn, and George Graham. 'Reconceiving Delusion'. *International Review of Psychiatry* 16, no. 3 (2004): 236–41.

Steup, Matthias. 'Doxastic Voluntarism and Epistemic Deontology'. *Acta Analytica* 15, no. 1 (2000): 25–56.

Stoljar, Natalie. 'Autonomy and the Feminist Intuition'. In *Relational Autonomy: Feminist Perspectives on Autonomy, Agency, and the Social Self*, edited by Catriona Mackenzie and Natalie Stoljar, 94–111. Oxford: Oxford University Press, 2000.

Strawson, Galen. 'Hume on Himself'. In *Essays in Practical Philosophy: From Action to Values*, edited by D. Egonsson, J. Josefsson, B. Petersson, and T. Rønnow-Rasmussen, 69–94. Aldershot: Ashgate, 2001.

Strawson, Galen. 'The Self'. In *Models of the Self*, edited by J. Shear and Shaun Gallagher. Thorverton: Academic Imprint, 1999.

Strohminger, Nina, Joshua Knobe, and George Newman. 'The True Self: A Psychological Concept Distinct from the Self'. *Perspectives on Psychological Science* 12, no. 4 (2017): 551–60.

Sumner, L. W. *Welfare, Happiness, and Ethics*. Oxford: Oxford University Press, 1996.

Sunstein, Cass R. 'Probability Neglect: Emotions, Worst Cases, and Law'. *The Yale Law Journal* 112, no. 1 (2002): 61–107.

Sunstein, Cass R. *Risk and Reason: Safety, Law, and the Environment*. Cambridge: Cambridge University Press, 2002.

Suntharalingam, Ganesh, Meghan R. Perry, Stephen Ward, Stephen J. Brett, Andrew Castello-Cortes, Michael D. Brunner, and Nicki Panoskaltsis. 'Cytokine Storm in a Phase 1 Trial of the Anti-CD28 Monoclonal Antibody TGN1412'. *New England Journal of Medicine* 355, no. 10 (2006): 1018–28.

Szasz, Thomas. *Insanity: The Idea and Its Consequences*. Syracuse, NY: Syracuse University Press, 1997.

Szmukler, George, and Frank Holloway. 'Mental Health Legislation Is Now a Harmful Anachronism'. *The Psychiatrist* 22, no. 11 (1998): 662–5.

Talbert, Matthew. 'Implanted Desires, Self-Formation and Blame'. *Journal of Ethics and Social Philosophy* 3, no. 2 (2009): 1–18.

Tan, Jacinta, and Martin Elphick. 'Competency and Use of the Mental Health Act—a Matrix to Aid Decision-Making'. *Psychiatric Bulletin* 26, no. 3 (2002): 104–6.

Tan, Jacinta, Anne Stewart, Ray Fitzpatrick, and R. A. Hope. 'Competence to Make Treatment Decisions in Anorexia Nervosa: Thinking Processes and Values'. *Philosophy, Psychiatry, & Psychology* 13, no. 4 (2007): 267–82.

Tappolet, Christine. 'Emotions, Reasons, and Autonomy'. In *Autonomy, Oppression and Gender*, edited by Andrea Veltman and Mark Piper, 163–80. Oxford: Oxford University Press, 2014.

Taylor, Charles. *The Ethics of Authenticity*. Cambridge, MA: Harvard University Press. 1992.

Taylor, James Stacey. *Practical Autonomy and Bioethics*. London: Routledge, 2009.

Taylor, James Stacey. *Stakes and Kidneys: Why Markets in Human Body Parts Are Morally Imperative*. Aldershot: Ashgate, 2005.

Thalberg, Irving. 'Hierarchical Analyses of Unfree Action'. *Canadian Journal of Philosophy* 8, no. 2 (1978): 211–26.

Thaler, Richard H., and Cass R. Sunstein. *Nudge: Improving Decisions about Health, Wealth and Happiness*, revised edition. London: Penguin Books, 2009.
The Belmont Report. Text. HHS.gov, 28 January 2010. http://www.hhs.gov/ohrp/regulations-and-policy/belmont-report/index.html.
Thibaut, Florence, Flora De La Barra, Harvey Gordon, Paul Cosyns, and John M. W. Bradford. 'The World Federation of Societies of Biological Psychiatry (WFSBP) Guidelines for the Biological Treatment of Paraphilias'. *The World Journal of Biological Psychiatry: The Official Journal of the World Federation of Societies of Biological Psychiatry* 11, no. 4 (2010): 604–55.
Thompson, Paul D., Barry A. Franklin, Gary J. Balady, Steven N. Blair, Domenico Corrado, N. A. Mark Estes, Janet E. Fulton, et al. 'Exercise and Acute Cardiovascular Events: Placing the Risks into Perspective. A Scientific Statement from the American Heart Association Council on Nutrition, Physical Activity, and Metabolism and the Council on Clinical Cardiology'. *Circulation* 115, no. 17 (2007): 2358–68.
Thomson, Judith Jarvis. *The Realm of Rights*. Cambridge, MA: Harvard University Press, 1990.
Turri, John. 'On the Relationship between Propositional and Doxastic Justification'. *Philosophy and Phenomenological Research* 80, no. 2 (2010): 312–26.
UK Department of Health. Mental Health Act 1983 (Revised 2007). Text, 2007. http://www.legislation.gov.uk/ukpga/1983/20/contents.
Valdman, Mikhail. 'Outsourcing Self-Government'. *Ethics* 120, no. 4 (2010): 761–90.
Varelius, Jukka. 'The Value of Autonomy in Medical Ethics'. *Medicine, Health Care, and Philosophy* 9, no. 3 (2006): 377–88.
Veatch, Robert M. 'Abandoning Informed Consent'. *The Hastings Center Report* 25, no. 2 (1995): 5–12.
Velleman, J. David. 'A Right of Self-Termination?' *Ethics* 109, no. 3 (1999): 606–28.
Velleman, J. David. 'Against the Right to Die'. *The Journal of Medicine and Philosophy* 17, no. 6 (1992): 665–81.
Velleman, J. David. *How We Get Along*. Cambridge: Cambridge University Press, 2009.
Velleman, J. David. 'The Possibility of Practical Reason'. *Ethics* 106, no. 4 (1996): 694–726.
Velleman, J. David. 'What Happens When Someone Acts?' *Mind* 101, no. 403 (1992): 461–81.
Vincent, Nicole. *Enhancing Responsibility*. TedX Talks, 2014. https://tedxsydney.com/talk/enhancing-responsibility-nicole-vincent/.
Vollmann, Jochen. '"But I Don't Feel It": Values and Emotions in the Assessment of Competence in Patients with Anorexia Nervosa'. *Philosophy, Psychiatry, & Psychology* 13, no. 4 (2007): 289–91.
Walker, Rebecca L. 'Medical Ethics Needs a New View of Autonomy'. *The Journal of Medicine and Philosophy* 33, no. 6 (2008): 594–608.
Walker, Rebecca L. 'Respect for Rational Autonomy'. *Kennedy Institute of Ethics Journal* 19, no. 4 (2009): 339–66.
Walker, Tom. 'Informed Consent and the Requirement to Ensure Understanding'. *Journal of Applied Philosophy* 29, no. 1 (2012): 50–62.
Wall, Steven. *Liberalism, Perfectionism and Restraint*. Cambridge: Cambridge University Press, 1998.
Waller, Bruce N. 'Natural Autonomy and Alternative Possibilities'. *American Philosophical Quarterly* 30, no. 1 (1993): 73–81.
Warburton, Darren E. R., Crystal Whitney Nicol, and Shannon S. D. Bredin. 'Health Benefits of Physical Activity: The Evidence'. *CMAJ: Canadian Medical Association Journal* 174, no. 6 (2006): 801–9.
Ware, Alan. 'The Concept of Manipulation: Its Relation to Democracy and Power'. *British Journal of Political Science* 11, no. 2 (1981): 163–81.
Watson, Gary. 'Free Agency'. *The Journal of Philosophy* 72, no. 8 (1975): 205–20.

Watson, Gary. 'Two Faces of Responsibility'. In *Agency and Answerability: Selected Essays*, 260–88. Oxford: Oxford University Press, 2004.

Weatherson, Brian. 'Deontology and Descartes's Demon'. *The Journal of Philosophy* 105, no. 9 (2008): 540–69.

Wenar, Leif. 'The Nature of Rights'. *Philosophy & Public Affairs* 33, no. 3 (2005): 223–52.

Wertheimer, Alan. *Coercion*, 2nd edition. Princeton, NJ: Princeton University Press, 2014.

Wertheimer, Alan. 'Voluntary Consent: Why a Value-Neutral Concept Won't Work'. *The Journal of Medicine and Philosophy* 37, no. 3 (2012): 226–54.

Wertheimer, Alan, and Franklin G. Miller. 'Payment for Research Participation: A Coercive Offer?' *Journal of Medical Ethics* 34, no. 5 (2008): 389–92.

Westlund, Andrea C. 'Rethinking Relational Autonomy'. *Hypatia* 24, no. 4 (2009): 26–49.

Westlund, Andrea C. 'Selflessness and Responsibility for Self: Is Deference Compatible with Autonomy?' *The Philosophical Review* 112, no. 4 (2003): 483–523.

Wicclair, Mark R. 'Justifying Conscience Clauses'. *The Hastings Center Report* 48, no. 5 (2018): 22–5.

Wicclair, Mark R. 'Patient Decision-Making Capacity and Risk'. *Bioethics* 5, no. 2 (1991): 91–104.

Widdershoven, Guy A. M., and Tineke A. Abma. 'Autonomy, Dialogue, and Practical Rationality'. In *Autonomy and Mental Disorder*, edited by Lubomira Radoilska, 217–32. Oxford: Oxford University Press, 2012.

Widdows, Heather. *Perfect Me*. Princeton, NJ: Princeton University Press, 2018.

Wilkinson, Martin, and Andrew Moore. 'Inducement in Research'. *Bioethics* 11, no. 5 (1997): 373–89.

Wilkinson, Stephen. 'Biomedical Research and the Commercial Exploitation of Human Tissue'. *Genomics, Society and Policy* 1, no. 1 (2005): 27–40.

Wilkinson, Stephen. *Bodies for Sale: Ethics and Exploitation in the Human Body Trade*. London: Routledge, 2003.

Wilkinson, T. M. 'Nudging and Manipulation'. *Political Studies* 61, no. 2 (2013): 341–55.

Williams, Bernard. 'Deciding to Believe'. In *Problems of the Self: Philosophical Papers 1956–1972*, 136–51. Cambridge: Cambridge University Press, 1973.

Williams, Bernard. *Moral Luck: Philosophical Papers, 1973–1980*. Cambridge: Cambridge University Press, 1981.

Winters, Barbara. 'Believing at Will'. *The Journal of Philosophy* 76, no. 5 (1979): 243–56.

Wolf, Susan R. *Freedom within Reason*. Oxford: Oxford University Press, 1990.

Wolff, Robert Paul. *In Defense of Anarchism*. Berkeley, CA: University of California Press, 1998.

Wood, Allen W. 'Coercion, Manipulation, Exploitation'. In *Manipulation: Theory and Practice*, edited by Christian Coons and Michael Weber, 17–50. New York: Oxford University Press, 2014.

Woodard, Christopher. 'Classifying Theories of Welfare'. *Philosophical Studies* 165, no. 3 (2013): 787–803.

World Medical Association Declaration of Helsinki. 'Ethical Principles for Medical Research Involving Human Subjects'. *JAMA* 310, no. 20 (2013): 2191–4.

Yaffe, Gideon. 'Indoctrination, Coercion and Freedom of Will'. *Philosophy and Phenomenological Research* 67, no. 2 (2003): 335–56.

Yang, Jingqing. 'Serve the People: Understanding Ideology and Professional Ethics of Medicine in China'. *Health Care Analysis* 18, no. 3 (2010): 294–309.

Young, Robert. 'Informed Consent and Patient Autonomy'. In *A Companion to Bioethics*, edited by Helga Kuhse and Peter Singer. Oxford: Blackwell, 2001.

Young, Robert. *Personal Autonomy: Beyond Negative and Positive Liberty*. London: Croom Helm, 1986.
Young, Robert. 'The Value of Autonomy'. *The Philosophical Quarterly* 32, no. 126 (1982): 35–44.
Zimmerman, David. 'Coercive Wage Offers'. *Philosophy & Public Affairs* 10, no. 2 (1981): 121–45.
Zimmerman, David. 'That Was Then, This Is Now: Personal History vs. Psychological Structure in Compatibilist Theories of Autonomous Agency'. *Noûs* 37, no. 4 (2003): 638–71.
Zohny, Hazem. 'The Myth of Cognitive Enhancement Drugs'. *Neuroethics* 8, no. 3 (2015): 257–69.

Index

Note: Figures are indicated by an italic '*f*' following the page number.

For the benefit of digital users, indexed terms that span two pages (e.g., 52–53) may, on occasion, appear on only one of those pages.

The manufacturer's authorised representative in the EU for product safety is Oxford University Press España S.A. of el Parque Empresarial San Fernando de Henares, Avenida de Castilla, 2 – 28830 Madrid (www.oup.es/en or product.safety@oup.com). OUP España S.A. also acts as importer into Spain of products made by the manufacturer.

www.ingramcontent.com/pod-product-compliance
Lightning Source LLC
LaVergne TN
LVHW011820200926
848484LV00005B/1253